Diagnostic Criteria in Neurology

CURRENT CLINICAL NEUROLOGY

Daniel Tarsy, MD, SERIES EDITOR

Diagnostic Criteria in Neurology

Edited By

Alan J. Lerner, MD

Departments of Neurology
University Hospitals of Cleveland
and
Case Western Reserve University
Cleveland, OH

HUMANA PRESS ✳ TOTOWA, NEW JERSEY

© 2006 Humana Press Inc.
999 Riverview Drive, Suite 208
Totowa, New Jersey 07512

www.humanapress.com

Due diligence has been taken by the publishers, editors, and authors of this book to assure the accuracy of the information published and to describe generally accepted practices. The contributors herein have carefully checked to ensure that the drug selections and dosages set forth in this text are accurate and in accord with the standards accepted at the time of publication. Notwithstanding, as new research, changes in government regulations, and knowledge from clinical experience relating to drug therapy and drug reactions constantly occurs, the reader is advised to check the product information provided by the manufacturer of each drug for any change in dosages or for additional warnings and contraindications. This is of utmost importance when the recommended drug herein is a new or infrequently used drug. It is the responsibility of the treating physician to determine dosages and treatment strategies for individual patients. Further it is the responsibility of the health care provider to ascertain the Food and Drug Administration status of each drug or device used in their clinical practice. The publisher, editors, and authors are not responsible for errors or omissions or for any consequences from the application of the information presented in this book and make no warranty, express or implied, with respect to the contents in this publication.

This publication is printed on acid-free paper. ∞
ANSI Z39.48-1984 (American Standards Institute) Permanence of Paper for Printed Library Materials.

Production Editor: Amy Thau

Cover design by Patricia F. Cleary

For additional copies, pricing for bulk purchases, and/or information about other Humana titles, contact Humana at the above address or at any of the following numbers: Tel.: 973-256-1699; Fax: 973-256-8314; E-mail: humana@humanapr.com, or visit our Website: http://humanapress.com

Printed in the United States of America. 10 9 8 7 6 5 4 3 2 1
eISBN: 1-59745-078-2
Library of Congress Cataloging in Publication Data
Lerner, Alan J. Diagnostic criteria in neurology / by Alan J. Lerner.
    p. ; cm. -- (Current clinical neurology)
 Includes bibliographical references and index.
ISBN 1-58829-482-X (alk. paper)
1. Neurologic examination. 2. Nervous system--Diseases--Diagnosis.
 [DNLM: 1. Diagnostic Techniques, Neurological. 2. Nervous System
Diseases--diagnosis. WL 141 L6165d 2006] I. Title. II. Series.
 RC348.L47 2006
 616.8'0475--dc22
                    2005029553

Dedication

...and whatever the man called the living creature, that remained its name. And the man assigned names to all of the cattle, and to the birds of the sky, and to every beast of the field...
—Genesis 2:19–20

Dedicated to my family, friends, and patients

Series Editor Introduction

It should be obvious that diagnosis is the first and foremost responsibility of the physician. Although the somewhat obsolete term "diagnostician" is no longer used, it did at one time convey the very special importance of this aspect of medical care. It should also be self-evident that accurate diagnosis comes before treatment. Too often patients with a symptom complex that fails to suggest an obvious diagnosis receive inadequate or inappropriate treatment. Of course, not infrequently, diagnosis may elude the treating physician, especially in the case of rare and unusual neurological disorders, but also in the case of the more common conditions. In his very insightful chapter, Dr. Brent Graham provides a useful introspective look at exactly what constitutes the diagnostic process. As he states, a diagnosis is merely a label provided by the clinician. As such, one should always be prepared to confirm it or drop it as indicated by the available clinical data. Ideally, lack of a satisfactory diagnosis should then stimulate further thought on the part of the treating physician and, if necessary, consultation with a specialist who may or may not be better equipped to arrive at a correct diagnosis.

The elated "high" that accompanies arrival at a diagnosis, especially when dealing with an unusual condition, is well known to all physicians. The patient's satisfaction at learning the diagnosis that explains their symptoms is equally powerful. As Dr. Alan Lerner points out in his preface, simply providing a name for the condition provides a large measure of relief in the patient's effort to gain control over their illness and understand their prognosis. In *Diagnostic Criteria in Neurology*, Dr. Lerner provides handy access to the latest available diagnostic criteria for a diverse group of neurological conditions. These are derived from authoritative sources and are the best that are currently available. Importantly, the dazzling array of useful tables concerns both common and uncommon neurological conditions. Used properly, this resource should greatly assist the diagnostic process. It should, of course, be remembered that sets of criteria usually represent consensus statements of experts reflecting the existing knowledge base of the time, subject to a constant process of revision. The individual clinician must reserve the prerogative to view these criteria with a critical eye as they determine their applicability to their own patient.

Daniel Tarsy, MD
Beth Israel Deaconess Medical Center
Harvard Medical School
Boston, MA

Preface

The word *diagnosis* derives from the Greek words of *dia-*, "thoroughly" and *-gnosis*, "to come to know." *Criterion* is from the Greek *krinein*, meaning "to judge" or "to separate." Therefore, literally, diagnostic criteria are a metaprocess of judging the judgment.

What these words do not convey is the emotion associated with the process of diagnosis, or the feelings of both patient and physician associated with the diagnosis, or the inability to reach a clinical conclusion based on signs and symptoms. *Diagnostic Criteria in Neurology* has been compiled in order to guide clinicians with this process by compiling sets of diagnostic criteria derived from the medical literature. In this process, I have endeavored not to be the final arbiter of diagnostic criteria, but to show the diversity of criteria that have been proposed, and to study their various extents. Thus, *Diagnostic Criteria in Neurology* may be viewed as a "cento," a text composed of pieces gathered from the works of other authors. In the process, I have purposely excluded conditions whose diagnosis depends solely on histopathology (e.g., brain tumors).

Another root for the genesis of *Diagnostic Criteria in Neurology* is the long-term observation regarding the statistical nature of medical diagnosis. One can imagine that diagnosis is a matching process of assigning a patient's symptoms and illnesses to a particular category or set of categories, and then proceeding to narrow the search based on additional information. However, this overlooks the probabilistic nature of all diagnoses. When we say that a patient has X, what we are really saying is, "to the limit of medical certainty [to borrow a term from the medico-legal arena], the patient fulfills the criteria I utilize for making a given diagnosis."

What happens when the diagnosis suggests a rarer entity? The individual practitioner has several routes of action. From a pragmatic standpoint, one approach is to refer the patient to a colleague, or an "expert," in the hope that the patient will become their problem to solve. Frequently, this does not result in learning for the referring practitioner, and may increase patient frustration as he or she wait for the next health care encounter.

A second approach is to stick too tightly to one's initial impressions or to provide only a diagnosis that refers to specific symptoms. Although this may satisfy some, it may lack intellectual rigor if it does not result in the acquisition of additional information that will help create appropriate, meaningful diagnostic information for both patient and physician.

Another approach would be to create the resource for the practitioner to consult the formal diagnostic criteria in the medical literature. Although one aim of medical training is to provide this comfort level with common illnesses, the ability to diagnose according to generally accepted criteria, even within one's stated specialties, has become a challenge.

In notable cases, such as multiple sclerosis, the diagnostic criteria have changed with time. There may also be regional differences in criteria depending on the source. Some diagnoses have shifted categories with time. Tourette syndrome was once considered primarily a psychiatric disorder, but today has roots in genetics, immunology, neurology, and psychiatry and could be considered in texts on all of these subjects.

I have also purposely and specifically not included the literature that surrounds every set of diagnostic criteria. Issues of sensitivity, specificity, and positive and negative predictive values are inherent in any signal detection system. This should be an issue for authors of diagnostic criteria because the utility of their work will depend on its operational usefulness.

The utility of diagnostic criteria may also depend on the underlying distribution of diseases in the differential diagnosis. Just as it takes little skill to forecast a sunny day in Los Angeles during the summer, the practitioner can achieve high degrees of success with limited heuristics. Diagnosing Alzheimer's disease in every older individual with cognitive impairment will result in a high "hit rate" of correct diagnoses. However, this approach runs counter to significant trends in science. We do not, ultimately, do our patients a service by utilizing generic diagnosis. One could not treat leukemia today without reference to cell types and genetic markers, despite their once being lumped into larger categories. We should not be satisfied with this approach within our own specialty.

I am often reminded of the story drawn from the Book of Genesis. Man's first act is to name the animals. Although open to many interpretations, one concept is that we gain control over the unknown and the emotionally terrifying through the process of naming. This process has ancient roots and I hope that *Diagnostic Criteria in Neurology* will help physicians in this ongoing task.

Please also keep in mind that this book is available as a personal digital assistant (PDA) product for easy and efficient clinical use. To obtain the PDA, please contact the publisher, Humana Press (www.humanapress.com).

Alan J. Lerner, MD

Acknowledgments

The biggest debt of gratitude for this volume belongs to the many authors of the sets of criteria entered into this volume. Without their effort in assembling the data, formulating criteria, publishing and disseminating this information, this volume would not be possible. I would like to thank Jan Toms, Sue Champa, and Adrienne Childs for their secretarial help. Zachary Lerner assisted in literature research and the word derivations from Greek. My colleagues, Robert Friedland, Henry Kaminski, Bashar Katirji, David Preston, and Barbara Shapiro gave important advice and encouragement. The staff and editors at Humana Press are also acknowledged for their time and patience and with nurturing this project to fruition.

Contents

1

Consensus, Disagreement, and Diagnostic Labels

Brent Graham

DIAGNOSES AND DIAGNOSTIC CRITERIA

Diagnosis is a fundamental activity of the physician and most other health care professionals. Therapeutic efforts to treat, prognosticate, palliate, or counsel logically emanate from knowledge of the nature of the patient's disease, or at least, the symptoms and objective physical signs produced by that condition. In general, the medical model uses the term *disease* in referring to conditions with adverse outcomes *(1)*. The manifestations of disease constitute the *illness* reported by the patient and observed by the physician in the course of taking a history and conducting a physical examination *(2)*. A *diagnosis* is the label given the patient's illness or disease by the clinician.

Sackett et al. *(2)* summarize the diagnostic process as classification, the goal of which is "to recognize the class or group to which a patient's illness belongs so that, based on our prior experience with that class, the subsequent acts we...carry out...maximize the patient's health." This description of the diagnostic paradigm underlines its principal function as a process for the labeling of both diseases and illnesses. The diagnostic label also facilitates the exchange of information and knowledge between clinicians about individuals or groups of patients with the same diagnosis because of an implicit assumption that the content and meaning of the information conveyed by the diagnosis is agreed on by the discussants. In other words, the acceptance of a diagnostic label to describe either a disease or an illness implies that there is consensus on the criteria to be met for using the term. In most instances, however, diagnostic criteria have not been formally stated, and operational definitions are lacking. Where there is disagreement regarding the criteria for establishing a diagnosis, there is likely to be poor reliability for use of the label.

The criteria used for a diagnostic label vary. The diagnoses of certain diseases are linked to the demonstration of an "essential" lesion. For example, many malignant conditions will be diagnosed based on histopathological findings from a tissue biopsy. Even though the diagnosis of tumors may appear to be relatively objective, consensus is still required on the specific aspects of the histological appearance of malignancy, such as the number and nature of mitotic figures. Thus, agreement may be variable depending on the tissue examined.

The diagnosis of other conditions is based on the measurement of a specific attribute. For example, the diagnosis of hypertension is made when measurements of blood pressure are observed to exceed a certain threshold. For the diagnosis to be reliable, there must be consensus on where the threshold for defining hypertension lies. Diabetes is another condition where measurement of an attribute—in this case blood glucose level—is compared with a threshold value considered by consensus to be "normal."

From: *Current Clinical Neurology: Diagnostic Criteria in Neurology*
Edited by: A. J. Lerner © Humana Press Inc., Totowa, NJ

Finally, the criteria for other diagnostic labels are based entirely on the symptoms and clinical findings that encompass the patient's illness. Although the reliability of the clinically acquired data may vary, the establishment of consensus on the diagnostic meaning of the findings is a key consideration determining the usefulness of the diagnostic term.

In the absence of consensus for identifying medical conditions, substantial variations in practice are observed. For example, Crombie et al. *(3)* have shown that variations among primary care physicians in the recording of International Statistical Classification of Diseases and Related Health Problems 9 codes are largely because of idiosyncratic patterns of diagnostic labeling. The loss of reliability that results from these differing patterns of practice may be at least partly responsible for regional differences observed for disease prevalence, outcomes of treatment, and resource utilization.

Variations in diagnostic practices can occur on several levels. As previously discussed, one important factor is the lack of consensus among clinicians on the criteria to be met for a given diagnosis. However, even where there is some agreement on the factors that should be considered in establishing a certain diagnosis, there may be substantial variance with respect to the way in which these criteria are applied. In addition, the reliability of agreed-upon diagnostic criteria may decline because of variation in the actual process of history taking or in the technique of physical examination *(4)*. Even reliably obtained clinical data may be utilized or interpreted differently by individual clinicians. This may be especially true with respect to the emphasis or importance placed on various factors. Finally, there may be variations in the way in which clinical material is combined, so that the same data lead to different diagnoses. For example, in the diagnosis of carpal tunnel syndrome, there is general agreement that certain symptoms, physical signs, and electrodiagnostic findings are commonly encountered; however, the manner in which this information is integrated into a diagnostic decision varies widely among clinicians.

DIAGNOSIS AS AN INDUCTIVE OR DEDUCTIVE PROCESS

The term *gold standard* usually implies a criterion that definitively identifies a diagnosis. However, a gold standard exists only by consensus. The term originated in the early era of standardization of the measurement of length. The gold standard refers to bars of gold, which, by consensus, served as standards of length and weight. Where there is no consensus, a standard cannot be established. This is equally true of gold standards for diagnostic criteria in medicine. The existence of agreement is the key issue, because the diagnostic label itself should essentially represent a way of summarizing the clinical facts observed in the condition.

The diagnoses of conditions that are characterized by an agreed-upon essential lesion is an inductive process. Recognition of the presence of the essential lesion is equated with definitive identification of the diagnosis itself. The tissue diagnosis of a malignancy is an example of the demonstration of an essential lesion that leads to this type of inductive diagnostic conclusion. The biopsy that demonstrates the essential lesion is a diagnostic gold standard test as long as there is agreement as to the meaning of the pathological findings.

Most medical conditions are not associated with a widely accepted essential lesion. Diagnosis in these conditions is a deductive process. Information from the history, physical examination, and from diagnostic tests is used by the clinician to identify one or more potential diagnoses as the explanation of the patient's complaints. The traditional exercise of establishing a differential diagnosis orders the potential diagnostic labels by the likelihood that each one is accurate. Implicit to this process is an intuitive acceptance of the probabilistic nature of the diagnostic process. Sheps and Schecter *(5)* state, "In the diagnostic context patients do not have disease, only a probability of disease."

Given the deductive nature of diagnosis in most clinical settings, a reasonable paradigm for logical practice would dictate that the clinician should use the history and physical examination in order to establish an *ad hoc* probability for each diagnostic possibility. Distinguishing between the possible diagnoses explaining the clinical observations may require that additional information be obtained from investigations like laboratory tests or diagnostic imaging. This probability for each diagnosis is then revised up or down as the new information becomes available and is integrated into the deductive diagnostic process *(5)*.

THE CONTEXT OF DIAGNOSTIC LABELS

The context in which the diagnosis is made must be considered when giving a label to a health state. Where the focus is on establishing population-based information regarding a condition, a diagnostic label that conveys precise clinical information may not be as relevant as it might be in the management of an individual patient. For example, the diagnostic label *hip fracture* might be useful in epidemiological studies where the objective is to define the burden of disease in a population. Usually, the specific details of the nature of the hip fracture are of less importance. This term might even be sufficiently descriptive for clinical usage in some settings, such as primary care, where the details of the surgical management are not of critical importance. Terms that classify the main condition, such as *subcapital*, *intertrochanteric*, and *subtrochanteric*, supplement the generic term hip fracture for effective communication among surgeons. The same contextual considerations might apply to the relationship between the terms *inflammatory bowel disease*, *Crohn's disease*, and *ulcerative colitis*.

The interaction between the extent and magnitude of clinical findings and labeling of the condition may be complex and highly variable between clinicians. Indications of disease severity like *mild*, *moderate*, and *severe* may be useful, but are not usually operationally defined. Even where these terms may be used, the threshold for applying the diagnostic label may vary significantly. *Ad hoc* descriptors of clinical activity, such as *burned out* rheumatoid arthritis, may also develop and add to the imprecision of classifying the current disease state.

Changes in clinically apparent disease activity may also be observed in instances where the condition is intermittent or manifests only under certain circumstances. For example, the diagnosis of asthma is usually applied to the pathophysiological state of reversible airway obstruction that generally occurs in response to environmental exposures that may be relatively well defined both temporally and qualitatively. In between attacks, the patient may be labeled *asthmatic*, a term that connotes a currently quiescent disease state. Similarly, *epilepsy* indicates a convulsive disorder of frequently unknown etiology. The use of the term *epileptic* has the same connotation as the label asthmatic, but may have a significant impact on the individual's ability to hold a driver's license or engage in certain occupations because the label implies a risk of relapse to the active disease state. This example shows how the capacity of the diagnostic label to accommodate variability in disease activity may be limited.

A further example would be conditions thought to be associated with an occupational exposure where diagnostic labels do not reflect potential variations in disease activity. For example, workers diagnosed with carpal tunnel syndrome may claim that the workplace caused the condition. Even when the symptoms of carpal tunnel syndrome have been successfully treated, the diagnostic label may remain and disqualify the patient from a return to certain activities. This situation may have significant ramifications for both insurers and beneficiaries.

Diagnostic labeling in patients who have undergone apparently curative therapy for a malignancy may also be inadequate for describing disease activity. Operationally defined interim diagnostic labels may be given to define *disease-free intervals*, implying the continued presence of the disease in a quiescent state. This incomplete understanding of prognosis may complicate defining the prevalence of cancer in a population, especially where therapies evolve rapidly. There are also psychological implications for patients, as well as considerations related to insurability and employability.

Finally, a fuller understanding of the genetic basis of certain conditions has further implications for the process of diagnostic labeling. The discovery of the *BRCA* gene in a currently asymptomatic individual is a marker for the potential development of breast cancer. An estimate of the probability for developing clinically identifiable cancer may be made, but what remains unclear is the point at which the transformation between carrier and patient takes place. Women carrying this gene who elect to undergo bilateral prophylactic mastectomies are, for all purposes, patients with breast tissue that is in a precancerous state despite the absence of a tissue diagnosis other than the genetic marker. Diagnostic paradoxes of this nature are likely to increase with further advances in technology and in our understanding of the etiological basis of diseases. Methods for identification and labeling of medical conditions that are both flexible and robust must be developed to meet the challenges posed by these discoveries and the resulting evolution in our concept of illness and disease.

MODELING THE DIAGNOSTIC PROCESS AND THE ESTABLISHMENT OF STANDARDIZED DIAGNOSTIC CRITERIA

Diagnostic criteria are usually based on traditional teaching that may be influenced through time by the literature. The literature often reflects an informal distillation of diagnostic concepts held by clinical experts in the field. However, a few examples exist where an *ad hoc* declaration of diagnostic criteria for a condition have been widely accepted. For instance, the Jones criteria for the diagnosis of rheumatic fever, although revised intermittently *(6)*, have been the accepted standard for the identification of this disease entity for more than 50 years *(7)*. Other examples include the criteria used for the diagnosis of essential hypertension *(8)* and systemic lupus erythematosus *(9,10)*.

The durability of the diagnostic criteria for these conditions suggests that there is a consensus as to their usefulness, although no formal means of obtaining agreement among the users of the criteria was used during their development. A widely accepted methodology for the establishment of diagnostic criteria in conditions lacking an accepted gold standard criterion has not been developed *(8,11–13)*.

An exception to this has been the *Diagnostic and Statistical Manual of Mental Disorders* (DSM), currently in its fourth edition *(14)*, which drew heavily on the use of expert panels during its development. The diagnostic criteria in the DSM-IV were established originally under the sponsorship of a national academic organization, the American Psychiatric Association. Committees of the American Psychiatric Association were created, comprising members from the research and clinical communities, including subspecialty interests. The panels functioned as consensus groups with the objective of establishing diagnostic criteria for psychiatric disorders within a framework of optimizing clinical usefulness, reliability, and compatibility with the International Statistical Classification of Diseases and Related Health Problems. Given the unique nature of mental disease, most of these diagnostic criteria have been based primarily on clinical judgment. Revisions of earlier drafts of the DSM have resulted from extensive field-testing and the process of refining the diagnostic criteria is an ongoing process. The DSM has become the reference standard for the labeling of psychiatric conditions.

The methodology used for the DSM represents a useful model for the development of diagnostic criteria that should be used more widely in clinical medicine. The key elements to its success appear to have been (1) the sponsorship of a well-respected national organization, (2) the use of a broadly based pool of credible experts functioning within the methodology of a group process, (3) a focus on clinical judgment, and (4) a continual process of field-testing and revision. Wherever feasible, the task of establishing diagnostic criteria should use this framework within the standard methodology for the creation of measurement scales. In other words, experts should be used in the process of item generation, item reduction, and validation. The focus should be on establishing consensus, using the various types of group process. In general, a more meaningful consensus will be likely if there is an avoidance of a geographic bias and all clinical groups that normally evaluate the condition participate in developing the criteria.

BARRIERS TO THE DEVELOPMENT OF UNIFORM DIAGNOSTIC CRITERIA

No justification is required for efforts to improve diagnostic practices. It can be assumed that this goal is worthwhile. However, significant obstacles, both practical and philosophical, stand in the way of this objective. The question could be asked: "What is meant by 'improvement' with respect to diagnostic practices?" Clearly, a fundamental goal of diagnosis is to match optimally treatments and prognoses to symptoms and complaints presented by patients. However, it might be argued that uniformity among diagnosticians in the manner in which diagnoses are made is of secondary importance. This assumes that as long as the treatment is appropriate, both the "correctness" of the diagnosis and the method of arriving at the diagnosis are less important.

This argument can be refuted on a number of different levels. The most basic issue relates to the validity of the diagnosis itself. In many cases, it may be impossible to determine if a diagnosis is correct. A successful outcome using an accepted treatment is often tacitly accepted as proof of the proposed diagnosis. However, there are many instances in which the relationship between diagnosis and treatment is unclear. For example, the natural history of a condition may result in improvement whether or not treatment is instituted. Improvement may occur in spite of treatment that is inappropriately recommended. Placebo effects may be operating so that treatment given for a wrong diagnosis is still associated with improvement in the patient's symptoms *(15)*. Conversely, there may be cases where treatment expected to succeed fails in the presence of a possible influential factor, such as a workers' compensation claim. Consequently, where it is difficult or impossible to confirm a diagnosis, there is even a greater need for uniform diagnostic criteria.

Second, if a diagnosis can be applied consistently, then better understanding of the condition and its current treatment may be gained. For example, a consensus on the diagnostic criteria for fibromyalgia has become more or less established *(16)*. The result is that rheumatologists make the diagnosis with moderate reliability *(17–19)*. Hopefully, this will have the effect of delineating a relatively uniform patient population so that the syndrome, its natural history, and appropriate treatment become better known.

Third, just as treatments may evolve over time, so too might the diagnostic criteria for a given condition. Implicit in the argument for consensus and uniformity in diagnostic practices is the recognition that the process of diagnosis will still be flawed and unreliable to a certain extent, even when widely agreed-upon criteria are met. As the ongoing process of validation of existing criteria continues, revisions are likely as new information and technology becomes available *(20)*. However, this cannot take place in the absence of an agreed-upon starting point for a diagnostic standard or without accepted methodological practices for establishing diagnostic criteria.

Clinicians themselves may resist a system of consensus-based diagnostic practices, even if the process used to develop the criteria is methodologically sound. An unwillingness to adopt standards of this nature has already been reflected in the slow acceptance of clinical practice guidelines. The basis of this reluctance appears to be related to the ingrained inviolability of expert clinical judgment *(21–24)*. The main argument made against actuarial systems of judgment is that they are inadequately flexible in dealing with the individual variations exhibited by patients in everyday practice. There may also be concerns related to the medico-legal implications of functioning outside a practice guideline related to diagnostic criteria if these become established.

In fact, the literature indicates that the principle advantage of actuarial systems is that they are more reliable than clinical judgments. Given the same input data, the same output will result. Expert clinicians have been shown to be much less consistent in their judgments. This may be related to the difficulty with which content experts explain how they accomplish the task of diagnosis *(25)*. The challenge in developing diagnostic criteria is in meeting the need to incorporate flexibility so that unusual observations or clinical manifestations can be included in the assessment. The objective should be to allow latitude for clinical judgment within the context of the diagnostic guideline. Expression of the diagnosis in probabilistic terms may meet this need where an instrument comprising items of varying reliability may be felt to be inaccurate by a clinician in a particular circumstance. Although the introduction of an "X-factor" to account for clinician intuition may subtract from the inherent reliability of a diagnostic scale, it might improve the likelihood that the instrument is used.

DEVELOPMENT OF A DIAGNOSTIC MEASUREMENT INSTRUMENT

Eddy and Clanton *(26)* have identified six steps expert clinicians take in making a diagnosis: (1) aggregation of groups of findings into patterns, (2) selection of a "pivot" or key finding, (3) generation of a potential cause list, (4) pruning of the cause list, (5) selection of a diagnosis, and (6) validation of the diagnosis. The process of aggregation may allow a number of smaller individual findings to be subsumed under one construct. For example, in carpal tunnel syndrome the symptoms of "numbness in the middle finger," "tingling in the thumb," and "pain in the hand" may be considered by the experienced diagnostician to be manifestations of the same physiological phenomenon: median nerve compression in the carnal canal. This linkage between knowledge of biology and the symptoms of the patient is an example of the diagnostic label as an *explanatory idea (2)*.

The seasoned clinician identifies key points and emphasizes them, temporarily ignoring all other findings *(26)*. For the example of carpal tunnel syndrome, symptoms and physical signs, such as nocturnal numbness, sensory splitting of the ring finger, a loss of two-point discrimination restricted to the median nerve distribution in the hand, and the presence of thenar atrophy, may achieve the status of a pivotal finding. The absence of one of these key symptoms or physical signs may, in some circumstances, strongly mitigate against the diagnosis of carpal tunnel syndrome, even if other weaker indicators are present. As a result, these findings should be considered especially pivotal, because they influence the likelihood of the diagnosis by either their presence or absence.

The intellectual analysis used by physicians to make diagnoses may be the result of one or more type(s) of reasoning, described by Murphy et al. *(27)* as deduction, inference, and illation. The illative process integrates the elements of the case that may be based on deduction or inference into a larger concept of disease. In this regard, they state: "a useful diagnosis has meaning that transcends the total facts on which it is based."

The breadth and differing nature of diagnostic problems in medicine dictates the need for a flexible system of logic that is appropriate to a given situation *(28)*. The substantialist and nominalist models of diagnostic reasoning may be contrasted in the following way *(28,29)*: the substantialist model integrates the clinical manifestations of a condition that itself cannot be directly observed, and acknowledges that other data may also contribute to the diagnosis of the disease. This illative process has, as its basis, a Bayesian approach.

Murphy's nominalist model focuses on abnormal data. For example, in the case of carpal tunnel syndrome, the result of electrodiagnostic testing is taken at face value. Findings that exceed an established threshold of normality are considered indicative of the diagnosis of carpal tunnel syndrome, and no other information is necessary to reach this conclusion.

The manner in which a diagnostic statement can be expressed is variable and at least partially dependent on whether the substantialist or nominalist model is the basis of the diagnostic process. The nominalist approach implies a binary outcome: the diagnosis is present or absent according to the result of a critical clinical or laboratory test. All inferences focus on determining where the test result lies in relation to the threshold for declaring the diagnosis. In contrast, the substantialist model represents a probability argument for a diagnosis that relies on the presence or absence of a number of clinical findings and test results of variable importance. The weighting of the clinical variables is a subjective judgment that converts the process to one of illation. Sometimes, it may be possible to refine the probability of a given diagnosis to a numerical estimate, whereas in other cases, the best resolution may be to an ordinal scale, such as low, medium, or high probability.

To summarize, the diagnostic process may utilize a system of logic that varies in different situations. The resulting diagnostic conclusion may be expressed as a binary or ordinal statement or as a probability. The best method for establishing the diagnostic criteria for a particular condition depends on the goal and the setting for which they are intended.

PROBABILISTIC MODELS OF DIAGNOSIS

Whether or not consciously acknowledged, most diagnoses made by clinicians actually represent probabilistic statements explaining clinical findings. When the diagnosis leads to an action, such as a therapeutic intervention, the diagnosis is treated like a certainty because the next step in the diagnosis/therapy linkage is triggered. Of course, a threshold effect is implicitly active and therapy, especially if it is dangerous or uncomfortable, is only started when the probability of the diagnosis passes a threshold at which the clinician determines the potential benefit of treatment exceeds its risk.

Despite the pervasiveness of this internalized concept of a probabilistic model of diagnosis, few diagnostic scales with a probability-based output have been developed *(30,31)*. There are several potential disadvantages to the expression of a diagnosis in probabilistic terms. First, stating a diagnosis as a probability may concern some clinicians because of the uncertainty patients may experience in the absence of a definitive declaration of the cause of their illness. Some patients may find this unsettling, and in many cases, an inability to grasp adequately the concept of probability may adversely affect their capacity for making informed decisions regarding their health.

Second, scales that express their output in probabilistic terms are often based on logistic regression models *(32,33)*. The use of these models is subject to the usual risks of overfitting that may result in a failure to validate in new samples. It is essential that these models be validated externally in order to ensure that they can be safely and effectively implemented on a broad scale.

The third point is that clinicians frequently desire a binary concept in diagnostic labeling because of the important role played by the diagnosis in guiding treatment. Expression of the diagnosis in probabilistic terms may be seen as complicating the decision to treat.

Diagnostic instruments in which the output is probabilistic have several advantages. First, in the absence of a consensus on diagnostic criteria that are reliable, the diagnosis represents an educated guess as to the true nature of the patient's symptoms *(5)*. The ability to state the expected accuracy of that guess by attaching to it an estimate of probability may allow clearer decisions to be made in relation to the treatment and prognosis that flow from the diagnostic label. This additional information may also provide greater insight to both patients and insurers as they make treatment decisions together with their physician.

Second, a probabilistic expression of diagnosis may better inform the use of diagnostic investigations. Laboratory tests and imaging studies presently play an important role in establishing many diagnoses. However, as the cost of advanced investigation escalates, the value added to a clinical diagnosis by various tests is likely to come under increasing scrutiny. Although laboratory tests are sometimes diagnostic themselves, in other instances they may only incrementally increase the probability of a diagnosis made on a clinical basis. Bayesian principles of probability-based decisions can guide the use of laboratory tests in the most cost-effective manner *(34,35)*. Even without the pressures of cost-containment however, the physician has a responsibility to limit testing that is time-consuming, inconvenient, uncomfortable, or even dangerous, where the result of the test has little or no bearing on the probability of the diagnosis in question. Once again, conceptualizing diagnosis in probabilistic terms is a key consideration in changing the way in which medical tests are used.

Third, the description of diagnoses in probabilistic terms may actually help guide health care planning. Decision analyses, cost–benefit evaluation, and other activities related to forecasting the direction of future health care interventions are likely to become increasingly important to health care policy makers. Most of these analyses require knowledge of the probability of various indicators in large health care systems, arguably the most fundamental of which is the diagnostic label. The comprehensive use of probabilities to describe diagnoses would require substantial changes to current methods of collecting and analyzing data related to utilization and cost.

Finally, scales that express their output in probabilistic terms may have an added element of versatility with respect to the setting in which they are used. The threshold for establishing a diagnosis may be adjusted according to need. For example, in using an instrument to identify a requirement for further investigation, to direct treatment, or to determine prognosis in an individual, there would likely be a requirement for both sensitivity and specificity in setting a threshold for defining the diagnosis. However, in a screening situation, the emphasis would be on sensitivity. In setting a low threshold, in probabilistic terms, for identifying the condition, effective screening could occur by applying the same instrument used for the evaluation of individual cases in which the probability of disease required to trigger treatment may be much higher.

SUMMARY

The development of diagnostic criteria for a given condition should consider the both objective and context in which the criteria will be used (e.g., establishment of treatment or prognosis, screening, measurement of prevalence, etc.) and the form or output that the criteria should take in determining the diagnosis. Related issues to consider would include the spectrum of clinicians expected to use the criteria, existing diagnostic criteria, and the relative roles of clinical evaluations and laboratory tests. If the objective is to create a diagnostic scale, then these considerations should be superimposed on the methodology used for the development of any measurement instrument: item generation, item reduction, and validation *(36)*.

REFERENCES

1. Temple L. An evaluation of the role of genetic testing in hereditary non-polyposis colorectal cancer (1-INPCC). MSc, University of Toronto, ON, 1998.
2. Sackett D, Haynes RB, Guyatt GH, Tugwell P. Clinical Epidemiology, A Basic Science for Clinical Medicine, 2nd ed. Toronto: Little, Brown, 1991.
3. Crombie DL, Cross KW, Fleming DM. The problem of diagnostic variability in general practice. J Epid Comm Health 1992;46:447–454.
4. Wright JG, Treble N, Feinstein AR. Measurement of lower limb alignment using long radiographs. J Bone Joint Surg Br 1991;73:721–723.
5. Sheps SB, Schechter MT. The assessment of diagnostic tests. A survey of current medical research. JAMA 1984;252: 2418–2422.
6. Stollerman GH, Siegel AC, Johnson EE. Variable epidemiology of streptococcal disease and the changing pattern of rheumatic fever. Mod Concepts Cardiovasc Dis 1965;34:45–48.
7. Shiffman RN. Guideline maintenance and revision. 50 years of the Jones criteria for diagnosis of rheumatic fever. Arch Pediatr Adolesc Med 1995;149:727–732.
8. Reeves RA. Does this patient have hypertension? How to measure blood pressure. JAMA 1995;273:1211–1218.
9. Smith EL, Shmerling RH. The American College of Rheumatology criteria for the classification of systemic lupus erythematosus: strengths, weaknesses, and opportunities for improvement. Lupus 1999;8:586–595.
10. Hochberg MC. Updating the American College of Rheumatology revised criteria for the classification of systemic lupus erythematosus. Arthritis Rheum 1997;40:1725.
11. Knottnerus JA. Diagnostic prediction rules: principles, requirements and pitfalls. Primary Care 1995;22:341–360.
12. Ebell M. Using decision rules in primary clinical practice. Primary Care 1995;22:319–329.
13. Bergus GR, Hamm RM. Clinical practice: how physicians make medical decisions and why medical decision making can help. Primary Care 1995;22:167–180.
14. DSM-IV. Diagnostic and Statistical Manual of Mental Disorders: DSM-IV, 4th ed. Washington, DC: American Psychiatric Association, 1994.
15. de Craen AJ, Kaptchuk TJ, Tijssen JG, Kleijnen J. Placebos and placebo effects in medicine: historical overview. J R Soc Med 1999;92:511–515.
16. Wolfe F, Smythe HA, Yunus MB, et al. The American College of Rheumatology 1990 criteria for the classification of fibromyalgia. Report of the Multicenter Criteria Committee. Arthritis Rheum 1990;33:160–172.
17. Tunks E, McCain GA, Hart LE, et al. The reliability of examination for tenderness in patients with myofascial pain, chronic fibromyalgia and controls. J Rheumatol 1995;22:944–952.
18. Wolfe F. Interrater reliability of the tender point criterion for fibromyalgia. J Rheumatol 1994;21:370, 371.
19. Cott A, Parkinson W, Bell MJ, et al. Interrater reliability of the tender point criterion for fibromyalgia. J Rheumatol 1992;19:1955–1959.
20. Browman GP, Levine MN, Mohide A, et al. The practice guidelines development cycle: a conceptual tool for practice guidelines development and implementation. J Clin Oncol 1995;13:502–512.
21. Cameron C, Naylor CD. No impact from active dissemination of the Ottawa Ankle Rules: further evidence of the need for local implementation of practice guidelines. CMAJ 1999;160:1165–1168.
22. Bloch DA, Michel BA, Hunder GG, et al. The American College of Rheumatology 1990 criteria for the classification of vasculitis. Arthritis Rheum 1990;33:1068–1073.
23. Forrest D, Hoskins A, Hussey R. Clinical guidelines and their implementation. Postgrad Med J 1996;72:19–22.
24. Lipman T. Discrepancies exist between general practitioners' clinical work and a guidelines implementation programme. BMJ 1998;317:604.
25. Kirwan JR, Chaput de Saintonge DM, Joyce CRB, Holmes J, Curry HLF. Inability of rheumatologists to describe their true policies for assessing rheumatoid arthritis. Ann. Rheum. Dis 1986;45:156–161.
26. Eddy DM, Clanton CH. The art of diagnosis: solving the clinicopathological exercise. N Engl J Med 1982;306:1263–1268.

27. Murphy EA, Rosell EM, Rosell MI. Deduction, inference, illation. Theoret Med 1986;7:329–353.
28. Scadding JG. Essentialism and nominalism in medicine: logic of diagnosis in disease terminology. Lancet 1996;348: 594–596.
29. Murphy EA. The logic of medicine. Am J Med 1979;66:907–909.
30. Poses RM, Cebul RD, Collins M, Fager SS. The importance of disease prevalence in transporting clinical prediction rules. The case of streptococcal pharyngitis. Ann Intern Med 1986;105:586–591.
31. Wigton RS, Hoellerich VL, Ornato JP, Leu V, Mazzotta LA, Cheng IH. Use of clinical findings in the diagnosis of urinary tract infection in women. Arch Intern Med 1985;145:2222–2227.
32. Diegpen TL, Sauerbrei W, Fartasch M. Development and validation of diagnostic scores for atopic dermatitis incorporating criteria of data quality and practical usefulness. J Clin Epid 1996;49:1031–1038.
33. Hamberg KJ, Carstensen B, Sorensen TI, Eghoje K. Accuracy of clinical diagnosis of cirrhosis among alcohol-abusing men. J Clin Epidemiol 1996;49:1295–1301.
34. Jones H. Bayesian analysis: an objective, scientific approach to better decisions. Clin Lab Manage Rev 1999;13:148–153.
35. van der Schouw YT, Verbeek AL, Ruijs SH. Guidelines for the assessment of new diagnostic tests. Invest Radiol 1995;30:334–340.
36. Graham B. The Development of Diagnostic Criteria for Carpal Tunnel Syndrome. University of Toronto, 2003.

2

Cerebrovascular Diseases

CEREBRAL AUTOSOMAL-DOMINANT ARTERIOPATHY WITH SUBCORTICAL INFARCTS AND LEUKOENCEPHALOPATHY

Cerebral autosomal-dominant arteriopathy with subcortical infarcts and leukoencephalopathy (CADASIL) is associated with mutations in the NOTCH 3 protein, which maps to chromosome 19q12. NOTCH signaling is important in development, but in adults, NOTCH 3 expression is limited to vascular smooth muscle cells, where its function is unknown. Pathologically, there are granular deposits in small cerebral arteries producing ischemic stroke because of vessel wall thickening, fibrosis, and occlusion. These deposits are found in small arteries throughout the body, and diagnosis may be confirmed by the presence of the osmiophilic granules in the basement membrane of vascular smooth muscle cells on skin biopsies.

CADASIL differs from other causes of diffuse subcortical ischemia, such as Binswanger's disease, by the frequent presence of migraine with or without aura, and individuals with CADASIL are not usually hypertensive. Occasionally, diagnostic confusion may occur with patients with multiple sclerosis, especially the primary progressive type, with the appearance of multiple white matter lesions.

CADASIL often presents in early adulthood, and most affected individuals show symptoms by age 60. In addition to migraine with or without aura, there may be depression and mood disturbances, focal neurological deficits, pseudobulbar palsy, and dementia. Approximately 10% of patients have seizures.

Davous, reviewing extent cases in 1998, proposed clinical diagnostic criteria to formalize the clinical data (Table 1).

PERIVENTRICULAR LEUKOMALACIA

Periventricular leukomalacia consists of multiple ischemic lesions in the periventricular white matter, and is considered to be the main factor responsible for spastic cerebral palsy in premature infants. Diagnostic criteria are in Table 2.

STROKE

The recommended standard World Health Organization definition of stroke is "a focal (or at times global) neurological impairment of sudden onset, and lasting more than 24 hours (or leading to death), and of presumed vascular origin."

This definition has been employed for decades in many different settings, and has proven to be a valuable tool that may be used irrespective of access to technological equipment. Although many countries have already invested in diagnostic tools, such as neuroimaging, enabling subtyping and more detailed descriptions, the clinical definition remains the standard and is suitable for future studies of stroke. The definition excludes transient ischemic attack, which is defined as focal neurological symptoms lasting less than 24 hours. Subdural or epidural hematoma, poisoning, and symptoms caused by trauma are also excluded.

From: *Current Clinical Neurology: Diagnostic Criteria in Neurology*
Edited by: A. J. Lerner © Humana Press Inc., Totowa, NJ

Table 1

Proposed Diagnostic Criteria for Cerebral Autosomal-Dominant Arteriopathy With Subcortical Infarcts and Leukoencephalopathy

1. Probable cerebral autosomal-dominant arteriopathy with subcortical infarcts and leukoencephalopathy (CADASIL):
   a. Young age at onset (≤50 years of age).
   b. At least two of the following:
      i. Clinical stroke-like episodes with permanent neurological signs.
      ii. Migraine.
      iii. Major mood disturbances.
      iv. "Subcortical-type" dementia.
   c. No vascular risk factor etiologically related to the deficit.
   d. Evidence of an inherited autosomal-dominant transmission.
   e. Abnormal magnetic resonance imaging (MRI) imaging of the white matter without cortical infarcts.
2. Definite CADASIL:
   a. Criteria of probable CADASIL associated with linkage to NOTCH 3 mutation, and/or
   b. Pathological findings demonstrating small vessel arteriopathy with granular osmiophilic material.
3. Possible CADASIL:
   a. Late age at onset (≤50).
   b. Stroke-like episodes without permanent signs, minor mood disturbances, global dementia.
   c. Minor vascular risk factors, such as mild hypertension, mild hyperlipidemia, smoking, and/or use of oral contraceptives.
   d. Unknown or incomplete family pedigree.
   e. Atypical MRI imaging of the white matter.
4. Exclusion criteria:
   a. Age at onset over 70 years.
   b. Severe hypertension or complicated heart or systemic vascular disease.
   c. Absence of any other case in a documented pedigree.
   d. Normal MRI imaging, age over 35 years.

Adapted with permission from Davous P. CADASIL: a review with proposed diagnostic criteria. Eur J Neurol 1998;5:230.

Table 2

Criteria for the Neuroimaging Diagnosis of Periventricular Leukomalacia

I. Serial ultrasonography:
   A. Cyst formation in periventricular area.
   B. Periventricular ultrasonographic echodensity greater than choroid plexus echogenicity.
   C. Findings of B prolonged over 3 weeks with irregularity of lateral ventricular walls and/or less uniform echodensity.

Findings of B or C indicate periventricular leukomalacia, whereas a finding of C indicates possible periventricular leukomalacia.

II. Computed tomography examination:
   A. At 40 weeks, corrected postlast menstrual period, a low density of the periventricular area, and/or centrum semiovale with dilatation and irregularity of lateral ventricle wall suggests periventricular leukomalacia.
III. Magnetic resonance imaging:
   B. After age 11 months, periventricular hypodensities (with dilatation and/or irregularity of lateral ventricular walls) on spin echo T2-weighted image and proton density image are consistent with the diagnosis of periventricular leukomalacia.

Adapted from Hashimoto K, Hasegawa H, Kida Y, Takeuchi Y. Correlation between neuroimaging and neurologic outcome in periventricular leukomalacia: diagnostic criteria. Pediatr Int 2001;43:244.

Occasionally, a focal brain lesion compatible with a previous stroke is randomly found in patients undergoing neuroimaging for reasons other than stroke. Because *stroke* is a clinical diagnosis, not based on purely radiological findings, this is usually referred to as *silent cerebral infarction*. Thus, if there is no history of corresponding symptoms, the diagnosis of stroke is not met.

Table 3
Stroke Subtypes

Subarachnoid hemorrhage

Symptoms: Abrupt onset of severe headache or unconsciousness or both. Signs of meningeal irritation (stiff neck, Kernig, and Brudzinski signs). Focal neurological deficits are usually not present.

Findings: At least one of the following must be present in addition to typical symptoms:

1. Necropsy—evidence of recent subarachnoid hemorrhage and an aneurysm or arteriovenous malformation.
2. Computed tomography (CT)—evidence of blood in the Sylvian fissure or between the frontal lobes or in the basal cistern or in cerebral ventricles.
3. Blood-stained cerebrospinal fluid (CSF; >2000 red blood cells per mm^3) and an aneurysm or an arteriovenous malformation found on angiography.
4. Blood-stained CSF (>2000 red blood cells per mm^3) that is also xanthochromic and intracerebral hemorrhage excluded by necropsy or CT examination.

Intracerebral hemorrhage

Symptoms: Usually sudden onset during activities. Often rapidly developing coma, but a small hemorrhage can present with no disturbance of consciousness.

Findings: CSF often, but not always, bloody or xanthochromic. Often, severe hypertension is present. Intracerebral hemorrhage must be confirmed by necropsy or by CT examination.

Brain infarction because of cerebral thrombosis/embolism

Symptoms: The defining characteristic is acute onset. Headache may be present during acute onset; it often occurs during sleep. Consciousness may be disturbed if stroke is large, bihemispheric, or involves brainstem structures. A transient ischemic attack can often be detected in history. Often, other symptoms of atherosclerosis (congenital heart disease, peripheral arterial disease) or underlying diseases (hypertension, diabetes) are also present.

Findings: Brain infarction in the necropsy or in the CT examination and no evidence for an embolic origin, or CT scan of satisfactory quality showing no recent brain lesion, although clinical criteria of stroke are fulfilled.

Investigations

Most studies that classify strokes into subcategories are likely to use brain imaging.

Adapted from World Health Organization. STEPS—Stroke Manual (version 1.2): The WHO STEPwise Approach to Stroke Surveillance.

Types of Stroke

There are three major stroke subgroups: ischemic stroke, intracerebral hemorrhage, and subarachnoid hemorrhage. Each of the types can produce clinical symptoms that fulfill the definition of stroke; however, they differ with respect to survival and long-term disability.

Ischemic stroke is caused by a sudden occlusion of arteries supplying the brain. The occlusion may either be because of a thrombus formed directly at the site of occlusion (thrombotic ischemic stroke) or be a thrombus formed in another part of the circulation that follows the blood stream until it obstructs arteries in the brain (embolic ischemic stroke). The diagnosis of ischemic stroke is usually based on neuroimaging recordings, but it may not be possible to decide clinically or radiologically whether it is a thrombotic or embolic ischemic stroke.

Intracerebral hemorrhage is a bleeding from one of the brain's arteries into the brain tissue. The lesion causes symptoms that mimic those seen for ischemic stroke. A diagnosis of intracerebral hemorrhage depends on access to neuroimaging, where it can be differentiated from ischemic stroke. Spontaneous intracerebral hemorrhage may be more prevalent in developing countries than in developed countries. The reasons for such differences remain unclear, but variations in diet, physical activity, treatment of hypertension, and genetic predisposition may be responsible.

Subarachnoid hemorrhage is characterized by arterial bleeding in the space between the pia mater and arachnoid layers of the meninges. Typical symptoms are sudden onset of severe headache and usually, impaired consciousness. Symptoms that mimic stroke may occur, but are rare. The diagnosis can be established either by neuroimaging or lumbar puncture.

Table 4
Classification of Acute Ischemic Cerebrovascular Syndrome

Category	Definition	Examples
Definite acute ischemic cerebrovascular syndrome (AICS)	Acute onset of neurological dysfunction of any severity consistent with focal brain ischemia *and* imaging/laboratory confirmation of an acute vascular ischemic pathology.[a]	1. Sudden onset of right hemiparesis and aphasia persisting for 3 hours with diffusion-weighted brain imaging (DWI) showing acute ischemic changes. 2. Twenty-minute episode of left hemisensory loss, which resolved, with acute right thalamic ischemic lesion confirmed on DWI.
Probable AICS	Acute onset of neurological dysfunction of any severity suggestive of focal brain ischemic syndrome but *without* imaging/laboratory *confirmation* of acute ischemic pathology[a] (diagnostic studies were negative but *insensitive* for ischemic pathology of the given duration, severity, and location). Imaging, laboratory, and clinical data studies do not suggest nonischemic etiology: possible alternative etiologies are ruled out.	1. Sudden onset of pure motor hemiplegia that persists with normal computed tomography (CT) at 12 hours after onset. Magnetic resonance imaging (MRI) was not performed. 2. Ten-minute episode of aphasia and right hemiparesis in a patient with atrial fibrillation and subtherapeutic international normalized ratio. MRI, including DWI, was negative.
Possible AICS	Acute neurological dysfunction of any duration or severity possibly consistent with focal brain ischemia *without* imaging/laboratory *confirmation* of acute ischemic pathology[a] (diagnostic studies were not performed or were negative and *sensitive* for ischemic pathology of the given duration, severity and location). Possible alternative etiologies are *not* ruled out. Symptoms may be nonfocal or difficult to localize.	1. Two-hour episode of isolated vertigo and headache in a 50-year-old man with a history of hypertension; symptoms resolved at time of imaging. MRI, including DWI, was negative. 2. Twenty-minute episode of isolated word-finding difficulty in 85-year-old woman with a history of dementia and coronary artery disease. Head CT was negative, and MRI was not performed.
Not AICS	Acute onset of neurological dysfunction with imaging/laboratory *confirmation* of *nonischemic* pathology[a] (including normal). Imaging/laboratory studies that are highly sensitive for ischemic pathology of the given duration, severity, and location) as the cause of the neurological syndrome.	1. Sudden onset of left hemiparesis and hemineglect. MRI showed right frontoparietal intracerebral hemorrhage. Imaging/laboratory studies that are highly sensitive for ischemic pathology of the given duration, severity, and location) as the cause of the neurological syndrome. 2. Thirty-year-old man with known seizure disorder found with altered mental status and right hemiplegia. Normal diffusion, perfusion-weighted MRI, and magnetic resonance angiography were acquired while symptoms were still present. Electro-encephalogram showed left temporal spikes.

[a]Imaging/laboratory confirmation includes neuroimaging studies demonstrating recent, appropriately located ischemic lesion (DWI, CT), vascular imaging demonstrating an acute arterial occlusion or stenosis appropriate to the clinical syndrome (transcranial Doppler, magnetic resonance angiography, CT angiography, conventional angiography), or perfusion technique demonstrating a perfusion deficit in an appropriately located vascular distribution (perfusion-weighted MRI, perfusion CT, single photon-emission CT, positron-emission tomography, xenon CT). In the future, additional neuroimaging techniques, such as magnetic resonance spectroscopy or serum/plasma biomarkers specific to acute ischemia, may be identified and could potentially provide similar laboratory confirmation.

(Adapted with permission from Kidwell CS, Warach S. Acute ischemic cerebrovascular syndrome: diagnostic criteria. Stroke 2003; 34:2995–2998.)

Further Definition of Stroke Subtypes

Classification of the stroke events into ischemic or hemorrhagic subtypes relies on access to laboratories and imaging technology. The benefit of using neuroimaging is that some misclassification will occur if clinical assessment alone is used. For example, cancer in the brain may mimic a stroke. Whether an event is hemorrhagic vs ischemic is also of importance from a clinical perspective, as aspirin or other antiplatelet or anticoagulant medication should not be given to patients with hemorrhagic stroke. Studies that include computed tomography (CT) scans in their surveillance system should register days between onset and investigation of the stroke. Preferably, the scan should be conducted within the first 2 weeks, as minor bleedings otherwise may have been absorbed, leading to incorrect classification of the event as ischemic stroke.

An alternative classification of "acute ischemic cerebrovascular syndrome" has been published. It attempts to incorporate imaging findings and laboratory results with clinical findings. This schemata is presented in Table 4.

VASCULAR DEMENTIA

The core of vascular dementia is the presence of dementia and its relationship to cerebrovascular disease (*see* Table 5). Evaluation of the former is straightforward, but what constitutes vascular disease and what its relationship is to clinical syndromes can be more perplexing. For example, many patients have magnetic resonance imaging findings of periventricular white matter signal change (leukoaraiosis, such as seen in Binswanger's disease). In the presence of a progressive dementia typical of Alzheimer's disease, the clinical picture may be interpreted as vascular dementia owing to small vessel ischemia, or Alzheimer's disease with "nonspecific" white matter findings. Another example of an unclear case would be an individual, again with findings of progressive dementia, but a single lacunar infarct on neuroimaging. Some clinicians would consider the location of the infarct, with regard to whether it is in an area important for memory dysfunction, whereas others may diagnose a mixed dementing disorder. Because vascular dementia may be the result of a single lesion, the term *multi-infarct dementia* is not synonymous with vascular dementia.

Overall vascular dementia accounts for 10–20% of all dementia, depending on the population studied. The most common criteria used for diagnosis is the National Institute of Neurological Disorders and Stroke-Associated Internationale pour la Reserche et l'Enseignement en Neurosciences (NINDS-AIREN) criteria (*see* Table 6). Other criteria included here are the *Diagnostic and Statistical Manual of Mental Disorders, 4th edition* (DSM-IV), and the Hachinski Ischemia Scale (*see* Table 7).

The NINDS-AIREN criteria stress the importance of the temporal relation between the vascular event and the onset of dementia. One of the major difficulties with implementing these vascular dementia guidelines is relatively poor interrater agreement in interpretation of neuroimaging studies. Holmes et al. found the sensitivity of the NINDS-AIREN criteria to be only 43%, whereas it had high specificity of 95%.

The DSM-IV guidelines are simpler to follow, but are vague in their requirements for temporal relationships and neuroimaging requirement. It is also unclear whether the presence of a focal deficit, such as aphasia, would be able to be counted in both criterions 1 and 3 because it represents a focal deficit.

The Hachinski criteria were developed using clinical criteria to separate vascular disease from primary degenerative dementia. It was developed at the time when CT scanning was being introduced, and thus has no imaging component. Some studies, particularly those emanating from the Alzheimer's disease literature, have used different cutoffs in excluding patients. The weighting system has been studied, and Molsa et al. reported that differentiation between populations could be enhanced by assigning varying weights to the variables with the highest discriminatory ability. However, the Hachinski Ischemia Score, as modified by Rosen, remains quite good in distinguishing patients with at least some vascular pathology, as determined in autopsy-based studies.

Table 5
DSM-IV Criteria for the Diagnosis of Vascular Dementia

1. The development of multiple cognitive deficits manifested by both memory impairment (impaired ability to learn new information or to recall previously learned information) and one or more of the following cognitive disturbances:
   a. Aphasia (language disturbance).
   b. Apraxia (impaired ability to carry out motor activities despite intact motor function).
   c. Agnosia (failure to recognize or identify objects despite intact sensory function).
   d. Disturbance in executive functioning (i.e., planning, organizing, sequencing, abstracting).
2. The cognitive deficits in criteria 1a and 1b each cause significant impairment in social or occupational functioning and represent a significant decline from a previous level of functioning.
3. Focal neurological signs and symptoms (e.g., exaggeration of deep tendon reflexes, extensor plantar response, pseudobulbar palsy, gait abnormalities, weakness of an extremity), or laboratory evidence indicative of cerebrovascular disease (e.g., multiple infarctions involving cortex and underlying white matter) that are judged to be etiologically related to the disturbance.
4. The deficits do not occur exclusively during the course of a delirium.

Adapted from American Psychiatric Association: Diagnostic and Statistical Manual of Mental Disorders, 4th rev. ed. Washington, DC: American Psychiatric Association, 1994.

Table 6
NINDS-AIREN Criteria for the Diagnosis of Vascular Dementia

I. The criteria for the clinical diagnosis of *probable* vascular dementia include *all* of the following:
   A. *Dementia*, defined by cognitive decline from a previously higher level of functioning and manifested by impairment of memory and of two or more cognitive domains (orientation, attention, language, visuospatial functions, executive functions, motor control, and praxis), preferably established by clinical examination and documented by neuropsychological testing; deficits should be severe enough to interfere with activities of daily living not because of physical effects of stroke alone. *Exclusion criteria*: cases with disturbance of consciousness, delirium, psychosis, severe aphasia, or major sensorimotor impairment precluding neuropsychological testing. Also excluded are systemic disorders or other brain diseases (such as Alzheimer's disease [AD]) that in and of themselves could account for deficits in memory and cognition.
   B. *Cerebrovascular disease*, defined by the presence of focal signs on neurological examination, such as hemiparesis, lower facial weakness, Babinski sign, sensory deficit, hemianopia, and dysarthria consistent with stroke (with or without history of stroke), and evidence of relevant cerebrovascular disease (CVD) by brain imaging (computed tomography or magnetic resonance imaging [MRI]) including *multiple large-vessel infarcts* or a *single strategically placed infarct* (angular gyrus, thalamus, basal forebrain, or posterior cerebral artery or anterior cerebral artery territories), as well as *multiple basal ganglia* and *white matter lacunes*, or *extensive periventricular white matter lesions*, or combinations thereof.
   C. *A relationship between the above two disorders*, manifested or inferred by the presence of one or more of the following:
      a. Onset of dementia within 3 months following a recognized stroke.
      b. Abrupt deterioration in cognitive functions.
      c. Fluctuating, stepwise progression of cognitive deficits.
II. Clinical features consistent with the diagnosis of *probable* vascular dementia include the following:
   A. Early presence of gait disturbance (small-step gait or marche a petits pas, or magnetic, apraxic-ataxic or parkinsonian gait).
   B. History of unsteadiness and frequent, unprovoked falls.
   C. Early urinary frequency, urgency, and other urinary symptoms not explained by urological disease.
   D. Pseudobulbar palsy.
   E. Personality and mood changes, abulia, depression, emotional incontinence, or other subcortical deficits including psychomotor retardation and abnormal executive function.

(Continued)

Table 6 (*Continued*)

III. Features that make the diagnosis of vascular dementia uncertain or unlikely include the following:
   A. Early onset of memory deficit and progressive worsening of memory deficit and progressive worsening of memory and other cognitive functions, such as language (transcortical sensory aphasia), motor skills (apraxia), and perception (agnosia), in the absence of corresponding focal lesions on brain imaging.
   B. Absence of focal neurological signs, other than cognitive disturbance.
   C. Absence of cerebrovascular lesions on brain CT or MRI.
IV. Clinical diagnosis of *possible* vascular dementia may be made in the presence of dementia (section I-A) with focal neurological signs in patients in whom brain imaging studies to confirm definite CVD are missing; or in the absence of clear temporal relationship between dementia and stroke; or in patients with subtle onset and variable course (plateau or improvement) of cognitive deficits and evidence of relevant CVD.
V. Criteria for diagnosis of *definite* vascular dementia are:
   A. Clinical criteria for *probable* vascular dementia.
   B. Histopathological evidence of CVD obtained from biopsy or autopsy.
   C. Absence of neurofibrillary tangles and neuritic plaques exceeding those expected for age.
   D. Absence of other clinical or pathological disorder capable of producing dementia.
VI. Classification of vascular dementia for research purposes may be made based on clinical, radiological, and neuropathological features, for subcategories or defined conditions, such as cortical vascular dementia, subcortical vascular dementia, Binswanger's disease, and thalamic dementia.

The term *AD with CVD* should be reserved to classify patients fulfilling the clinical criteria for possible AD and who also present clinical or brain imaging evidence of relevant CVD. Traditionally, these patients have been included with vascular dementia in epidemiological studies. The term *mixed dementia*, used hitherto, should be avoided.

Table 7
Hachinski Ischemia Score

Feature	Score
Abrupt onset	2
Stepwise deterioration	1
luctuating course	2
Nocturnal confusion	1
Relative preservation of personality	1
Depression	1
Somatic complaints	1
Emotional incontinence	1
History of hypertension	1
History of strokes	2
Evidence of associated atherosclerosis	1
Focal neurological symptoms	2
Focal neurological signs	2
Total score:	____

Adapted with permission from Rosen WG, Terry RD, Fuld PA, et al. Pathological verification of ischemic score in differentiation of dementias. Ann Neurol 1980;7:486–488.

Imaging in Stroke

Diagnostic criteria from the American Heart Association developed as part of comprehensive standards for the evaluation of transient ischemic attacks and stroke (Tables 8–10).

Table 8
Diagnostic Criteria for Acute Cerebral Infarction, Using Computed Tomography Imaging of the Brain

- Infarction: a focal hypodense area, in cortical, subcortical, or deep gray or white matter, following a vascular territory, or in a "watershed" (also known as "borderzone") distribution. Early subtle findings may

(*Continued*)

Table 8 *(Continued)*

include blurring of gray/white matter differentiation, effacement of sulci because of early edema or findings such as "insular ribbon."

- Hemorrhage: hyperdense image in white or deep gray matter, with or without involvement of cortical surface (40 to 90 Hounsfield units [HU]). "Petechial" refers to scattered hyperdense points, coalescing to form irregularly hyperdense areas with hypodense interruptions. "Hematoma" refers to a solid, homogeneously hyperdense image.
- Hyperdense image in major intracranial artery: suggestive of vascular embolic material (such as the dense middle cerebral artery sign).
- Calcification: hyperdense image within or attached to vessel wall (>120 HU).
- Incidental: silent infarct, subdural collection, tumor, giant aneurysm, arteriovenous malformation.

Adapted from Culebras A, Kase CS, Masdeu JC, et al. Practice guidelines for the use of imaging in transient ischemic attacks and acute stroke. A report of the Stroke Council, American Heart Association. Stroke 1997;28:1480–1497.

Table 9
Infarction of the Brain in Magnetic Resonance Imaging in Acute Stroke

- Acute: Subtle, low signal (hypointense) on T1-weighted images, often difficult to see at this stage, and high signal (hyperintense) on spin density and/or T2-weighted and proton density-weighted images starting 8 hours after onset; should follow vascular distribution. Mass effect maximal at 24 hours, sometimes starting 2 hours after onset, even in the absence of parenchymal signal changes. No parenchymal enhancement with a paramagnetic contrast agent, such as gadolinium. Territorial intravascular paramagnetic contrast enhancement of "slow-flow" arteries in hyperacute infarcts; at 48 hours, parenchymal and meningeal enhancement can be expected.
- Subacute (1 week or older): Low signal on T1-weighted images, high signal on T2-weighted images. Follows vascular distribution. Revascularization and blood–brain barrier breakdown may cause parenchymal enhancement with contrast agents.
- Old (several weeks to years): Low signal on T1-weighted images, high signal on T2-weighted images. Mass effect generally disappears after 1 month. Loss of tissue with large infarcts. Parenchymal enhancement fades after several months.

Adapted from Culebras A, Kase CS, Masdeu JC, et al. Practice guidelines for the use of imaging in transient ischemic attacks and acute stroke. A report of the Stroke Council, American Heart Association. Stroke 1997;28:1480–1497.

Table 10
Hemorrhage in Magnetic Resonance Imaging of the Brain

	Age	*T1-weighted*	*T2-weighted*
Hyperacute	Hours old, mainly oxyhemoglobin with surrounding edema	Hypointense	Hyperintense
Acute	Days old, mainly deoxyhemoglobin with surrounding edema	Hypointense	Hypointense, surrounded by hyperintense margin
Subacute	Weeks old, mainly methemoglobin	Hyperintense	Hypointense, early subacute with predominantly intracellular methemoglobin. Hyperintense, late subacute with predominantly extracellular methemoglobin
Chronic	Years old, hemosiderin slit or hemosiderin margin surrounding fluid cavity	Hypointense	Hypointense slit, or hypointense margin surrounding hyperintense fluid cavity

Adapted from Culebras A, Kase CS, Masdeu JC, et al. Practice guidelines for the use of imaging in transient ischemic attacks and acute stroke. A report of the Stroke Council, American Heart Association. Stroke 1997;28:1480–1497.

SOURCES

Cerebral Autosomal-Dominant Arteriopathy With Subcortical Infarcts and Leukoencephalopathy

Davous P. CADASIL: a review with proposed diagnostic criteria. Eur J Neurol 1998;5:219–233.

Desmond DW, Moroney JT, Lynch T, et al. CADASIL in a North American family: clinical, pathologic, and radiologic findings. Neurology 1998;51:844–849.

Dichgans M, Mayer M, Uttner I, et al. The phenotypic spectrum of CADASIL: clinical findings in 102 cases. Ann Neurol 1998;44:731–739.

Kalimo H, Ruchoux MM, Viitanen M, Kalaria RN. CADASIL: a common form of hereditary arteriopathy causing brain infarcts and dementia. Brain Pathol 2002;12:371–384.

Stroke

Culebras A, Kase CS, Masdeu JC, et al. Practice guidelines for the use of imaging in transient ischemic attacks and acute stroke. A report of the Stroke Council, American Heart Association. Stroke 1997;28:1480–1497.

Kidwell CS, Warach S. Acute ischemic cerebrovascular syndrome: diagnostic criteria. Stroke 2003;34:2995–2998.

Sherman DG. Reconsideration of TIA diagnostic criteria. Neurology 2004;62(Suppl):S20–S21.

World Health Organization. STEPS—Stroke Manual (version 1.2): The WHO STEPwise Approach to Stroke Surveillance.

Periventricular Leukomalacia

Hashimoto K, Hasegawa H, Kida Y, Takeuchi Y. Correlation between neuroimaging and neurological outcome in periventricular leukomalacia: diagnostic criteria. Pediatr Int 2001;43:240–245.

Vascular Dementia

American Psychiatric Association: Diagnostic and Statistical Manual of Mental Disorders, 4th ed., text revision. Washington, DC: American Psychiatric Association, 2000.

Hachinski VC, Iliff LD, Zilhka E, et al. Cerebral blood flow in dementia. Arch Neurol 1975;32:632–637.

Holmes C, Cairns N, Lantos P, et al. Validity of current clinical criteria for Alzheimer's disease, vascular dementia and dementia with Lewy bodies. Br J Psychiatry 1999;174:45–50.

Knopman DS, Dekosky ST, Cummings J, et al. Practice parameter: diagnosis of dementia (an evidence-based review) Neurology 2001;56:1143–1153.

Molsa PK, Paljarvi L, Rinne JO, Rinne UK, Sako E. Validity of clinical diagnosis in dementia: a prospective clinicopathological study. J Neurol Neurosurg Psychiatry 1985;48:1085–1090.

Moroney JT, Bagiella E, Desmond DW, et al. Meta-analysis of the Hachinski Ischemic Score in pathologically verified dementias. Neurology 1997;49:1096–1105.

Mungas D, Reed BR, Jagust WJ, et al. Volumetric MRI predicts rate of cognitive decline related to AD and cerebrovascular disease. Neurology 2002;59:867–873.

Roman GC, Tatemichi KT, Erkinjuntti T, et al. Vascular dementia: diagnostic criteria for research studies. Report of the NINDS-AIREN International Workshop. Neurology 1993;250–260.

Rosen WG, Terry RD, Fuld PA, et al. Pathological verification of ischemic score in differentiation of dementias. Ann Neurol 1980;7:486–488.

Tullberg M, Fletcher E, DeCarli C, et al. White matter lesions impair frontal lobe function regardless of their location. Neurology. 2004;63:246–253.

van Straaten EC, Scheltens P, Knol DL, et al. Operational definitions for the NINDS-AIREN criteria for vascular dementia: an interobserver study. Stroke 2003;34:1907–1912.

3

Dementias and Behavioral Disorders

ALCOHOL-RELATED DEMENTIA

The existence of alcohol-related dementia is complicated by the various syndromes described in individuals who abuse alcohol, as well as other possible comorbidities contributing to cognitive dysfunction in these individuals (vitamin B_{12} deficiency, subdural hematomas and head injuries, cerebrovascular disease, etc.). Knowledge about whether alcohol abuse may be a risk factor for other dementias is also sparse.

The *Diagnostic and Statistical Manual of Mental Disorders, 4th edition* (DSM-IV), classification relies on alcohol use to identify alcohol-related dementia, a process that may be subjective or based on limited information. Oslin et al. propose diagnostic criteria following the model used in the National Institute of Neurological and Communicative Diseases and Stroke/Alzheimer's Disease and Related Disorders Association (NINCDS/ADRDA) criteria for Alzheimer's disease (AD). It also uses cutoffs for "heavy drinking" of 28 drinks per week for women and 35 for men. As the authors state, these cutoffs are based on previous surveys of cognitive effects from alcohol rather than strict biological criteria. Furthermore, it acknowledges the possibility that multiple pathologies may be present, and incorporates some neuroimaging details, such as cortical atrophy or atrophy of the cerebellum, especially the cerebellar vermis, into the proposed criteria.

ALZHEIMER'S DISEASE

AD is the most common form of dementia, accounting for an estimated 65–75% of cases of dementia, especially in aged individuals. Dementia itself is a symptom, not a diagnosis. *Dementia* is defined as acquired loss of cognitive functioning, and occurs in clear consciousness. This distinguishes it from mental retardation/developmental delay and cases where consciousness is fluctuating or impaired, such as delirium or coma.

AD was also one of the first neurological disorders to have a set of codified diagnostic criteria based on the work of McKhann and others, who published their criteria in 1984. The NINCDS/ADRDA criteria have also served as the model for many later published criteria, with their emphasis on probable as opposed to possible or definite AD. Since then, many studies have looked at the sensitivity and specificity of these clinical criteria, correlation with autopsy studies to define accuracy, and the ability of other sets of criteria for dementing illnesses to distinguish their cases from AD cases.

The criteria contrast sharply with the criteria for mild cognitive impairment, and have overlaps with criteria for other dementing illnesses in their requirement for significant cognitive impairment. The NINCDS/ADRDA criteria differ from the DSM-IV criteria in only specifying that "two or more" areas of cognition be impaired, whereas the DSM-IV requires memory and one other impaired area of cognition. Particularly in studies that identify AD based on memory, the latter criteria may skew the results by excluding cases that do not have any, or prominent, memory impairment. It also underscores that the criteria for mild cognitive impairment also highlight memory, and the condition is often

From: *Current Clinical Neurology: Diagnostic Criteria in Neurology*
Edited by: A. J. Lerner © Humana Press Inc., Totowa, NJ

Table 1
Classification of Alcohol-Related Dementia

Dementia

Dementia is defined as a significant deterioration of cognitive function sufficient to interfere in social or occupational functioning.

As defined by the *Diagnostic and Statistical Manual of Mental Disorders, 4th edition*, this requires a deterioration in memory and at least one other area of intellectual functioning. Moreover, the cognitive changes are not attributable to the presence of delirium or substance-induced intoxication or withdrawal.

Definite Alcohol-Related Dementia

At the current time, there are no acceptable criteria to define definitively alcohol-related dementia.

Probable Alcohol-Related Dementia

I. The criteria for the clinical diagnosis of probable alcohol-related dementia include the following:
   a. A clinical diagnosis of dementia at least 60 days after the last exposure to alcohol.
   b. Significant alcohol use as defined by a minimum average of 35 standard drinks per week for men and 28 for women for a period greater than 5 years. The period of significant alcohol use must occur within 3 years of the initial onset of dementia.

II. The diagnosis of alcohol-related dementia is supported by the presence of any of the following:
   a. Alcohol-related hepatic, pancreatic, gastrointestinal, cardiovascular, or renal disease, i.e., other end-organ damage.
   b. Ataxia or peripheral sensory polyneuropathy (not attributable to other specific causes).
   c. Beyond 60 days of abstinence, the cognitive impairment stabilizes or improves.
   d. After 60 days of abstinence, any neuroimaging evidence of ventricular or sulcal dilatation improves.
   e. Neuroimaging evidence of cerebellar atrophy, especially of the vermis.

III. The following clinical features cast doubt on the diagnosis of alcohol-related dementia:
   a. The presence of language impairment, especially dysnomia or anomia.
   b. The presence of focal neurological signs or symptoms (except ataxia or peripheral sensory polyneuropathy).
   c. Neuroimaging evidence for cortical or subcortical infarction, subdural hematoma, or other focal brain pathology.
   d. Elevated Hachinski Ischemia Scale score.

IV. Clinical features that are neither supportive nor cast doubt on the diagnosis of alcohol-related dementia include the following:
   a. Neuroimaging evidence of cortical atrophy.
   b. The presence of periventricular or deep white matter lesions on neuroimaging in the absence of focal infarct(s).
   c. The presence of the ApolipoproteinE ε4 allele.

V. The diagnosis of possible alcohol-related dementia may be made when there are
   a. A clinical diagnosis of dementia at least 60 days after the last exposure to alcohol; and
   b. Either:
      1. *Significant alcohol use,* as defined by a minimum average of 35 standard drinks per week for men and 28 for women for 5 or more years; however, the period of significant alcohol use occurred more than 3 years but less than 10 years before the initial onset of cognitive deficits; or
      2. *Possibly significant alcohol use,* as defined by a minimum average of 21 standard drinks per week for men and 14 for women but no more than 34 drinks per week for men and 27 for women for 5 years. The period of significant alcohol use must have occurred within 3 years of the onset of cognitive deficits.

Mixed Dementia

A diagnosis of *mixed dementia* is reserved for clinical cases that appear to have more than one cause for dementia. The classification of probable or possible should continue to be used to convey the certainty of the diagnosis of alcohol-related dementia. The classification of mixed dementia should not be used to convey uncertainty of the diagnosis or to imply a differential diagnosis.

Alcohol as a Contributing Factor in the Development or Course of Dementia

The designation of alcohol as a contributing factor is used for the situation in which alcohol is used, but not to the degree required or within the time required to meet the classification of probable or possible alcohol-related dementia. This designation should not preclude the use of probable vascular dementia or dementia of the Alzheimer's type.

Adapted from Oslin D, Atkinson RM, Smith DM, Hendrie H. Alcohol related dementia: proposed clinical criteria. Int J Geriatr Psychiatr 1998;13:203–220.

summarized as memory impairment without dementia, i.e., the individual is not impaired in social or occupational functioning and has intact activities of daily living.

Because these criteria have been so influential in terms of serving as a template for others, it is important to look closely at the terminology used. In order to have probable AD, one must have "deficits in at least two areas of cognition." The authors did not specify what constitutes a "deficit" or "dysfunction," leaving it open to some degree of interpretation.

The relationship of behavioral disturbances to the core criteria for AD diagnosis should also be considered. Behavioral disturbances are mentioned as supportive of the diagnosis but are not listed as critical to the clinical diagnosis. Regardless of the affect of depression, anxiety, and psychotic behavior on patients and their families, this approach suggests that such severe cognitive problems may be dissociated from behavioral disturbances. It is impossible to distinguish between the two, especially as AD progresses. If one cannot remember a recent question that has been answered, is it not logical to ask the question again? And, as the process escalates to agitation on the part of the patient with AD who feels that information is being withheld, it becomes increasingly difficult to separate the emotional and cognitive components of behavior. On a more practical level, it is noted that the major criteria for the approval of a pharmacological agent for the treatment of AD in the United States includes a cognitive test and a global rating scale; behavior *per se* may not factor significantly into this process.

The relationship to vascular disease is also worthy of scrutiny. Features with sudden onset are clearly excluded as are early focal findings. Nonetheless, AD may present with lateralizing, if not localizing, features, such as a progressive aphasia or complex visual disturbances, such as Balint's syndrome. Many early studies rigorously excluded individuals with significant vascular disease as determined by the Hachinski Ischemia Scale. However, the issue of diagnosis has become more difficult because of the ready availability of magnetic resonance imaging. Should individuals with "nonspecific" white matter hyperintensities be excluded from AD, or labeled *vascular dementia* or *mixed dementia*? Conversely, how shall we classify an individual with a given stroke, either in a location felt to be unrelated to cognitive functioning (such as a subcortical lacunar stroke in motor pathways), or with a stable deficit whose cognition worsens over a period of months or years?

The strict age cutoffs no longer seem as imperative to the diagnosis, although they serve as useful guideposts. Genetic testing is now available for the young-onset familial cases that may have mutations in the amyloid precursor protein (chromosome 21), or mutation *f* the presenilin-1 or -2 genes (chromosomes 14 and 1, respectively). Genetic studies including the Apolipoprotein E (*APOE*) genotype are still not seen as central to the diagnosis of AD. This stems from the rarity of early-onset familial forms in clinical practice. Possession of one or more *APOE* ε4 alleles increases AD risk, but it is not a deterministic gene. The majority of patients with AD do not possess one or more *APOE* ε4 alleles. When compared with *APOE* testing, clinical examination remains the basis for diagnosis.

With the revolution in neuroimaging, we may expect that the next generation of AD criteria to incorporate additional imaging features and possibly quantitative measures, such as hippocampal volumetry.

ATTENTION DEFICIT HYPERACTIVITY DISORDER

Attention deficit hyperactivity disorder (ADHD) and its variants are disorders of unknown etiology, but with a strong familial component and a higher incidence in males. It is being increasingly recognized in adults, but no criteria specific to this population have been proposed. By definition, it begins in childhood, helping to differentiate ADHD from many disorders of attention that may arise in adulthood. Examples of the latter include attentional problems because of head trauma, substance abuse, depression, or causes of encephalopathy.

AUTISTIC SPECTRUM DISORDERS

Austism is now recognized as a spectrum of disorders, the diagnostic criteria of which have emerged from the DSM-IV as the standard for clinical purposes.

Table 2
Probable Alzheimer's Disease According to NINCDS-ADRDA Criteria

I. Criteria for the clinical diagnosis of *probable* Alzheimer's disease:
   a. Dementia established by clinical examination and documented by the mini-mental test, Blessed Dementia Scale, or some similar examination, and confirmed by neuropsychological tests.
   b. Deficits in two or more areas of cognition.
   c. Progressive worsening of memory and other cognitive functions.
   d. No disturbance of consciousness.
   e. Onset between ages 40 and 90, most often after age 65.
   f. Absence of systemic disorders or other brain diseases that in and of themselves could account for the progressive deficits in memory and cognition.
II. The diagnosis of *probable* Alzheimer's disease is supported by the following:
   a. Progressive deterioration of specific cognitive functions such as language (aphasia), motor skills (apraxia), and perceptions (agnosia).
   b. Impaired activities of daily living and altered patterns of behavior.
   c. Family history of similar disorders, particularly if confirmed neuropathologically.
   d. Laboratory results of:
      1. Normal lumbar puncture as evaluated by standard techniques.
      2. Normal pattern or nonspecific changes in electroencephalogram, such as increased slow-wave activity.
      3. Evidence of cerebral atrophy on computed tomography with progression documented by serial observation.
III. Other clinical features consistent with the diagnosis of *probable* Alzheimer's disease, after exclusion of causes of dementia other than Alzheimer's disease, include the following:
   a. Plateaus in the course of progression of the illness.
   b. Associated symptoms of depression, insomnia, incontinence, delusions, illusions, hallucinations, catastrophic verbal, emotional, or physical outbursts, sexual disorders, and weight loss.
   c. Other neurological abnormalities in some patients, especially with more advanced disease and including motor signs, such as increased muscle tone, myoclonus, or gait disorder.
   d. Seizures in advanced disease.
   e. Computed tomography normal for age.
IV. Features that make the diagnosis of *probable* Alzheimer's disease uncertain or unlikely include the following:
   a. Sudden, apoplectic onset.
   b. Focal neurological findings such as hemiparesis, sensory loss, visual field deficits, and incoordination early in the course of the illness.
   c. Seizures or gait disturbances at the onset or very early in the course of the illness.

Adapted from McKhann G, Drachman D, Folstein M, Katzman R, Price D, Stadlan EM. Clinical diagnosis of Alzheimer's disease: report of the NINCDS-ADRDA Work Group under the auspices of Department of Health and Human Services Task Force on Alzheimer's Disease. Neurology 1984;34:939–944.

Asperger's Syndrome

Asperger's syndrome is a condition along the autistic spectrum, now being more frequently recognized in adults, but with onset obligately in childhood.

Rett's Disorder

A disorder primarily affecting females, the genetic basis of Rett's disorder is being unraveled, and genetic testing may supplant clinical criteria. A more detailed listing of diagnostic criteria is listed in Chapter 7. It is included here because Rett's syndrome, aside from its genetic roots, is often classified among the autistic spectrum disorders, at least according to the standard DSM-IV scheme.

Childhood Disintegrative Disorder

The roots of this diagnosis may be traced back to Heller, who, in 1908, described several cases he termed *dementia infantalis*. As is now known, childhood disintegrative disorder is a rare condition, affecting less than 1 in 10,000 children, although limited epidemiological data are available. In the

Table 3
DSM-IV Revised Criteria for Diagnostic Criteria for Dementia of the Alzheimer's Type

A. The development of multiple cognitive deficits manifested by both
  1. Memory impairment (impaired ability to learn new information or to recall previously learned information).
  2. One (or more) of the following cognitive disturbances:
    a. Aphasia (language disturbance).
    b. Apraxia.
    c. Agnosia.
    d. Disturbance in executive functioning (i.e., planning, organizing, sequencing, abstracting).
B. The cognitive deficits in criteria A1 and A2 each cause significant impairment in social or occupational functioning and represent a significant decline from a previous level of functioning.
C. The course is characterized by gradual onset and continuing cognitive decline.
D. The cognitive deficits in criteria A1 and A2 are not caused by any of the following:
  1. Other central nervous system conditions that cause progressive deficits in memory and cognition (e.g., cerebrovascular disease, Parkinson's disease, Huntington's disease, subdural hematoma, normal-pressure hydrocephalus, brain tumor).
  2. Systemic conditions that are known to cause dementia (e.g., hypothyroidism, vitamin B or folic acid deficiency, niacin deficiency, hypercalcemia, neurosyphilis, HIV infection).

Adapted from Diagnostic and Statistical Manual of Mental Disorders, 4th rev. ed. Washington, DC: American Psychiatric Association, 1994.

Table 4
DSM-IV Criteria for Diagnosis of Attention Deficit Hyperactivity Disorder

A. Either 1 or 2:
  1. Six or more of the following symptoms of inattention have persisted for at least 6 months to a degree that is maladaptive and inconsistent with developmental level:
  Inattention
    • Often fails to give close attention to details or makes careless mistakes in schoolwork, work, or other activities.
    • Often has difficulty sustaining attention in tasks or play.
    • Often does not seem to listen when spoken to directly.
    • Often does not follow through on instructions and fails to finish schoolwork, chores, or duties in the workplace (not because of oppositional behavior or failure to understand instructions).
    • Often has difficulty organizing tasks and activities.
    • Often avoids, dislikes, or is reluctant to engage in tasks that require sustained mental effort (such as schoolwork or homework).
    • Often loses things necessary for tasks or activities (e.g., toys, school assignments, pencils, books, or tools).
    • Is often easily distracted by extraneous stimuli.
    • Is often forgetful in daily activities.
  2. Six or more of the following symptoms of hyperactivity/impulsivity have persisted for at least 6 months to a degree that is maladaptive and inconsistent with developmental level:
  Hyperactivity
    • Often fidgets with hands or feet or squirms in seat.
    • Often leaves seat in classroom or in other situations in which remaining seated is expected.
    • Often runs about or climbs excessively in situations in which it is inappropriate (in adolescents or adults, may be limited to subjective feelings of restlessness).
    • Often has difficulty playing or engaging in leisure activities quietly.
    • Is often "on the go" or often acts as if "driven by a motor."
    • Often talks excessively.
  Impulsivity
    • Often blurts out answers before questions have been completed.
    • Often has difficulty awaiting turn.
    • Often interrupts or intrudes on others (e.g., butts into conversations or games).
B. Some hyperactive, impulsive, or inattentive symptoms that caused impairment were present before 7 years of age.

(Continued)

Table 4 *(Continued)*

C. Some impairment from the symptoms is present in two or more settings (e.g., at school, work, and at home).
D. There must be clear evidence of clinically significant impairment in social, academic, or occupational functioning.
E. The symptoms do not occur exclusively during the course of a pervasive developmental disorder, schizophrenia, or other psychotic disorder, and are not better accounted for by another mental disorder.

Adapted from American Psychiatric Association. Diagnostic and Statistical Manual of Mental Disorders, 4th rev. ed. Washington, DC: American Psychiatric Association, 1994.

Table 5
Diagnostic Criteria for Autistic Disorder

A. A total of six (or more) items from criteria 1, 2, and 3, with at least two from criterion 1, and one each from criteria 2 and 3:
　1. Qualitative impairment in social interaction, as manifested by at least two of the following:
　　a. Marked impairment in the use of multiple nonverbal behaviors, such as eye-to-eye gaze, facial expression, body postures, and gestures to regulate social interaction.
　　b. Failure to develop peer relationships appropriate to developmental level.
　　c. A lack of spontaneous seeking to share enjoyment, interests, or achievements with other people (e.g., by a lack of showing, bringing, or pointing out objects of interest).
　　d. Lack of social or emotional reciprocity.
　2. Qualitative impairments in communication, as manifested by at least one of the following:
　　a. Delay in, or total lack of, the development of spoken language (not accompanied by an attempt to compensate through alternative modes of communication, such as gesture or mime).
　　b. In individuals with adequate speech, marked impairment in the ability to initiate or sustain a conversation with others.
　　c. Stereotyped and repetitive use of language or idiosyncratic language.
　　d. Lack of varied, spontaneous make-believe play or social imitative play appropriate to developmental level.
　3. Restricted, repetitive, and stereotyped patterns of behavior, interests, and activities as manifested by at least one of the following:
　　a. Encompassing preoccupation with one or more stereotyped and restricted patterns of interest that is abnormal either in intensity or focus.
　　b. Apparently inflexible adherence to specific, nonfunctional routines or rituals.
　　c. Stereotyped and repetitive motor mannerisms (e.g., hand or finger flapping or twisting or complex whole-body movements).
　　d. Persistent preoccupation with parts of objects.
B. Delays or abnormal functioning in at least one of the following areas, with onset before 3 years of age:
　1. Social interaction.
　2. Language as used in social communication.
　3. Symbolic or imaginative play.
C. The disturbance is not better accounted for by Rett's disorder or childhood disintegrative disorder.

Adapted from American Psychiatric Association. Diagnostic and Statistical Manual of Mental Disorders, 4th rev. ed. Washington, DC: American Psychiatric Association, 1994.

literature, this condition has been termed *dementia infantilis*, *Heller's syndrome*, *progressive disintegrative psychosis*, *disintegrative psychosis*, and *pervasive disintegrative disorder*.

Childhood disintegrative disorder is nonspecific in terms of etiology. Children or adolescents with "typical" autism may regress in terms of previously developed skills. One should be careful in applying this diagnosis without a substantial search for more specific genetic, metabolic, toxic, or traumatic conditions that may incidentally fulfill the following diagnostic criteria. As the age of presentation of the regression increases, the likelihood of a diagnosable neurological disorder also increases. In addition to autism with regression, differential diagnosis includes Rett's disorder, Landau-Kleffner syndrome, or other epileptic disorders.

Table 6
Diagnostic Criteria for Asperger's Syndrome

A. There is a qualitative impairment in social interaction, as manifested by at least two of the following:
   1. Marked impairment in the use of multiple nonverbal behaviors, such as eye contact, facial expression, body postures, and gestures to regulate social interaction.
   2. Failure to develop peer relationships appropriate to developmental level.
   3. A lack of spontaneous seeking to share enjoyment, interests, or achievements with other people (e.g., by a lack of showing, bringing, or pointing out objects of interest to other people).
   4. Lack of social or emotional reciprocity.
B. Restricted, repetitive, and stereotyped patterns of behavior, interests, and activities, as manifested by at least one of the following:
   1. Encompassing preoccupation with one or more stereotyped and restricted patterns of interest that is abnormal *either* in intensity or focus.
   2. Apparently inflexible adherence to specific, nonfunctional routines or rituals.
   3. Stereotyped and repetitive motor mannerisms (e.g., hand or finger flapping or twisting, or complex whole-body movements).
   4. Persistent preoccupation with parts of objects.
C. The disturbance causes clinically significant impairment in social, occupational, or other important areas of functioning.
D. There is no clinically significant general delay in language.
E. There is no clinically significant delay in cognitive development or in the development of age-appropriate self-help skills, adaptive behavior (other than in social interaction), and curiosity about the environment in childhood.
F. Criteria are not met for another specific pervasive developmental disorder or schizophrenia.

Adapted from American Psychiatric Association. Diagnostic and Statistical Manual of Mental Disorders, 4th rev. ed. Washington, DC: American Psychiatric Association, 1994.

Table 7
DSM-IV Diagnostic Criteria for Rett's Disorder

A. All of the following:
   1. Apparently normal prenatal and perinatal development.
   2. Apparently normal psychomotor development through the first 5 months after birth.
   3. Normal head circumference at birth.
B. Onset of all of the following after the period of normal development:
   1. Deceleration of head growth between ages 5 and 48 months.
   2. Loss of previously acquired purposeful hand skills between ages 5 and 30 months, with the subsequent development of stereotyped hand movements (i.e., hand wringing or hand washing).
   3. Loss of social engagement early in the course (although often social interaction develops later).
   4. Appearance of poorly coordinated gait or trunk movements.
   5. Severely impaired expressive and receptive language development with severe psychomotor retardation.

Adapted from American Psychiatric Association. Diagnostic and Statistical Manual of Mental Disorders, 4th rev ed. Washington, DC: American Psychiatric Association, 1994.

Pervasive Developmental Disorder Not Otherwise Specified

This disorder is diagnosed when there is a severe and pervasive impairment in the development of reciprocal social interaction or verbal and nonverbal communication skills, or when stereotyped behavior, interests, and activities are present. However, the criteria are not met for a specific pervasive developmental disorder, schizophrenia, schizotypal personality disorder, or avoidant personality disorder. This category includes "atypical autism"—presentations that do not meet the criteria for autistic disorder because of late age of onset, atypical symptomatology, or subthreshold symptomatology, or all of these.

Table 8
DSM-IV Diagnostic Criteria for Childhood Disintegrative Disorder

A. Apparently normal development for at least the first 2 years after birth as manifested by the presence of age-appropriate verbal and nonverbal communication, social relationships, play, and adaptive behavior.
B. Clinically significant loss of previously acquired skills (before age 10 years) in at least two of the following areas:
   1. Expressive or receptive language.
   2. Social skills or adaptive behavior.
   3. Bowel or bladder control.
   4. Play.
   5. Motor skills.
C. Abnormalities of functioning in at least two of the following areas:
   1. Qualitative impairment in social interaction (e.g., impairment in nonverbal behaviors, failure to develop peer relationships, lack of social or emotional reciprocity).
   2. Qualitative impairments in communication (e.g., delay or lack of spoken language, inability to initiate or sustain a conversation, stereotyped and repetitive use of language, lack of varied make-believe play).
   3. Restricted, repetitive, and stereotyped patterns of behavior, interests, and activities, including motor stereotypies and mannerisms.
D. The disturbance is not better accounted for by another specific pervasive developmental disorder or by schizophrenia.

Adapted from American Psychiatric Association. Diagnostic and Statistical Manual of Mental Disorders, 4th rev. ed. Washington, DC: American Psychiatric Association, 1994.

CONVERSION DISORDER

Table 9
DSM-IV Diagnostic Criteria for Conversion Disorder

A. One or more symptoms or deficits affecting voluntary motor or sensory function suggest(s) a neurological or other general medical condition.
B. Psychological factors are judged to be associated with the symptom or deficit because the initiation or exacerbation of the symptom or deficit is preceded by conflicts or other stressors.
C. The symptom or deficit is not intentionally produced or feigned (as in factitious disorder or malingering).
D. The symptom or deficit cannot, after appropriate investigation, be explained fully by a general medical condition, or by the direct effects of a substance, or as a culturally sanctioned behavior or experience.
E. The symptom or deficit causes clinically significant distress or impairment in social, occupational, or other important areas of functioning or warrants medical evaluation.
F. The symptom or deficit is not limited to pain or sexual dysfunction, does not occur exclusively during the course of the somatization disorder, and is not better accounted for by another mental disorder.

Adapted from American Psychiatric Association. Diagnostic and Statistical Manual of Mental Disorders, 4th rev. ed. Washington, DC: American Psychiatric Association, 1994.

CREUTZFELDT-JAKOB DISEASE

The spectrum of prion-mediated disorders has increased over the years, with the recognition of familial Creutzfeldt-Jakob disease, new-variant Creutzfeldt-Jakob disease, fatal familial insomnia, and other disorders. The optimal method for diagnosis remains tissue histopathology, and the relative accuracy of the 14-3-3 protein and neuroimaging remains to be fully defined. Table 10 lists diagnostic criteria proposed by the World Health Organization and is supplemented by Tables 11–16.

DELIRIUM AND INTOXICATIONS

Delirium is also known as the acute confusional state, and is a nonspecific syndrome. It may be the result of a medical condition, such as major organ failure (e.g., hepatic encephalopathy or sepsis), or

Table 10
World Health Organization Diagnostic Criteria for Creutzfeldt-Jakob Disease

1. Creutzfeldt-Jakob Disease (CJD) clinical diagnosis:
   Criteria for *probable* sporadic CJD: The clinical diagnosis of CJD is currently based on the combination of progressive dementia, myoclonus, and multifocal neurological dysfunction, associated with a characteristic periodic electroencephalogram (EEG). However, new variant CJD, most growth hormone-related iatrogenic cases, and up to 40% of sporadic cases are not noted to have the characteristic EEG appearance. This hampers clinical diagnosis, and hence surveillance, and illustrates the need for additional diagnostic tests. Proposed criteria for *probable* sporadic CJD:
   a. Progressive dementia.
      and
   b. At least two out of the following four clinical features:
      i. Myoclonus.
      ii. Visual or cerebellar disturbance.
      iii. Pyramidal/extrapyramidal dysfunction.
      iv. Akinetic mutism.
      and
2. A typical EEG during an illness of any duration.
   and/or
3. A positive 14-3-3 cerebral spinal fluid assay and a clinical duration to death less than 2 years.
4. Routine investigations should not suggest an alternative diagnosis.

Note: Results from a recent study suggest that the detection of high signal from the basal ganglia on T2- and proton-density-weighted magnetic resonance imaging support the diagnosis of sporadic CJD. These abnormalities can be particularly prominent if a fluid-attenuated inversion recovery sequence or diffusion-weighted images are obtained.
(Adapted from World Health Organization. Human transmissable spongiform encephalopathies. Wkly Epidemiol Rec 1998;73:361–365.)

Table 11
Electroencephalogram Interpretation in Creutzfeldt-Jakob Disease

No widely agreed and validated definition of a diagnostic electroencephalogram tracing is available, leading to potential inconsistencies in case ascertainment between centers. To enhance Creutzfeldt-Jakob disease surveillance, a workable definition of a *diagnostic* electroencephalogram is required.
The following criteria devised by Steinhoff and Knight are suggested for use now, with results being evaluated further:
1. Strictly periodic activity:
   a. Variability of intercomplex intervals is less than 500 ms.
   b. Periodic activity is continuous for at least one 10-second period.
2. Bi- or triphasic morphology of periodic complexes.
3. Duration of majority of complexes ranges from 100 to 600 ms.
4. Periodic complexes may be generalized or lateralized, but not regional or asynchronous.

Adapted from World Health Organization. Human transmissable spongiform encephalopathies. Wkly Epidemiol Rec 1998;73:361–365.

of the effects of intoxication (e.g., alcohol or phencyclidine, etc.). The cardinal finding in delirium is altered mental status, which helps distinguish it from dementia, generally conceived of as occurring in clear consciousness. Not all individuals with delirium are agitated or hyperexcitable. In that regard, there is broad overlap with conditions capable of causing stupor or coma. The evaluation and differential diagnosis of delirium is essentially the same as evaluation of the comatose individual with consideration to signs, symptoms, and etiologies.

It should also be borne in mind that dementia itself is a risk factor for delirium, but should not be diagnosed when the mental status changes of dementia occur exclusively during a delirious episode.

The DSM-IV diagnostic criteria for delirium because of a general medical condition are presented in Table 17. The section on intoxications is drawn from the International Statistical Classification of Diseases and Related Health Problems, 10th edition, classification scheme.

Table 12
New-Variant Creutzfeldt-Jakob Disease: Suspect Case Definition

New-variant Creutzfeldt-Jakob disease (nvCJD) cannot be diagnosed with certainty on clinical criteria alone at present. However, based on the 23 neuropathologically confirmed cases, the diagnosis of nvCJD should be considered as a possibility in a patient with a progressive neuropsychiatric disorder, with at least five out of the following six List 1 clinical features. The suspicion of nvCJD is strengthened by the following criteria in List 2. A patient with a progressive neuropsychiatric disorder and five out of the six clinical features in List 1 and all of the criteria in List 2 should be considered as a suspect case of nvCJD for surveillance purposes.

List 1
1. Early psychiatric symptoms.
2. Early persistent parasthesias/dysesthesias.
3. Ataxia.
4. Chorea/dystonia or myoclonus.
5. Dementia.
6. Akinetic mutism.

List 2
1. The absence of a history of potential iatrogenic exposure.
2. Clinical duration more than 6 months.
3. Age at onset less than 50 years.
4. The absence of a *PrP* gene mutation.
5. The EEG does not show the typical periodic appearance.
6. Routine investigations that do not suggest an alternative diagnosis.
7. A magnetic resonance image showing abnormal bilateral high signal from the pulvinar on axial T2- and/or proton-density-weighted images.

Adapted from World Health Organization. Human transmissable spongiform encephalopathies. Wkly Epidemiol Rec 1998;73:361–365.

Table 13
Revised World Health Organization Definition of Creutzfeldt-Jakob Disease Subtypes

Sporadic CJD	
1. Definite	Diagnosed by standard neuropathological techniques and/or immunocytochemically and/or Western blot-confirmed protease-resistant PrP and/or presence of scrapie-associated fibrils.
2. Probable	a. Progressive dementia and at least two out of the following four clinical features: • Myoclonus. • Visual or cerebellar disturbance. • Pyramidal/extrapyramidal dysfunction. • Akinetic mutism. and b. A typical EEG during an illness of any duration and/or c. A positive 14-3-3 CSF assay and a clinical duration to death less than 2 years. d. Routine investigations should not suggest an alternative diagnosis.
3. Possible	Same clinical criteria as definite but no, or atypical, EEG and duration less than 2 years
Iatrogenic CJD	Progressive cerebellar syndrome in a recipient of human cadaveric-derived pituitary hormone; or Sporadic CJD with a recognized exposure risk, e.g., antecedent neurosurgery with dura mater graft
Familial CJD	Definite or probable CJD plus definite or probable CJD in a first-degree relative and/or Neuropsychiatric disorder plus disease-specific *PrP* gene mutation

CJD, Creutzfeldt-Jakob Disease; PrP, prion protein; EEG, electroencephalogram; CSF, cerebrospinal fluid.

Table 14
Neuropathological Criteria for Creutzfeldt-Jakob Disease and Other Human Transmissible Spongiform Encephalopathies

1. Creutzfeldt-Jakob disease (CJD)—*sporadic, iatrogenic* (recognized risk) or *familial* (same disease in first-degree relative or disease-associated *PrP* gene mutation): Spongiform encephalopathy in cerebral and/or cerebellar cortex and/or subcortical gray matter; and/or encephalopathy with prion protein (PrP) immunoreactivity (plaque and/or diffuse synaptic and/or patchy/perivacuolar types).
2. New-variant CJD: Spongiform encephalopathy with abundant PrP deposition; in particular, multiple fibrillary PrP plaques surrounded by a halo of spongiform vacuoles ("florid" plaques, "daisy-like" plaques) and other PrP plaques, and amorphous pericellular and perivascular PrP deposits; especially prominent in the cerebellar molecular layer.
3. Gerstmann-Sträussler-Scheinker disease (in family with dominantly inherited progressive ataxia and/or dementia and one of a variety of *PrP* gene mutations): Encephalo(myelo)pathy with multicentric PrP plaques.
4. Familial fatal insomnia (in member of a family with a *PrP* gene mutation at codon 178 in frame with methionine at codon 129): Thalamic degeneration, variable spongiform change in cerebrum.
5. Kuru: Spongiform encephalopathy in the Fore population of Papua New Guinea.

Additional information:

1. Genetic analysis

   Screening cases of CJD for the mutations associated with the hereditary forms of disease raises ethical and logistic concerns. Written consent for genetic testing is considered mandatory in many countries, but may be culturally unacceptable in others. The World Health Organization Consultation Diagnostic Procedures for Transmissible Spongiform Encephalopathies recommends that genetic counseling of patients and/or their families should be performed before any *PrP* gene analysis and that ideally written consent, but if not documented, oral consent should be obtained. The genetic counselor should be provided with information on the genetics of human transmissible spongiform encephalopathy to be used when seeking consent.

2. Electroencephalogram interpretation

   a. Preliminary notes:

      i. The finding of a characteristic periodic EEG pattern is very helpful in the diagnosis of sporadic CJD.

      ii. Some cases of sporadic CJD never show this pattern. A "negative" result cannot exclude the diagnosis.

      iii. A periodic EEG, such as that seen in CJD, may rarely be found in a number of other conditions, and these must be considered in the clinical context. A list of these conditions is given in Table 15.

      iv. The EEG changes in CJD undergo evolution. A periodic pattern may not be seen in the early phases of disease. The EEG may progress from showing nonspecific abnormalities to the characteristic appearance within days. Therefore, frequent serial EEG recordings should be undertaken whenever possible.

      v. If a typical periodic EEG is obtained, then it is not absolutely necessary to repeat it, although this should be considered if there is any clinical doubt about other possible causes of the EEG pattern (such as metabolic factors).

      vi. A repeatedly normal EEG is not consistent with a diagnosis of sporadic CJD.

   b. Technical notes:

      i. Bipolar montages including the vertex should be used.

      ii. Referential montages including vertex and CZ reference electrodes should be used.

      iii. The ECG should be coregistered.

      iv. External alerting stimuli should be used.

      v. The whole record should be viewed whenever possible, and a 2-minute continuous sequence used as a minimum.

Adapted from Budka H, Agguzi A, Brown P, et al. Neuropathological diagnostic criteria for Creutzfeldt-Jakob disease and other human spongiform encephalopathies [prion diseases]. Brain Pathol 1995;5:459–466.

Table 15
Conditions That May Cause a Creutzfeldt-Jakob Disease-Like Electroencephalogram

Alzheimer's disease
Hyperammonemia
Lewy body disease
Binswanger's disease
AIDS dementia
Hyperparathyroidism
Hypo- and hypernatremia
Hypoglycemia
Multiple cerebral abscesses
MELAS syndrome
Hepatic encephalopathy
Baclofen, mianserin, metrizamide, and lithium toxicity
Postanoxic encephalopathy

MELAS, mitochondrial encephalopathy, lactic acidosis, and stroke-like episodes.

(Adapted from Global surveillance, diagnosis and therapy of human transmissible spongiform encephalopathies: Report of a WHO consultation. Geneva, Switzerland, 9–11 February 1998.)

Table 16
Conditions Other Than Creutzfeldt-Jakob Disease That Can Have a Positive 14-3-3 Result

Herpes simplex and other encephalitides
Stroke (especially recent)
Subarachnoid hemorrhage
Hypoxic/Ischemic encephalopathy
Barbiturate intoxication
Glioblastoma
Carcinomatous meningitis (especially small-cell lung carcinoma)
Paraneoplastic encephalopathy
Corticobasal degeneration

Adapted from Global surveillance, diagnosis and therapy of human transmissible spongiform encephalopathies: Report of a WHO consultation. Geneva, Switzerland, 9–11 February 1998.

Table 17
DSM-IV Diagnostic Criteria for Delirium Caused by a General Medical Condition

A. Disturbance of consciousness (i.e., reduced clarity of awareness of the environment) with reduced ability to focus, sustain, or shift attention.
B. A change in cognition (such as memory disturbance, disorientation, language disturbance) or the development of a perceptual disturbance that is not better accounted for by a preexisting, established, or evolving dementia.
C. The disturbance develops over a short time (usually hours to days) and tends to fluctuate during the course of the day.
D. There is evidence from the history, physical examination, or laboratory findings that the disturbance is caused by the direct physiological consequences of a general medical condition.

Adapted from American Psychiatric Association. Diagnostic and Statistical Manual of Mental Disorders, 4th rev. ed. Washington, DC: American Psychiatric Association, 1994.

The International Statistical Classification of Diseases and Related Health Problems, 10th Edition, Classification of Mental and Behavioral Disorders: Diagnostic Criteria for Research (Tables 18–45)

Table 18
Intoxication

1. There must be clear evidence of recent use of a psychoactive substance (or substances) at sufficiently high-dose levels to be consistent with intoxication.
2. There must be symptoms or signs of intoxication compatible with the known actions of the particular substance (or substances), such as specified in Table 19, and of sufficient severity to produce disturbances in the level of consciousness, cognition, perception, affect, or behavior that are of clinical importance.
3. The symptoms or signs present cannot be accounted for by a medical disorder unrelated to substance use, and not better accounted for by another mental or behavioral disorder.

Acute intoxication frequently occurs in persons who have more persistent alcohol- or drug-related problems as well. Where there are such problems, e.g., harmful use, dependence syndrome, or psychotic disorder, they should also be recorded.

Table 19
Acute Intoxication Owing to Alcohol Use

A. The general criteria for acute intoxication must be met.
B. There must be dysfunctional behavior, as evidenced by at least one of the following:
   1. Disinhibition.
   2. Argumentativeness.
   3. Aggression.
   4. Lability of mood.
   5. Impaired attention.
   6. Impaired judgment.
   7. Interference with personal functioning.
C. At least one of the following signs must be present:
   1. Unsteady gait.
   2. Difficulty in standing.
   3. Slurred speech.
   4. Nystagmus.
   5. Decreased level of consciousness (e.g., stupor, coma).
   6. Flushed face.
   7. Conjunctival injection.

   Comment: When severe, acute alcohol intoxication may be accompanied by hypotension, hypothermia, and depression of the gag reflex.

Table 20
Pathological Alcohol Intoxication

A. The general criteria for acute intoxication must be met, with the exception that pathological intoxication occurs after drinking amounts of alcohol insufficient to cause intoxication in most people.
B. There is verbally aggressive or physically violent behavior that is not typical of the person when sober.
C. The intoxication occurs very soon (usually a few minutes) after consumption of alcohol.
D. There is no evidence of organic cerebral disorder or other mental disorders.

   Note: The status of this condition is being examined. These research criteria must be regarded as tentative.
   Comment: This is an uncommon condition. The blood alcohol levels found in this disorder are lower than those that would cause acute intoxication in most people, i.e., lower than 40 mg/100 mL.

DEMENTIA WITH LEWY BODIES

Combining both features of a primary degenerative dementia and an akinetic-rigid, parkinsonian syndrome with prominent behavioral features, dementia with Lewy bodies (DLB) illustrates some of the

Table 21
Acute Intoxication Owing to Opioid Use

A. The general criteria for acute intoxication must be met.
B. There must be dysfunctional behavior, as evidenced by at least one of the following:
   1. Apathy and sedation.
   2. Disinhibition.
   3. Psychomotor retardation.
   4. Impaired attention.
   5. Impaired judgment.
   6. Interference with personal functioning.
C. At least one of the following signs must be present:
   1. Drowsiness.
   2. Slurred speech.
   3. Pupillary constriction (except in anoxia from severe overdose, when pupillary dilatation occurs).
   4. Decreased level of consciousness (e.g., stupor, coma).

Comment: When severe, acute opioid intoxication may be accompanied by respiratory depression (and hypoxia), hypotension, and hypothermia.

Table 22
Acute Intoxication Owing to Cannabinoid Use

A. The general criteria for acute intoxication must be met.
B. There must be dysfunctional behavior or perceptual abnormalities, including at least one of the following:
   1. Euphoria and disinhibition.
   2. Anxiety or agitation.
   3. Suspiciousness or paranoid ideation.
   4. Temporal showing (a sense that time is passing very slowly, and/or the person is experiencing a rapid flow of ideas).
   5. Impaired judgment.
   6. Impaired attention.
   7. Impaired reaction time.
   8. Auditory, visual, or tactile illusions.
   9. Hallucinations with preserved orientation.
   10. Depersonalization.
   11. Derealization.
   12. Interference with personal functioning.
C. At least one of the following signs must be present:
   1. Increased appetite.
   2. Dry mouth.
   3. Conjunctival injection.
   4. Tachycardia.

shortcomings of current nosological schemata. Lewy bodies are the pathological hallmark of Parkinson's disease, where they are primarily restricted to substantia nigra and pigmented brainstem nuclei. However, the presence of Lewy bodies in the cerebral cortex coupled with behavioral symptoms, such as visual hallucinations, led to the recognition of DLB as a distinct syndrome. Complicating this assessment is the presence of AD pathology in about 50% of autopsies of clinically diagnosed cases of DLB, leading to the concept of a Lewy body variant of AD. A number of diagnostic criteria have been proposed and are summarized in Table 46. A number of studies, utilizing varying proportions of DLB cases have reported validity, and reliability of the clinical criteria of DLB, often in relation to populations of AD or other mixed dementia groups (summarized in Table 47). Because positive and negative predictive values will vary according to the prevalence in the population, the small sample sizes and possibly relatively high proportion of true DLB cases in the referenced studies may overestimate these values in routine clinical practice. At present, the most important and widely used set is that proposed by McKieth et al. in their 1996 revision of the consensus criteria (Table 48).

Table 23
Acute Intoxication Owing to Sedative or Hypnotics Use

A. The general criteria for acute intoxication must be met.
B. There is dysfunctional behavior, as evidenced by at least one of the following:
    1. Euphoria and disinhibition.
    2. Apathy and sedation.
    3. Abusiveness or aggression.
    4. Lability of mood.
    5. Impaired attention.
    6. Anterograde amnesia.
    7. Impaired psychomotor performance.
    8. Interference with personal functioning.
C. At least one of the following signs must be present:
    1. Unsteady gait.
    2. Difficulty in standing.
    3. Slurred speech.
    4. Nystagmus.
    5. Decreased level of consciousness (e.g., stupor, coma).
    6. Erythematous skin lesions or blisters.

Comment: When severe, acute intoxication from sedative or hypnotic drugs may be accompanied by hypotension, hypothermia, and depression of the gag reflex.

Table 24
Acute Intoxication Owing to Cocaine Use

A. The general criteria for acute intoxication must be met.
B. There must be dysfunctional behavior or perceptual abnormalities, as evidenced by at least one of the following:
    1. Euphoria and sensation of increased energy.
    2. Hypervigilance.
    3. Grandiose beliefs or actions.
    4. Abusiveness or aggression.
    5. Argumentativeness.
    6. Lability of mood.
    7. Repetitive stereotyped behaviors.
    8. Auditory, visual, or tactile illusions.
    9. Hallucinations, usually with intact orientation.
    10. Paranoid ideation.
    11. Interference with personal functioning.
C. At least two of the following signs must be present:
    1. Tachycardia (sometimes bradycardia).
    2. Cardiac arrhythmias.
    3. Hypertension (sometimes hypotension).
    4. Sweating and chills.
    5. Nausea and vomiting.
    6. Evidence of weight loss.
    7. Pupillary dilatation.
    8. Psychomotor agitation (sometimes retardation).
    9. Muscular weakness.
    10. Chest pain.
    11. Convulsions.

Comment: Interference with personal functioning is most readily apparent from the social interactions of cocaine users, which range from extreme gregariousness to social withdrawal.

Knopman, Boeve and Peterson present a modified version of DLB diagnostic criteria that are similar to the World Health Organization Consortium criteria, but do not specify a temporal relationship between onset of Parkinsonism and dementia, and include rapid eye movement sleep behavior disorder.

Table 25
Acute Intoxication Owing to Use of Other Stimulants, Including Caffeine

A. The general criteria for acute intoxication must be met.
B. There must be dysfunctional behavior or perceptual abnormalities, as evidenced by at least one of the following:
    1. Euphoria and sensation of increased energy.
    2. Hypervigilance.
    3. Grandiose beliefs or actions.
    4. Abusiveness or aggression.
    5. Argumentativeness.
    6. Lability of mood.
    7. Repetitive stereotyped behaviors.
    8. Auditory, visual, or tactile illusions.
    9. Hallucinations, usually with intact orientation.
    10. Paranoid ideation.
    11. Interference with personal functioning.
C. At least two of the following signs must be present:
    1. Tachycardia (sometimes bradycardia).
    2. Cardiac arrhythmias.
    3. Hypertension (sometimes hypotension).
    4. Sweating and chills.
    5. Nausea and vomiting.
    6. Evidence of weight loss.
    7. Pupillary dilatation.
    8. Psychomotor agitation (sometimes retardation).
    9. Muscular weakness.
    10. Chest pain.
    11. Convulsions.

Comment: Interference with personal functioning is most readily apparent from the social interactions of the substance users, which range from extreme gregariousness to social withdrawal.

Table 26
Acute Intoxication Owing to Hallucinogen Use

A. The general criteria for acute intoxication must be met.
B. There must be dysfunctional behavior or perceptual abnormalities, as evidenced by at least one of the following:
    1. Anxiety and fearfulness.
    2. Auditory, visual, or tactile illusions or hallucinations occurring in a state of full wakefulness and alertness.
    3. Depersonalization.
    4. Derealization.
    5. Paranoid ideation.
    6. Ideas of reference.
    7. Lability of mood.
    8. Hyperactivity.
    9. Impulsive acts.
    10. Impaired attention.
    11. Interference with personal functioning.
C. At least two of the following signs must be present:
    1. Tachycardia.
    2. Palpitations.
    3. Sweating and chills.
    4. Tremor.
    5. Blurring of vision.
    6. Pupillary dilatation.
    7. Incoordination.

Table 27
Acute Intoxication Because of Tobacco Use (Acute Nicotine Intoxication)

A. The general criteria for acute intoxication must be met.
B. There must be dysfunctional behavior or perceptual abnormalities, as evidenced by at least one of the following:
    1. Insomnia.
    2. Bizarre dreams.
    3. Lability of mood.
    4. Derealization.
    5. Interference with personal functioning.
C. At least one of the following signs must be present:
    1. Nausea or vomiting.
    2. Sweating.
    3. Tachycardia.
    4. Cardiac arrhythmias.

Table 28
Acute Intoxication Because of Volatile Solvent Use

A. The general criteria for intoxication must be met.
B. There must be dysfunctional behavior, evidenced by at least one of the following:
    1. Apathy and lethargy.
    2. Argumentativeness.
    3. Abusiveness or aggression.
    4. Lability of mood.
    5. Impaired judgment.
    6. Impaired attention and memory.
    7. Psychomotor retardation.
    8. Interference with personal functioning.
C. At least one of the following signs must be present:
    1. Unsteady gait.
    2. Difficulty in standing.
    3. Slurred speech.
    4. Nystagmus.
    5. Decreased level of consciousness (e.g., stupor, coma).
    6. Muscle weakness.
    7. Blurred vision or diplopia.

Comment: Acute intoxication from inhalation of substances other than solvents should also be coded here. When severe, acute intoxication from volatile solvents may be accompanied by hypotension, hypothermia, and depression of the gag reflex.

Table 29
Acute Intoxication Because of Multiple Drug Use and Use of Other Psychoactive Substances

This category should be used when there is evidence of intoxication caused by recent use of other psychoactive substances (e.g., phencyclidine) or of multiple psychoactive substances, where it is uncertain which substance has predominated.

Table 30
Definition of Harmful Use

A. There must be clear evidence that the substance use was responsible for (or substantially contributed to) physical or psychological harm, including impaired judgment or dysfunctional behavior, which may lead to disability or have adverse consequences for interpersonal relationships.
B. The nature of the harm should be clearly identifiable (and specified).
C. The pattern of use has persisted for at least 1 month or has occurred repeatedly within a 12-month period.
D. The disorder does not meet the criteria for any other mental or behavioral disorder related to the same drug in the same time period (except for acute intoxication).

Table 31
Definition of Dependence Syndrome

Three or more of the following manifestations should have occurred together for at least 1 month or, if persisting for periods of less than 1 month, should have occurred together repeatedly within a 12-month period:
1. A strong desire or sense of compulsion to take the substance.
2. Impaired capacity to control substance-taking behavior in terms of its onset, termination, or levels of use, as evidenced by the substance being often taken in larger amounts or over a longer period than intended, or by a persistent desire or unsuccessful efforts to reduce or control substance use.
3. A physiological withdrawal state when substance use is reduced or ceased, as evidenced by the characteristic withdrawal syndrome for the substance, or by use of the same (or closely related) substance with the intention of relieving or avoiding withdrawal symptoms.
4. Evidence of tolerance to the effects of the substance, such that there is a need for significantly increased amounts of the substance to achieve intoxication or the desired effect, or a markedly diminished effect with continued use of the same amount of the substance.
5. Preoccupation with substance use, as manifested by important alternative pleasures or interests being given up or reduced because of substance use or a great deal of time being spent in activities necessary to obtain, take, or recover from the effects of the substance.
6. Persistent substance use despite clear evidence of harmful consequences as evidenced by continued use when the individual is actually aware, or may be expected to be aware, of the nature and extent of harm.

Table 32
Definition of Withdrawal State

1. There must be clear evidence of recent cessation or reduction of substance use after repeated, and usually prolonged and/or high-dose use of that substance.
2. Symptoms and signs are compatible with the known features of a withdrawal state from the particular substance or substances.
3. Symptoms and signs are not accounted for by a medical disorder unrelated to substance use, and not better accounted for by another mental or behavioral disorder.

Table 33
Diagnostic Criteria for Alcohol Withdrawal State

A. The general criteria for withdrawal state must be met.
B. Any three of the following signs must be present:
    1. Tremor of the tongue, eyelids, or outstretched hands.
    2. Sweating.
    3. Nausea or vomiting.
    4. Tachycardia or hypertension.
    5. Psychomotor agitation.
    6. Headache.
    7. Insomnia.
    8. Malaise or weakness.
    9. Transient visual, tactile, or auditory hallucinations or illusions.
    10. Grand mal convulsions.

Comment: If delirium is present, the diagnosis should be "alcohol withdrawal state with delirium" (*delirium tremens*).

FRONTOTEMPORAL DEMENTIA

Frontotemporal dementia (FTD) is a term encompassing a number of disorders now grouped together on the basis both of clinical expression and pathology. Some of the disorders now included under FTD are Pick's disease, progressive nonfluent aphasia, and semantic dementia. About 15% of FTD cases are familial, associated with mutations in the microtubule-associated protein, tau, whose

Table 34
Opioid Withdrawal State

A. The general criteria for withdrawal state must be met.[a]
B. Any three of the following signs must be present:
    1. Craving for an opioid drug.
    2. Rhinorrhea or sneezing.
    3. Lacrimation.
    4. Muscle aches or cramps.
    5. Abdominal cramps.
    6. Nausea or vomiting.
    7. Diarrhea.
    8. Pupillary dilatation.
    9. Piloerection or recurrent chills.
    10. Tachycardia or hypertension.
    11. Yawning.
    12. Restless sleep.

[a]An opioid withdrawal state may also be induced by administration of an opioid antagonist after a brief period of opioid use.

Table 35
Cannabinoid Withdrawal State

This is an ill-defined syndrome for which definitive diagnostic criteria cannot be established at the present time. It occurs following cessation of prolonged high-dose use of cannabis. It has been reported variously as lasting from several hours to up to 7 days.
Symptoms and signs include anxiety, irritability, tremor of the outstretched hands, sweating, and muscle aches.

Table 36
Sedative or Hypnotic Withdrawal State

A. The general criteria for withdrawal state must be met.
B. Any three of the following signs must be present:
    1. Tremor of the tongue, eyelids, or outstretched hands.
    2. Nausea or vomiting.
    3. Tachycardia.
    4. Postural hypotension.
    5. Psychomotor agitation.
    6. Headache.
    7. Insomnia.
    8. Malaise or weakness.
    9. Transient visual, tactile, or auditory hallucinations or illusions.
    10. Paranoid ideation.
    11. Grand mal convulsions.

Comment: If delirium is present, the diagnosis should be "sedative or hypnotic withdrawal state with delirium."

Table 37
Cocaine Withdrawal State

A. The general criteria for withdrawal state must be met.
B. There is dysphoric mood (for instance, sadness, or anhedonia).
C. Any two of the following signs must be present:
    1. Lethargy and fatigue.
    2. Psychomotor retardation or agitation.
    3. Craving for cocaine.
    4. Increased appetite.
    5. Insomnia or hypersomnia.
    6. Bizarre or unpleasant dreams.

Table 38
Withdrawal State From Other Stimulants, Including Caffeine

A. The general criteria for withdrawal state must be met.
B. There is dysphoric mood (for instance, sadness, or anhedonia).
C. Any two of the following signs must be present:
    1. Lethargy and fatigue.
    2. Psychomotor retardation or agitation.
    3. Craving for stimulant drugs.
    4. Increased appetite.
    5. Insomnia or hypersomnia.
    6. Bizarre or unpleasant dreams.

Table 39
Hallucinogen Withdrawal State

There is no recognized hallucinogen withdrawal state.

Table 40
Tobacco Withdrawal State

A. The general criteria for withdrawal state must be met.
B. Any two of the following signs must be present:
    1. Craving for tobacco (or other nicotine-containing products).
    2. Malaise or weakness.
    3. Anxiety.
    4. Dysphoric mood.
    5. Irritability or restlessness.
    6. Insomnia.
    7. Increased appetite.
    8. Increased cough.
    9. Mouth ulceration.
    10. Difficulty in concentrating.

Table 41
Volatile Solvent Withdrawal State

There is inadequate information on withdrawal states from volatile solvents for research criteria to be formulated.

Table 42
Withdrawal State With Delirium

A. The general criteria for withdrawal state must be met.
B. The criteria for delirium must be met.

Table 43
Diagnostic Criteria for Psychotic Disorder

A. Onset of psychotic symptoms must occur during or within 2 weeks of substance use.
B. The psychotic symptoms must persist for more than 48 hours.
C. Duration of the disorder must not exceed 6 months.

Comment: For research purposes, it is recommended that change of the disorder from either a nonpsychotic to a clearly psychotic state be further specified as either abrupt (onset within 48 hours) or acute (onset in more than 48 hours but less than 2 weeks).

Table 44
Amnestic Syndrome

A. Memory impairment is manifest in both:
   1. A defect of recent memory (impaired learning of new material) to a degree sufficient to interfere with daily living.
   2. A reduced ability to recall past experiences.
B. All of the following are absent (or relatively absent):
   1. Defect in immediate recall (as tested, for example, by the digit span).
   2. Clouding of consciousness and disturbance of attention.
   3. Global intellectual decline (dementia).
C. There is no objective evidence from physical and neurological examination, laboratory tests, or history of a disorder or disease of the brain (especially involving bilaterally the diencephalic and medial temporal structures), other than that related to substance use, which can reasonably be presumed to be responsible for the clinical manifestations described under criterion A.

See also Table 61.

Table 45
Residual and Late-Onset Psychotic Disorder

A. Conditions and disorders meeting the criteria for the individual syndromes should be clearly related to substance use. Where onset of the condition or disorder occurs subsequent to use of psychoactive substances, strong evidence should be provided to demonstrate a link.
B. The general criteria for psychotic disorder must be met, except with regard to the onset of the disorder, which is more than 2 weeks but not more than 6 weeks after substance use.

Comments: In view of the considerable variation in this category, the characteristics of such residual states or conditions should be clearly documented in terms of their type, severity, and duration. For research purposes, full descriptive details should be specified.

Table 46
Consensus Criteria for the Clinical Diagnosis of Probable and Possible Dementia With Lewy Bodies

1. The central feature required for a diagnosis of dementia with Lewy bodies (DLB) is a progressive, cognitive decline of sufficient magnitude to interfere with normal social or occupational functioning. Prominent or persistent memory impairment may not necessarily occur in the early stages, but is usually evident with progression. Deficits on tests of attention and of frontal-subcortical skills and visuospatial ability may be especially prominent.
2. Two of the following core features are essential to a diagnosis of probable DLB:
   a. Fluctuating cognition with pronounced variations in attention and alertness.
   b. Recurrent visual hallucinations that are typically well formed and detailed.
   c. Spontaneous motor features of Parkinsonism.
3. Features supportive of the diagnosis:
   a. Repeated falls.
   b. Syncope.
   c. Transient loss of consciousness.
   d. Neuroleptic sensitivity.
   e. Systematic delusions.
   f. Hallucinations in other modalities.
4. A diagnosis of DLB is less likely in the presence of:
   a. Stroke, evident as focal neurological signs or on brain imaging; or
   b. Evidence on physical examination and investigation of any physical illness or other brain disorder sufficient to account for the clinical picture.

Adapted with permission from McKeith IG, Galasko D, Kosaka K, et al. Consensus guidelines for the clinical and pathologic diagnosis of dementia with Lewy bodies: report of the consortium on DLB international workshop. Neurology 1996;47:1113–1124.

Table 47
Published Diagnostic Criteria for Dementia With Lewy Bodies

Reference	Year	Derivation and use
Byrne et al.	1991	Criteria divided into probable and possible, Parkinsonism mandatory PDD included as a subtype of DLB.
McKeith et al.	1992	Retrospectively derived from review of 21 pathologically confirmed cases. Fluctuating cognition and one of three of visual hallucinations, Parkinsonism, and repeated falls, or disturbances of consciousness.
CERAD criteria, Hulette et al.	1995	Two of three of delusions or hallucinations, Parkinsonism, and unexplained falls or changes in consciousness.
Refined 1992 consensus criteria, McKeith et al.	1996	Require cognitive impairment with attentional and visuospatial deficits and two of three (probable DLB), one of three (possible DLB) of fluctuating cognition, visual hallucinations or Parkinsonism.
Luis et al.	1999	Empirically derived from review of 35 pathologically confirmed cases; three diagnostic categories (A,B,C) requiring one, two, or three of hallucinations, unspecified Parkinsonism, fluctuating course, or rapid progression.

PDD, Parkinsonism disease and dementia; DLB, dementia with Lewy bodies.

(Adapted with permission from Litvan I, Bhatia KP, Burn DJ, et al. SIC Task Force appraisal of clinical diagnostic criteria for Parkinsonian disorders. Mov Dis 2003;18:467–486.)

gene is located on chromosome 17. Because many other disorders have been associated with abnormalities in tau expression, it has been suggested that the clinical spectrum of FTD may involve disorders such as progressive supranuclear palsy and corticobasal degeneration. In AD, tau is associated with neurofibrillary tangles, implying a classification of the dementias based on understanding of molecular pathology may be forthcoming in the future.

FTD has two major clinical presentations. The most common form is a behavioral syndrome. Individuals develop early changes in social and personal functioning. Symptoms may include disinhibition, impulsive and inappropriate behavior, and breakdown of social conventions. There may be stereotyped or repetitive actions admixed with these aforementioned behaviors. Memory may be affected, but tends not to be (clinically) the most significant abnormality.

In the language variant, individuals with FTD may develop expressive language dysfunction, with frequent anomia. Problems in reading comprehension and written expression may follow. Eventually, such patients may be mute. Other patients may have pronounced difficulty with naming and verbal comprehension. Patients with FTD may also develop motor abnormalities including a motor neuron disease syndrome or Parkinsonism.

Possibly because the full extent of FTD is still evolving, several sets of diagnostic criteria have been proposed. McKhann et al. have proposed relatively simple clinical criteria, which are shown in Table 50. The same work group also described five basic patterns of neuropathological change, and gave appropriate neurological differential diagnosis for each type, summarized in Table 51. (Note that the wide variety of syndromic names and varying neuropathology may make identification of a patient's syndrome obscure even in well-studied cases. Despite the wide-ranging phenotypes, in a mixed dementia population [autopsy-defined], there was excellent inter-rater reliability of the FTD diagnostic criteria.)

The current criteria (Table 50) contrasts with the comprehensive criteria proposed by an international consortium (Tables 52–55). The Appendix contains explanations of the terms used in Table 55.

MILD COGNITIVE IMPAIRMENT

Mild cognitive impairment (MCI) describes a condition that lies intermediately between normal cognition and dementia, defined broadly as acquired loss of cognitive abilities. The major operational

Table 48
Validity and Reliability of Consensus Criteria for Dementia With Lewy Bodies

Reference	DLB cases/ all cases	Diagnostic criteria	Sens.	Spec.	PPV	NPV	κ	Comments and recommendations
Mega et al.	4 DLB/ 24 AD	Prob.	75	79	100	93	F = 0.25 H = 0.59	Retrospective; suggest four of six of H, C, R, B, N, and Fl.
		Poss.	N/A	N/A	N/A	N/A	P = 0.46	
Litvan et al.	14 DLB/ 105 PD, PSP, MSA, CBD, AD	[a]	18	99	75	89	0.19–0.38	Retrospective; no formal criteria for DLB used; comparison mainly with movement disorder patients.
Holmes et al.	9 DLB/ 80 AD, VaD	Prob. Poss.	22 N/A	1.00 N/A	100 N/A	91 N/A	N/A	Retrospective; no specific recs.; mixed pathology. cases hardest to diagnose.
Luis et al.	35 DLB/ 56 AD	Prob.	57	90	91	56	F = 0.30 H = 0.91	Retrospective; suggest H, P, Fl, and rapid progression.
		N/A	N/A	N/A	N/A	N/A	P = 0.61	
Verghese et al.	18 DLB/ 94 AD	Prob.	61	84	48	90	F = 0.57 H = 0.87	Retrospective; suggest three of six of P, Fl, H, N, D, and F.
		Poss.	89	28	23	91	P = 0.90	
Lopez et al.	28/40		0	100	0	80		Retrospective; probable DLB not diagnosed once by team of four raters; no specific recs.
Hohl et al.	5 DLB/ 10 AD	Prob. Poss.	100 100	8 0	83 N/A	100 N/A	N/A	Consensus criteria applied retrospectively; clinician diagnosis without World Health Organization Consensus criteria had PPV of 50.
McKeith et al.	29 DLB/ 50 AD, VaD	Prob. Poss.	83 N/A	95 N/A	96 N/A	80 N/A	N/A	Prospective; false-negatives associated with comorbid pathology.
Lopez et al.	13 DLB/ 26 AD	Prob. Poss.	23 N/A	100 N/A	100 N/A	43 N/A		Prospective, met NINCDS-ADRDA criteria for AD, only four of them met DLB criteria.

[a]No criteria applied, retrospective clinical diagnosis.

Validity values are given in percentages.

DLB, dementia with Lewy bodies; AD, Alzheimer's disease; PD, Parkinson's disease; PSP, progressive supranuclear palsy; MSA, multiple system atrophy; CBD, corticobasal degeneration; VaD, vascular dementia; Sens., sensitivity; Spec., specificity; PPV, positive predictive value; NPV, negative predictive value; κ, kappa statistic (inter-rater reliability); Prob., probable; Poss., possible; H, hallucinations; C, cogwheeling, R, rigidity; B, bradykinesia; N, neuroleptic sensitivity; Fl, fluctuation; D, delusions; F; falls; P, Parkinsonism; N/A, not available; NINCDS-ADRDA, National Institute of Neurological and Communicative Diseases and Stroke/Alzheimer's Disease and Related Disorders Association.

(Adapted with permission from Litvan I, Bhatia KP, Burn DJ, et al. SIC Task Force appraisal of clinical diagnostic criteria for Parkinsonian disorders. Mov Dis 2003;18:467–486.)

distinction is that individuals with MCI, although manifesting objective memory impairment, by either routine examination or neuropsychological testing, are not impaired in terms of social or occupational functioning or, more broadly, in terms of activities of daily living. MCI often progresses to frank dementia, with progression rates to full-blown AD (*see* Table 2) of about 15% per year.

Although there may be minor differences in definition, MCI has superseded previous entities, such as benign senescent forgetfulness or age-associated memory impairment. It may correspond to the

Table 49
Proposed Additional Diagnostic Criteria for Dementia With Lewy Bodies

A. On the basis of evidence from a patient's history and mental status examination, dementia with Lewy bodies is characterized by the presence of at least two of the following impairments:
  1. Impaired learning and impaired retention of new information.
  2. Impaired handling of complex tasks.
  3. Impaired reasoning ability.
  4. Impaired spatial ability and orientation.
  5. Impaired language.
B. The impairments in criterion A notably interfere with work or usual social activities or relationships with others.
C. The impairments in criterion A represent a notable decline from a previous level of functioning.
D. Dementia with Lewy bodies is characterized by the presence of at least two of the following symptoms:
  1. Parkinsonism (muscular rigidity, resting tremor, bradykinesia, postural instability, parkinsonian gait disorder).
  2. Prominent, fully formed visual hallucinations.
  3. Substantial fluctuations in alertness or cognition.
  4. Rapid eye movement sleep behavior disorder.
E. The impairments in criterion A do not occur exclusively during the course of delirium.
F. The impairments in criterion A are not better explained by a major psychiatric diagnosis.
G. The impairments in criterion A are not better explained by a systemic disease or another brain disease.

Diagnostic criteria for dementia with Lewy bodies is based on the World Health Organization Consortium on Dementia with Lewy Bodies but contain several important modifications. No limitations are based on the temporal relationship between onset of dementia and onset of Parkinsonism. Rapid eye movement sleep behavior disorder is an additional characteristic diagnostic feature.

(Adapted with permission from Knopman DS, Boeve BF, Petersen RC. Essentials of the proper diagnoses of mild cognitive impairment, dementia, and major subtypes of dementia. Mayo Clin Proc 2003;78:1290–1308.)

Table 50
Clinical Criteria for Frontotemporal Dementia

1. The development of behavioral or cognitive deficits manifested by either:
  a. Early and progressive change in personality, characterized by difficulty in modulating behavior, often resulting in inappropriate responses or activities.
  b. Early and progressive change in language, characterized by problems with expression of language or severe naming difficulty and problems with word meaning.
2. The deficits outlined in criterion 1a or 1b cause significant impairment in social or occupational functioning and represent a significant decline from a previous level of functioning.
3. The course is characterized by a gradual onset and continuing decline in function.
4. The deficits outlined in 1a or 1b are not the results of other nervous system conditions, systemic conditions, or substance-induced conditions.
5. The deficits do not occur exclusively during a delirium.
6. The disturbance is not better accounted for by a psychiatric diagnosis (e.g., depression).

Adapted with permission from Mckhann GH, Albert MS, Grossman M, Miller B, Dickson D, Trojanowski JQ. Clinical and pathological diagnosis of frontotemporal dementia: report of the work group on frontotemporal dementia and Pick's disease. Arch Neurol 2001;58:1803–1809, and from the American Medical Association.

rating of 0.5–1 on the Clinical Dementia Rating scale. Few neuropathological correlative studies are available, but some individuals with MCI have early AD neuropathology involving medial temporal structures, and a few may even meet neuropathological criteria for AD.

MUNCHAUSEN SYNDROME BY PROXY

Generally a pediatric diagnosis, Munchausen syndrome by proxy (MSBP) may be diagnosed both by inclusion and by exclusion. Table 57 identifies the specific criteria to be followed. Unfortunately,

Table 51
Neuropathological Subtypes in Frontotemporal Dementia

1. When the predominant neuropathological abnormalities are tau-positive inclusions (with associated neuron loss and gliosis), and insoluble tau has a predominance of tau with three microtubule-binding repeats, the most likely diagnoses are as follows:
   a. Pick's disease.
   b. Frontotemporal dementia with Parkinsonism linked to chromosome 17.
   c. Other as-yet-unidentified familial and sporadic frontotemporal disorders.
2. When the predominant neuropathological abnormalities are tau-positive inclusions (with associated neuron loss and gliosis), and insoluble tau has a predominance of four microtubule-binding repeats, the most likely diagnoses are as follows:
   a. Corticobasal degeneration.
   b. Progressive supranuclear palsy.
   c. Frontotemporal dementia with Parkinsonism linked to chromosome 17.
   d. Other as-yet-unidentified familial and sporadic frontotemporal disorders.
3. When the predominant neuropathological abnormalities are tau-positive inclusions (with associated neuron loss and gliosis), and insoluble tau has a predominance of three and four microtubule-binding repeats, the most likely diagnoses are as follows:
   a. Neurofibrillary tangle dementia.
   b. Frontotemporal dementia with Parkinsonism linked to chromosome 17.
   c. Other as-yet-unidentified familial and sporadic frontotemporal disorders.
4. When the predominant neuropathological abnormalities are frontotemporal neuronal loss and gliosis without tau- or ubiquitin-positive inclusions and without detectable amounts of insoluble tau, the most likely diagnoses areas follows:
   a. Frontotemporal lobar degeneration (also known as dementia lacking distinct histopathological features).
   b. Other as-yet-unidentified familial and sporadic frontotemporal disorders.
5. When the predominant neuropathological abnormalities are frontotemporal neuronal loss and gliosis with ubiquitin-positive, tau-negative inclusions and without detectable amounts of insoluble tau, with motor neuron disease (MND) or without MND but with MND-type inclusions, the most likely diagnoses areas follows:
   a. Frontotemporal lobar degeneration with MND.
   b. Frontotemporal lobar degeneration with MND-type inclusions but without MND.
   c. Other as-yet-unidentified familial and sporadic frontotemporal disorders.

Adapted from McKhann GH, Albert MS, Grossman M, Miller B, Dickson D, Trojanowski JQ. Clinical and pathological diagnosis of frontotemporal dementia: report of the work group on frontotemporal dementia and Pick's disease. Arch Neurol 2001;58:1803–1809.

Table 52
Consensus Diagnostic Criteria for Frontotemporal Lobar Degeneration

List 1: the clinical diagnostic features of frontotemporal dementia
Clinical profile
Character change and disordered social conduct are the dominant features initially and throughout the disease course. Instrumental functions of perception, spatial skills, praxis, and memory are intact or relatively well preserved.

 I. Core diagnostic features:
    A. Insidious onset and gradual progression.
    B. Early decline in social interpersonal conduct.
    C. Early impairment in regulation of personal conduct.
    D. Early emotional blunting.
    E. Early loss of insight.
 II. Supportive diagnostic features:
    A. Behavioral disorder:
       1. Decline in personal hygiene and grooming.
       2. Mental rigidity and inflexibility.
       3. Distractibility and impersistence.
       4. Hyperorality and dietary changes.

(Continued)

Table 52 (*Continued*)

      5. Perseverative and stereotyped behavior.

      6. Utilization behavior.

  B. Speech and language:

      1. Altered speech output.

        a. Aspontaneity and economy of speech.

        b. Press of speech.

      2. Stereotypy of speech.

      3. Echolalia.

      4. Perseveration.

      5. Mutism.

  C. Physical signs:

      1. Primitive reflexes.

      2. Incontinence.

      3. Akinesia, rigidity, and tremor.

      4. Low and labile blood pressure.

  D. Investigations:

      1. Neuropsychology: significant impairment on frontal lobe tests in the absence of severe amnesia, aphasia, or perceptuospatial disorder.

      2. Electroencephalography: normal on conventional electroencephalogram despite clinically evident dementia.

      3. Brain imaging (structural and/or functional): predominant frontal and/or anterior temporal abnormality.

Adapted with permission from Neary D, Snowden JS, Gustafson L, et al. Frontotemporal lobar degeneration: a consensus on clinical diagnostic criteria. Neurology 1998;51:1546–1554.

Table 53
Consensus Diagnostic Criteria for Frontotemporal Lobar Degeneration

List 2: the clinical diagnostic features of progressive nonfluent aphasia

Clinical profile

Disorder of expressive language is the dominant feature initially and throughout the disease course. Other aspects of cognition are intact or relatively well preserved.

  I. Core diagnostic features

    A. Insidious onset and gradual progression.

    B. Nonfluent spontaneous speech with at least one of the following: agrammatism, phonemic paraphasias, anomia.

  II. Supportive diagnostic features

    A. Speech and language:

      1. Stuttering or oral apraxia.

      2. Impaired repetition.

      3. Alexia, agraphia.

      4. Early preservation of word meaning.

      5. Late mutism.

    B. Behavior:

      1. Early preservation of social skills.

      2. Late behavioral changes similar to frontotemporal dementia.

    C. Physical signs: late contralateral primitive reflexes, akinesia, rigidity, and tremor.

    D. Investigations:

      1. Neuropsychology: nonfluent aphasia in the absence of severe amnesia or perceptuospatial disorder.

      2. Electroencephalography: normal or minor asymmetric slowing.

      3. Brain imaging (structural and/or functional): asymmetric abnormality predominantly affecting dominant (usually left) hemisphere.

Adapted with permission from Neary D, Snowden JS, Gustafson L, et al. Frontotemporal lobar degeneration: a consensus on clinical diagnostic criteria. Neurology 1998;51:1546–1554.

Table 54
Consensus Diagnostic Criteria for Frontotemporal Lobar Degeneration

List 3: consensus clinical diagnostic features of semantic aphasia and associative agnosia
Clinical profile
Semantic disorder (impaired understanding of word meaning and/or object identity) is the dominant feature initially and throughout the disease course. Other aspects of cognition, including autobiographic memory, are intact or relatively well preserved.

I. Core diagnostic features
   A. Insidious onset and gradual progression.
   B. Language disorder characterized by:
      1. Progressive, fluent, empty spontaneous speech.
      2. Loss of word meaning, manifest by impaired naming and comprehension.
      3. Semantic paraphasias and/or
   C. Perceptual disorder characterized by:
      1. Prosopagnosia: impaired recognition of identity of familiar faces and/or
      2. Associative agnosia: impaired recognition of object identity.
   D. Preserved perceptual matching and drawing reproduction.
   E. Preserved single-word repetition.
   F. Preserved ability to read aloud and write to dictation orthographically regular words.
II. Supportive diagnostic features
   A. Speech and language:
      1. Press of speech.
      2. Idiosyncratic word usage.
      3. Absence of phonemic paraphasias.
      4. Surface dyslexia and dysgraphia.
      5. Preserved calculation.
   B. Behavior:
      1. Loss of sympathy and empathy.
      2. Narrowed preoccupations.
      3. Parsimony.
   C. Physical signs:
      1. Absent or late primitive reflexes.
      2. Akinesia, rigidity, and tremor.
   D. Investigations:
   E. Neuropsychology:
      1. Profound semantic loss, manifest in failure of word comprehension and naming and/or face and object recognition.
      2. Preserved phonology and syntax, and elementary perceptual processing, spatial skills, and day-to-day memorizing.
   F. Electroencephalography: normal.
   G. Brain imaging (structural and/or functional): predominant anterior temporal abnormality (symmetric or asymmetric).

Adapted with permission from Neary D, Snowden JS, Gustafson L, et al. Frontotemporal lobar degeneration: a consensus on clinical diagnostic criteria. Neurology 1998;51:1546–1554.

Table 55
Consensus Diagnostic Criteria for Frontotemporal Lobar Degeneration

List 4: features common to the frontotemporal dementia syndromes
Features common to clinical syndromes of frontotemporal lobar degeneration (extension of Lists 1–3).

I. Supportive features
   A. Onset before 65 years: positive family history of similar disorder in first-degree relative.
   B. Bulbar palsy, muscular weakness and wasting, fasciculations (associated motor neuron disease present in a minority of patients).

(Continued)

Table 55 *(Continued)*

II. Diagnostic exclusion features
A. Historical and clinical:
1. Abrupt onset with ictal events.
2. Head trauma related to onset.
3. Early, severe amnesia.
4. Spatial disorientation.
5. Logoclonic, festinant speech with loss of train of thought.
6. Myoclonus.
7. Corticospinal weakness.
8. Cerebellar ataxia.
9. Choreoathetosis.
B. Investigations:
1. Brain imaging: predominant postcentral structural or functional deficit; multifocal lesions on computed tomography or magnetic resonance imaging.
2. Laboratory tests indicating brain involvement of metabolic or inflammatory disorder such as multiple sclerosis, syphilis, AIDS, and herpes simplex encephalitis.
III. Relative diagnostic exclusion features
A. Typical history of chronic alcoholism.
B. Sustained hypertension.
C. History of vascular disease (e.g., angina, claudication).

Adapted with permission from Neary D, Snowden JS, Gustafson L, et al. Frontotemporal lobar degeneration: a consensus on clinical diagnostic criteria. Neurology 1998;51:1546–1554.

See Appendix for further information.

Table 56
Diagnostic Criteria Used in Clinical Trials for Mild Cognitive Impairment

1. Subjective memory impairment, preferably corroborated by an informant.
2. Objective memory impairment when compared with persons of similar age and education (more than 1.5 standard deviations below the mean for control population).
3. Normal general cognitive function.
4. Normal activity of daily living.
5. Not demented.

Adapted with permission from Petersen RC, Smith GE, Waring SC, Ivnik RJ, Tangalos EG, Kokmen E. Mild cognitive impairment: clinical characterization and outcome. Arch Neurol 2001;56:303–308, and from the American Medical Association.

the diagnostic criteria do not account for cases where some or all criteria may not be present, suggesting a higher level of certainty needed to make the diagnosis compared with other medical conditions. (Note that "intent" is not a diagnostic criterion.)

The author of the criteria also includes a discussion of whether MSBP is *per se* a psychiatric diagnosis. This is rejected as not being hypothesis driven, and therefore not a testable conclusion, but rather an example of circular logic, i.e., only someone who is psychiatrically ill would do this; therefore, it is a psychiatric disorder. This would not be validated by the large number of individuals with all manners of psychopathology who do not commit acts of MSBP.

NORMAL PRESSURE HYDROCEPHALUS

Since its first descriptions in the early 1960s, normal pressure hydrocephalus (NPH) has been difficult to recognize, and conclusive diagnosis relied on response to cerebrospinal fluid shunting. The clinical manifestations classically consist of the triad of gait apraxia, urinary incontinence, and dementia.

Neuroimaging has made diagnosis of enlarged ventricles relatively easy, although distinguishing ventriculomegaly secondary to brain atrophy vs idiopathic NPH remains challenging. A variety of

Table 57
Diagnostic Criteria for Munchausen Syndrome by Proxy

Definite Munchausen syndrome by proxy (MSBP) by inclusion
1. Child has been repeatedly presented for medical care; and
2. Test/event is positive for tampering with child, or with the child's medical situation; and
3. Positivity of event is not credibly the result of test error or misinterpretation, nor of miscommunication or specimen mishandling; and
4. No explanation for the positive test/event other than illness falsification is medically possible; and
5. No findings credibly exclude illness falsification.

Definite MSBP by exclusion
1. Child has been repeatedly presented for medical care; and
2. All diagnoses other than illness falsification have been credibly eliminated, so that
   a. If the child is alive, the competing diagnoses are those that took into account the child's major medical findings and that account for the entirety of the child's presentation (a major medical finding is one that is objectively observed, sufficiently specific as to help formulate the range of diagnoses, and verifiable in the record); or
   b. If the child is alive, separation of the child from the alleged perpetrator results in resolution of the child's reversible medical problems, in accordance with their degree and speed of reversibility. No variable other than the separation can logically and fully account for the child's improvement; or
   c. If the child is dead, autopsy examination does not reveal a cause of death that is credibly accidental, natural, or suicidal in manner; and
3. No findings credibly exclude illness falsification.

Possible diagnosis of MSBP
1. Child has been repeatedly presented for medical care; and
2. Test/event is presumptively positive for tampering with the child, or with child's medical situation. No other explanation is readily apparent. No findings appear to exclude illness falsification; or
3. Child has a condition that cannot fully be explained medically, despite a respectable medical evaluation, at least. Cogent hypothesis suggests a faked medical condition. No findings appear to exclude illness falsification.

Inconclusive determination of MSBP
1. Child has been repeatedly presented for medical care; and
2. The relevant and available information has been reviewed, and the child is appropriately evaluated; and
3. One is left with a differential diagnosis rather than a single diagnosis; and
4. It is not possible to conclusively affirm one diagnosis; and
5. It is not possible to exclude conclusively all but one diagnosis on the differential diagnosis.

Definitely not MSBP
1. Child has been repeatedly presented for medical care; and
2. What had appeared to be possible falsification of illness has been wholly and credibly accounted for in some other way.

Adapted with permission from Rosenberg DA. Munchausen's syndrome by proxy: medical diagnostic criteria. Child Abuse Neglect 2003;27:421–430.

supplemental diagnostic tests have been used to help predict response to shunting. These include the high-volume lumbar puncture (50 mL), external lumbar drainage, radioisotope cisternography, CSF outflow resistance measurement, MRI-derived CSF flow voids, and intracranial pressure monitoring. The lumbar puncture remains the simplest of these techniques, but suffers from low sensitivity and the occurrence of equivocal or even false-positive results.

There have not been well-defined criteria for idiopathic (INPH) until recently. A set of proposed diagnostic criteria with operational definitions of the classical triad based on review of the published medical literature in Table 58.

OBSESSIVE-COMPULSIVE DISORDER

Obsessive-compulsive disorder, a primary psychiatric disorder, is included here because of its close relation to Tourette's syndrome, where more than half of affected individuals meet criteria for obsessive-compulsive disorder (*see* Table 59).

Table 58
Description of Idiopathic Normal Pressure Hydrocephalus Classification: Probable, Possible, and Unlikely Categories

Probable INPH

The diagnosis of probable INPH is based on clinical history, brain imaging, physical findings, and physiological criteria.

I. History

Reported symptoms should be corroborated by an informant familiar with the patient's premorbid and current condition, and must include the following:

a. Insidious onset (versus acute).
b. Origin after age 40 years.
c. A minimum duration of at least 3 to 6 months.
d. No evidence of an antecedent event, such as head trauma, intracerebral hemorrhage, meningitis, or other known causes of secondary hydrocephalus.
e. Progression over time.
f. No other neurological, psychiatric, or general medical conditions that sufficiently explain the presenting symptoms.

II. Brain imaging

A brain imaging study (CT or MRI) performed after onset of symptoms must show evidence of the following:

a. Ventricular enlargement not entirely attributable to cerebral atrophy or congenital enlargement (Evan's index ≥0.3 or comparable measure).
b. No macroscopic obstruction to CSF flow.
c. At least one of the following supportive features:
   i. Enlargement of the temporal horns of the lateral ventricles not entirely attributable to hippocampus atrophy.
   ii. Callosal angle of 40° or more.
   iii. Evidence of altered brain water content, including periventricular signal changes on CT and MRI not attributable to microvascular ischemic changes or demyelination.
   iv. An aqueductal or fourth ventricular flow void on MRI.

Other brain imaging findings, such as the following, may be supportive of an INPH diagnosis but are not required for a "probable" designation:

a. A brain imaging study performed before onset of symptoms showing smaller ventricular size or without evidence of hydrocephalus.
b. Radionuclide cisternogram showing delayed clearance of radiotracer over the cerebral convexities after 48–72 hours.
c. Cine MRI study or other technique showing increased ventricular flow rate.
d. A SPECT-acetazolamide challenge showing decreased periventricular perfusion that is not altered by acetazolamide.

III. Clinical

By classic definitions, findings of gait/balance disturbance must be present, plus at least one other area of impairment in cognition, urinary symptoms, or both. With respect to gait/balance, at least two of the following should be present and not be entirely attributable to other conditions:

a. Decreased step height.
b. Decreased step length.
c. Decreased cadence (speed of walking).
d. Increased trunk sway during walking.
e. Widened standing base.
f. Toes turned outward on walking.
g. Retropulsion (spontaneous or provoked).
h. *En bloc* turning (turning requiring three or more steps for 180°).
i. Impaired walking balance, as evidenced by two or more corrections out of eight steps on tandem gait testing.

With respect to cognition, there must be documented impairment (adjusted for age and educational attainment) and/or decrease in performance on a cognitive screening instrument (such as the Mini-Mental State Examination), or evidence of at least two of the following on examination that are not fully attributable to other conditions:

(Continued)

Table 58 *(Continued)*

a. Psychomotor slowing (increased response latency).
b. Decreased fine motor speed.
c. Decreased fine motor accuracy.
d. Difficulty dividing or maintaining attention.
e. Impaired recall, especially for recent events.
f. Executive dysfunction, such as impairment in multistep procedures, working memory, formulation of abstractions/similarities, insight.
g. Behavioral or personality changes.

To document symptoms in the domain of urinary continence, either one of the following should be present:

a. Episodic or persistent urinary incontinence not attributable to primary urological disorders.
b. Persistent urinary incontinence.
c. Urinary and fecal incontinence.

OR any two of the following should be present:

a. Urinary urgency, as defined by frequent perception of a pressing need to void.
b. Urinary frequency, as defined by more than six voiding episodes in an average 12-hour period despite normal fluid intake.
c. Nocturia, as defined by the need to urinate more than twice in an average night.

IV. Physiological

CSF opening pressure in the range of 5–18 mmHg (or 70–245 mmH$_2$O), as determined by a lumbar puncture or a comparable procedure. Appropriately measured pressures that are significantly higher or lower than this range are not consistent with a probable NPH diagnosis.

Possible INPH

A diagnosis of "possible INPH" is based on historical, brain imaging, and clinical and physiological criteria

I. History

Reported symptoms may:

a. Have a subacute or indeterminate mode of onset.
b. Begin at any age after childhood.
c. Last less than 3 months or indeterminate duration.
d. Follow events, such as mild head trauma, remote history of intracerebral hemorrhage, or childhood and adolescent meningitis or other conditions, that, in the judgment of the clinician, are not likely to be causally related.
e. Coexist with other neurological, psychiatric, or general medical disorders but, in the judgment of the clinician, may not be entirely attributable to these conditions.
f. Be nonprogressive or not clearly progressive.

II. Brain imaging

Ventricular enlargement consistent with hydrocephalus but associated with any of the following:

a. Evidence of cerebral atrophy of sufficient severity to potentially explain ventricular size.
b. Structural lesions that may influence ventricular size.

III. Clinical

Symptoms of either of the following:

a. Incontinence and/or cognitive impairment in the absence of an observable gait or balance disturbance.
b. Gait disturbance or dementia alone.

IV. Physiological

Opening pressure measurement not available or pressure outside the range required for probable INPH.

Unlikely INPH

a. No evidence of ventriculomegaly.
b. Signs of increased intracranial pressure, such as papilledema.
c. No component of the clinical triad of INPH is present.
d. Symptoms explained by other causes (e.g., spinal stenosis).

INPH, idiopathic normal-pressure hydrocephalus; CT, computed tomography; MRI, magnetic resonance imaging; CSF, cerebrospinal fluid; SPECT, single-photon emission computed tomography.

(Adapted from Relkin N, Marmarou A, Klinge P, Bergsneider M, Black, Peter McL. Diagnosing idiopathic normal-pressure hydrocephalus. Guidelines for the diagnosis and management of idiopathic normal-pressure hydrocephalus. Neurosurgery 2005;57:S2-4–S2-16.)

Table 59
DSM-IV Diagnostic Criteria for Obsessive-Compulsive Disorder

A. Either obsessions or compulsions:
    Obsessions as defined by the following:
    1. Recurrent and persistent thoughts, impulses, or images that are intrusive and inappropriate and that cause marked anxiety or distress.
    2. The thoughts, impulses, or images are not simply excessive worries about real-life problems.
    3. The person attempts to ignore or suppress such thoughts, impulses, or images, or to neutralize them with some other thought or action.
    4. The person recognizes that the obsessive thoughts, impulses, or images are a product of his or her own mind (not imposed from without as in thought insertion).
    Compulsions as defined by:
    1. Repetitive behaviors (e.g., hand washing, ordering, checking) or mental acts (e.g., praying, counting, repeating words silently) that the person feels driven to perform in response to an obsession, or according to rigidly applied rules.
    2. The behaviors or mental acts are aimed at preventing or reducing distress or preventing some dreaded event or situation; however, these behaviors or mental acts either are not connected in a realistic way with what they are designed to neutralize or prevent or are clearly excessive.
B. At some point during the course of the disorder, the person has recognized that the obsessions or compulsions are excessive or unreasonable. (**Note:** This does not apply to children.)
C. The obsessions or compulsions cause marked distress, are time-consuming (take more than 1 hour a day), or significantly interfere with the person's normal routine, occupational (or academic) functioning, or usual social activities or relationships.
D. If another DSM-defined Axis I disorder is present, the content of the obsessions or compulsions is not restricted to it (e.g., preoccupation with food in the presence of an eating disorder; hair pulling in the presence of trichotillomania; concern with appearance in the presence of body dysmorphic disorder; preoccupation with drugs in the presence of a substance use disorder; preoccupation with having a serious illness in the presence of hypochondriasis; preoccupation with sexual urges or fantasies in the presence of a paraphilia; or guilty ruminations in the presence of major depressive disorder).
E. The disturbance is not caused by the direct physiological effects of a substance or a general medical condition.

Adapted from American Psychiatric Association. Diagnostic and Statistical Manual of Mental Disorders, 4th rev. ed. Washington, DC: American Psychiatric Association, 1994.

OLFACTORY REFERENCE SYNDROME

Olfactory reference syndrome is an obscure neuropsychiatric disorder of unclear nosology, but has characteristic symptoms. It bears an uncertain relationship to major depression, anxiety disorders, and body dysmorphic disorder. The criteria are based on limited data, and have not been validated in a large clinical series.

PRIMARY PROGRESSIVE APHASIA

As originally formulated by Mesulam, primary progressive aphasia is recognized by the presence of aphasia dissociated from the general cognitive decline in other cognitive spheres characterizing the dementing illnesses. The original description emphasized the long clinical course, without progression to a more generalized dementia. Subsequent to that, cases progressing to dementia with wide variety of pathological entities have been described in case reports.

The diagnostic criteria proposed by Mesulam have been updated. His criteria are based on ongoing experience on defining the syndrome (Table 61). Generalized neuropsychological deficits may accumulate, but are generally not the limiting fact within the first 2 years of clinical illness, and aphasia remains the most severe deficit over the disease course.

TRANSIENT GLOBAL AMNESIA

Transient global amnesia was first described by Fisher and Adams in 1964 as a transient event in which there is altered behavior with prominent memory loss. Patients with this condition are typically

Table 60
Diagnostic Criteria for Olfactory Reference Syndrome

A.	A preoccupation with imagined body odor (including halitosis) persisting despite reassurance.
B.	At some point during the course of the disorder, the person recognizes that the preoccupation (obsession/compulsion) is excessive or unreasonable.
C.	The symptoms cause clinically significant distress or impairment in social, occupational, or other areas of functioning.
D.	Does not occur solely during the course of another disorder (e.g., body dysmorphic disorder, hypochondriasis, social anxiety disorder, mood disorder, and obsessive-compulsive disorder)
E.	The disturbance is not the result of the direct physiological effects of an exogenous substance or medication or a general medical condition (e.g., hyperthyroidism).

Reprinted with permission from Lochner C, Stein DJ. Olfactory reference syndrome: diagnostic criteria and differential diagnosis. Postgrad Med J 2003;49:328–331 and from BMJ Publishing Group.

Table 61
Diagnostic Criteria for Primary Progressive Aphasia

1. Insidious onset and gradual progression of word finding object naming, or word-comprehension impairments as manifested during spontaneous conversation or as assessed, through formal neuropsychological tests of language.
2. All limitation of daily living activities attributable to the language impairment, for at least 2 years after onset.
3. Intact premorbid language function (except for developmental dyslexia).
4. Absence of significant apathy, disinhibition, memory dysfunction for recent events, visuospatial impairment, visual recognition deficits, or sensory-motor dysfunction within the first 2 years of the illness. This criterion can be fulfilled by history, survey of daily living activities, or formal neuropsychological testing.
5. Acalculia and ideomotor apraxia may be present even in the first 2 years. Mild constructional deficits and perseveration (as assessed in the go/no-go task) are also acceptable as long as neither visuospatial deficits nor disinhibition influences daily living activities.
6. Other domains possibly affected after the first 2 years, but language remains the most impaired function throughout the course of the illness and deteriorates faster than other affected domains.
7. Absence of "specific" causes, such as stroke or tumor, as ascertained by neuroimaging.

Adapted with permission from Mesulam MM. Primary progressive aphasia. Ann Neurol 2001;49:425–432, and from John Wiley and Sons.

Table 62
Diagnostic Criteria for Transient Global Amnesia

1. Information should be available about the beginning of the attack from a capable observer.
2. The patient should be examined during the attack to be certain that neurological signs and symptoms do not accompany the amnesia.
3. There should be no accompanying neurological signs.
4. The memory loss should be transient.

Adapted from Caplan LR. Transient global amnesia. In: Vinken PJ, Bruyn GW, Klawans HL, eds. Handbook of Clinical Neurology, vol 1. Amsterdam: Elsevier Science, 1985;205–218.

agitated during the event, often asking repeated questions. The etiology of transient global amnesia is unknown, with theories ranging from cerebrovascular events, migrainous phenomena, and epilepsy being proffered. Recent studies with functional neuroimaging including single-photon emission computed tomography and diffusion-weighted magnetic resonance imaging have shown that regional blood flow and focal brain abnormalities occur during the attack. Many of the described cases in the literature consist of a transient global amnesia syndrome as the presenting feature of another disorder, or that resulted in permanent neurological deficits. A strict categorical definition was proposed by Caplan in 1985 in analysis of a large case series. Four points were central to the diagnosis in the ideal case and are listed in Table 62.

APPENDIX: DEFINITION OF TERMS FOR FRONTOTEMPORAL LOBE DEMENTIA IN TABLE 55

Exclusion Features Common to Each Clinical Syndrome

Clinical

All features (*see* Table 55) must be absent. Early severe amnesia, early spatial disorientation, logoclonic speech with loss of train of thought, and myoclonus are features designed to exclude Alzheimer's disease.

Investigations

All features should be absent (when the relevant information is available).

Relative Diagnostic Exclusion Features

These are features (*see* Table 55) that caution against, but do not firmly exclude, a diagnosis of frontotemporal lobar degeneration (FTLD). A history of alcohol abuse raises the possibility of an alcohol-related basis for a frontal lobe syndrome. However, excessive alcohol intake may also occur in patients with frontotemporal dementia (FTD) as a secondary manifestation of social disinhibition or hyperoral tendencies. The presence of vascular risk factors, such as hypertension, ought to alert investigators to a possible vascular etiology. Nevertheless, such risk factors are common in the general population and may be present coincidentally in some patients with FTLD, particularly in those of more advanced age.

Definitions of Clinical Features

This information is adapted from Neary D, Snowden JS, Gustafson L, et al. Frontotemporal lobar degeneration: a consensus on clinical diagnostic criteria. Neurology 1998;51:1546–1554. It gives operational definitions to the terms used in Lists 1–4.

Frontotemporal Dementia

See Table 52.

CORE FEATURES

Insidious Onset and Gradual Progression. There should be no evidence of an acute medical or traumatic event precipitating symptoms. Evidence for a gradually progressive course should be based on historic evidence of altered functional capacity (e.g., inability to work) over a period of at least 6 months, and may be supported by a decline in neuropsychological test performance. The degree of anticipated change is not specified, because it is highly variable. In some patients, change is dramatic over a 12-month period, whereas in others it is manifest only over a period of several years. Dramatic social and domestic events leading to perturbations in the patient's behavior must be distinguished from ictal occurrences of a neurological or psychological nature. Only the latter are grounds for exclusion.

Early Decline in Social Interpersonal Conduct. This refers to qualitative breaches of interpersonal etiquette that are incongruent with the patient's premorbid behavior. This includes decline in manners, social graces, and decorum (e.g., disinhibited speech and gestures, and violation of interpersonal space), as well as active antisocial and disinhibited verbal, physical, and sexual behavior (e.g., criminal acts, incontinence, sexual exposure, tactlessness, and offensiveness). "Early" for this and other features implies that the abnormality should be present at initial presentation of the patient.

Early Impaired Regulation of Personal Conduct. This refers to departures from customary behavior of a quantitative type, ranging from passivity, inertia, and inactivity to overactivity, pacing, and wandering; and increased talking, laughing, singing, sexuality, and aggression.

Early Emotional Blunting. This refers to an inappropriate emotional shallowness with unconcern and a loss of emotional warmth, empathy, and sympathy, and an indifference to others.

Early Loss of Insight. This is defined as a lack of awareness of mental symptoms, evidenced by frank denial of symptoms or unconcern about the social, occupational, and financial consequences of mental failure.

Supportive Features: Behavioral Disorder

Decline in Personal Hygiene and Grooming. The caregivers' accounts of failure to wash, bathe, groom, apply makeup, and dress appropriately as before are reinforced by clinical observations of unkemptness, body odor, clothing stains, garish makeup, and inappropriate clothing combinations.

Mental Rigidity and Inflexibility. This refers to egocentricity and loss of mental adaptability, evidenced by reports of any one of the following: the patient has to have his or her own way, is unable to see another person's point of view, adheres to routine, and is unable to adapt to novel circumstances.

Distractibility and Impersistence. These are reflected in failure to complete tasks and inappropriate digressions of attention to nonrelevant stimuli.

Hyperorality and Dietary Changes. This refers to overeating, bingeing, altered food preferences and food fads, excessive consumption of liquids, alcohol, and cigarettes, and the oral exploration of inanimate objects.

Perseverative and Stereotyped Behavior. This encompasses simple repetitive behaviors, such as hand rubbing and clapping, counting aloud, tune humming, giggling, and dancing, as well as complex behavioral routines, such as wandering a fixed route, collecting and hoarding objects, and rituals involving toileting and dressing.

Utilization Behavior. This is stimulus-bound behavior during which patients grasp and repeatedly use objects in their visual field, despite the objects' irrelevance to the task at hand (e.g., patients repeatedly switch lights on and off, open and close doors, or continue eating if unlimited supplies of food are within reach). During clinical interview, they may drink repeatedly from an empty cup or use scissors placed before them.

Speech and Language

Altered Speech Output. There are two types of altered speech output: aspontaneity and economy of utterance, and press of speech. In aspontaneity and economy of utterance, either the patient does not initiate conversation or output is limited to short phrases or stereotyped utterances. Responses to questions involve single-word replies or short, unelaborated phrases, such as "don't know." Encouragement to amplify responses are unsuccessful. In press of speech, the patient speaks interruptedly, monopolizing a conversational interchange.

Stereotypy of Speech. These are single words, phrases, or entire themes that the patient produces repeatedly and habitually either spontaneously or in response to questions, replacing appropriate conversational discourse.

Echolalia. Echolalia refers to a repetition of the utterances of others, either completely or in part, sometimes with change of syntax (e.g., Interviewer: "Did you go out yesterday?" Patient: "Did I go out yesterday") when this is a substitute for, and not a precursor to, an appropriate elaborated response.

Perseveration. "Perseveration" is defined as a repetition of a patient's own responses. It is a word or phrase that, once uttered, intrudes into the patient's subsequent utterances. It differs from a stereotypy in that the repeated word or phrase is not habitual. Perseverations may occur spontaneously in conversation or are elicited in naming tasks (e.g., the patient names scissors as "scissors" and later names a clock as "scissors"). Perseveration includes palilalia, in which there is immediate repetition of a word, phrase, or sentence (e.g., "I went down town, down town, down town").

Mutism. This is an absence of speech or speech sounds. Patients may pass through a transitional phase of "virtual mutism," during which they generate no propositional speech, yet echolalic responses and some automatic speech (e.g., "three" when prompted with "one, two") may still be present.

Physical Signs

Primitive Reflexes. At least one of the following is present: grasp, snout, sucking reflexes.

Incontinence. This refers to voiding of urine or feces without concern.

Neuropsychology

Significant Impairment on Frontal Lobe Tests in the Absence of Severe Amnesia, Aphasia, or Perceptuospatial Disorder. Impairment on frontal lobe tests is defined operationally as failures (scores lower than the fifth percentile) on conventional tests of frontal lobe function (e.g., Wisconsin/Nelson card sort, Stroop, Trail Making) in which a qualitative pattern of performance typically associated with frontal lobe dysfunction is demonstrated: concreteness, poor set shifting, perseveration, failure to use information from one trial to guide subsequent responses, inability to inhibit overlearned responses, and poor organization and temporal sequencing. Abnormal scores that arise secondary to memory, language, or perceptuospatial disorder (such as forgetting instructions or the inability to recognize or locate test stimuli) would not be accepted as evidence of impairment on frontal lobe tests as operationally defined.

Patients with FTD may perform inefficiently on formal memory, language, perceptual, and spatial tests as a secondary consequence of deficits associated with frontal lobe dysfunction, such as inattention, poor self-monitoring and checking, and a lack of concern for accuracy. Poor test scores *per se* would not therefore exclude a diagnosis of FTD. An absence of severe amnesia, aphasia, or perceptuospatial disorder would be demonstrated by patchiness or inconsistency in performance (e.g., failure on easy items and pass on more difficult items) or demonstration that correct responses can be elicited by cuing or by directing the patient's attention to test stimuli.

Electroencephalography

Normal Despite Clinically Evident Dementia. Conventional electroencephalogram reveals frequencies within the normal range for the patient's age (minimal θ would be considered within normal limits). There are no features of focal epileptiform activity.

Brain Imaging (Structural or Functional)

Predominant Frontal or Anterior Temporal Abnormality. Atrophy, in the case of structural imaging (computed tomography or magnetic resonance imaging), and tracer uptake abnormality, in the case of functional brain imaging (positron-emission tomography or single-photon emission computed tomography), is more marked in the frontal or anterior temporal lobes. Anterior hemisphere abnormalities may be bilaterally symmetric or asymmetric, affecting the left or right hemisphere disproportionately.

Progressive Nonfluent Aphasia

Definitions are for features (*see* Table 53) that differ from or are in addition to those of FTD.

Core Features

Nonfluent Spontaneous Speech With at Least One of the Following: Agrammatism, Phonemic Paraphasias, Anomia. Nonfluent speech is defined as hesitant, effortful production, with reduced rate of output. Agrammatism refers to the omission or incorrect use of grammatical terms, including articles, prepositions, auxiliary verbs, inflexions, and derivations (e.g., "man went town;" "he comed yesterday").

"Phonemic paraphasias" are sound-based errors that include incorrect phoneme use (e.g., "gat" for "cat") and phoneme transposition (e.g., "aminal" for "animal"). The frequency of such errors should exceed that reasonably attributed to normal slips of the tongue.

"Anomia" is defined as a difficulty in naming manifest by an inability to find the correct word, by prolonged word retrieval latencies relative to the norm, or by incorrect word production. The availability of partial knowledge of a word, such as the initial letter, would be consistent with anomia, as would several attempts to produce a word, each yielding a close approximation (e.g., "scinners... sivvers... scivvers... scissors").

SUPPORTIVE DIAGNOSTIC FEATURES: SPEECH AND LANGUAGE

Stuttering or Oral Apraxia. Articulation is effortful, and repetition of parts of a word, particularly the first consonant, occurs in the patient's effort to produce a complete utterance. (Developmental stuttering is excluded.)

Impaired Repetition. The patient has a reduced repetition span (less than five digits forward; less than four monosyllabic words) or makes phonemic paraphasias when attempting to repeat polysyllabic words, word sequences, or short phrases.

Alexia and Agraphia. Reading is nonfluent and effortful. Sound-based errors are produced (phonemic paralexias). Writing is effortful, contains spelling errors, and may show features of agrammatism.

Early Preservation of Word Meaning (Understanding Preserved at Single-Word Level). Patients should show an understanding of the nominal terms employed during a routine clinical examination. There should be a demonstrable discrepancy between word comprehension and naming: Patients should show understanding of words that they have difficulty retrieving.

BEHAVIOR

Early Preservation of Social Skills. The language disorder should be the presenting symptom. At the time of onset of language disorder, patients should demonstrate preserved interpersonal and personal conduct.

Late Behavioral Changes in FTD. The changes outlined for FTD in conduct, if they occur, should not be presenting symptoms. There should be a clear, documented period of circumscribed language disorder before their development.

NEUROPSYCHOLOGY

Nonfluent Aphasia in the Absence of Severe Amnesia or Perceptuospatial Disorder. There is difficulty in verbal expression. The language impairment may compromise performance on verbal memory tasks, so that poor scores on memory tests *per se* would not exclude a diagnosis of progressive aphasia. The presence of normal scores on one or more tests of visual memory, or a demonstration of normal rates of forgetting (i.e., no abnormal loss of information from immediate to delayed recall/recognition), would provide evidence for an absence of severe amnesia. An absence of a severe perceptual disorder would be demonstrated by accurate recognition of the line drawings employed during routine naming tasks, as determined by the patient's ability to produce a correct name, an approximation to the name, a functional description of the object's use, or a pertinent gesture or action pantomime. An absence of severe spatial disorder is demonstrated by normal performance on two or more spatial tasks, such as dot counting, line orientation, and drawing/copying.

Semantic Aphasia and Associative Agnosia

CORE FEATURES

Fluent, Empty, Spontaneous Speech. Speech production is effortless, without hesitancies, and the patient does not search for words. However, little information is conveyed, reflecting reduced use of precise nominal terms, and increased use of broad generic terms such as "thing." In the early stages of the disorder, the "empty" nature of the speech output may become apparent only on successive interviews, which reveal a limited and repetitive conversational repertoire.

Loss of Word Meaning. There must be evidence of a disorder both of single-word comprehension and naming. A semantic deficit may be alerted by patients' remarks of the type, "What's a ____? I don't know what that is." However, impairment may not be immediately apparent in conversation because the patient's effortless speech gives an impression of facility with language. Word comprehension impairment needs to be established by word definition and object-pointing tasks. A range of stimuli needs to be tested, both animate and inanimate, because meaning may be differentially affected for different material types.

Semantic Paraphasias. Semantically related words replace correct nominal terms. Although these may include superordinate category substitutions (e.g., "animal" for camel), coordinate category errors (e.g., "dog" for elephant; "sock" for glove) must be present to meet operational criteria.

Prosopagnosia. This is impaired recognition of familiar face identity, not attributable to anomia. It is demonstrated by the patient's inability to provide defining or contextual information about faces of acquaintances or well-known celebrities.

Associative Agnosia. This is an impairment of object identity present both on visual and tactile presentation that cannot be explained in terms of nominal difficulties. It is indicated historically by reports of misuse of objects or loss of knowledge of their function. It is demonstrated clinically by patients' reports of lack of recognition and by their inability to convey the use of an object either verbally or by action pantomime.

Preserved Perceptual Matching and Drawing Reproduction. There should be some demonstration that the patient's inability to recognize faces or objects does not arise at the level of elementary visual processing. Demonstration of an ability to match for identity (to identify identical object pairs, shapes, or letters) or to reproduce simple line drawings (e.g., of a clock face, a flower, or a simple abstract design) would provide the minimum requirement to fulfill criteria for diagnosis.

Preserved Single-Word Repetition. The relative preservation of repetition skills is a central feature of the disorder. This typically includes the ability to repeat short phrases and sequences of words, although for such complex material, errors may emerge ultimately in advanced disease in the context of severe semantic loss. Demonstration of accurate repetition at least at the level of a single polysyllabic word is required to fulfill criteria for diagnosis.

Preserved Ability to Read Aloud and to Write to Dictation Orthographically Regular Words. The ability to read without comprehension is central to the disorder. However, reading performance is not entirely error free. Orthographically irregular words commonly elicit "surface dyslexic"-type errors (e.g., "pint" read to rhyme with "mint;" "glove" to rhyme with "rove" and "strove"). Patients should demonstrate the ability to read aloud accurately at least one-syllable words with regular spelling-to-sound correspondence. Writing of orthographically irregular words also typically reveals regularization errors (e.g., "caught" written as "cort"). Patients should demonstrate accurate writing to dictation at least of one-syllable orthographically regular words.

SUPPORTIVE DIAGNOSTIC FEATURES: SPEECH AND LANGUAGE

Press of Speech. The patient speaks without interruption. This occurs in many, but not all, patients.

Idiosyncratic Word Usage. Vocabulary is used consistently but idiosyncratically. For example, the word "container" applied to small objects regardless of their facility to contain, and "on the side" applied to spatial locations, both near (e.g., on the table) and distant (e.g., in Australia). The semantic link between the adopted word or phrase and its referent may be tenuous or absent.

Absence of Phonemic Paraphasias in Spontaneous Speech. Sound-based errors are absent in conversational speech. The feature, although characteristic, is not included as a core feature because occasional phonemic errors may emerge in advanced disease in the context of a profound disorder of meaning.

Surface Dyslexia/Dysgraphia. The presence of surface dyslexic errors (described earlier) in reading and writing is a strong supportive feature.

Preserved Calculation. The preserved ability of patients to calculate (to carry out accurately two-digit written addition and subtraction) is characteristic. It is not included as a core feature because calculation skills may break down in advanced disease as a consequence of failure to recognize the identity of Arabic numerals.

BEHAVIOR

Loss of Sympathy and Empathy. Patients are regarded by relatives as self-centered, lacking in emotional warmth, and lacking awareness of the needs of others.

Narrowed Preoccupations. Patients are reported to have a narrowed range of interests that they pursue at the expense of routine daily activities (e.g., doing jigsaw puzzles all day and neglecting the housework).

Parsimony. Patients show an abnormal preoccupation with money or financial economy. This may be demonstrated by hoarding or constant counting of money, by patients' avoidance of spending their own money, by their purchase of the cheapest items regardless of quality, or by their attempts to restrain usage by other family members of household utilities (e.g., electricity and water).

NEUROPSYCHOLOGY

Profound Semantic Loss, Manifest in Failure of Word Comprehension and Naming or Face and Object Recognition; Preserved Phonology and Syntax, and Elementary Perceptual Processing, Spatial Skills, and Day-to-Day Memorizing. Significant impairment should be demonstrated on word comprehension and naming or famous face identification or object recognition tasks. It should be shown that poor scores arise at a semantic level and not at a more elementary level of verbal or visual processing by demonstrating that the patient can repeat words that are not understood, can match for identity, and can copy drawings of objects. Patients should demonstrate normal performance on two or more spatial tasks, such as dot counting and line orientation. Performance on formal memory tests (e.g., involving remembering words or faces) is compromised by patients' semantic disorder. Nevertheless, patients retain the ability to remember autobiographically relevant day-to-day events (e.g., that a grandchild visits on Saturdays). Such preservation is striking clinically but may be difficult to capture on formal tests, which by definition are divorced from daily life.

Features Common to Each Clinical Syndrome

DIAGNOSTIC EXCLUSION FEATURES

Early Severe Amnesia. Symptoms of poor memory may be present and inefficient performance demonstrated on memory tests; these may occur secondary to executive or language impairments. However, memory failures are patchy and inconsistent, and patients do not present a picture of classic amnesia. Demonstration that a patient is disoriented in both time and place and shows a consistent, pervasive amnesia for salient contemporary autobiographical events would be incompatible with the clinical syndromes of FTLD.

Spatial Disorientation. Patients with FTD who wander from a familiar environment may become lost because of failure of self-regulation of behavior (i.e., for reasons that are not primarily spatial). They do not exhibit spatial disorientation in familiar surroundings such as their own home. They negotiate their surroundings with ease, and localize objects in the environment with accurate reaching actions. Preservation of primary spatial skills is demonstrable even in patients with advanced disease by their capacity, for example, to align objects and to fold paper accurately. Evidence of poor spatial localization and disorientation in highly familiar surroundings would exclude clinical diagnoses of FTD, progressive nonfluent aphasia, or semantic aphasia and associative agnosia.

Logoclonic, Festinant Speech With Rapid Loss of Train of Thought. Logoclonia is defined as the effortless repetition of the final syllable of a word (e.g., Washington ton ton ton). Festinant speech refers to a rapid, effortless reiteration of individual phonemes. Logoclonic and festinant speech need to be distinguished from stuttering, which has an effortful quality and usually involves repetition of the first consonant or syllable. They need to be distinguished from palilalia, during which there is repetition of complete words and phrases. Loss of train of thought is a common feature of Alzheimer's disease: patients begin sentences that they fail to complete, not only because of word-finding difficulty but also because of rapid forgetting of the intended proposition. A demonstration in conversation that patients are rapidly losing track would be contrary to a diagnosis of FTLD.

SOURCES

Alcohol-Related Dementia

Oslin D, Atkinson RM, Smith DM, Hendrie H. Alcohol related dementia: proposed clinical criteria. Int J Geriatr Psychiatr 1998;13:203–220.

Alzheimer's Disease

American Psychiatric Association. Diagnostic and Statistical Manual of Mental Disorders, 4th rev. ed. Washington, DC: American Psychiatric Association, 1994.

McKhann G, Drachman D, Folstein M, Katzman R, Price D, Stadlan EM. Clinical diagnosis of Alzheimer's disease: report of the NINCDS-ADRDA Work Group under the auspices of Department of Health and Human Services Task Force on Alzheimer's Disease. Neurology 1984;34:939–944.

Petersen RC, Smith GE, Waring SC, Ivnik RJ, Tangalos EG, Kokmen E. Mild cognitive impairment: clinical characterisation and outcome. Arch Neurol 1999;56:303–308.

Attention Deficit Hyperactivity Disorder

American Psychiatric Association. Task Force on DSM-IV. Diagnostic and statistical manual of mental disorders: DSM-IV, 4th rev. ed. Washington, DC: American Psychiatric Association, 1994.

Autistic Spectrum Disorders

American Psychiatric Association. Task Force on DSM-IV. Diagnostic and Statistical Manual of Mental Disorders: DSM-IV, 4th ed. Washington, DC: American Psychiatric Association, 1994.

Mouridsen SE. Childhood disintegrative disorder. Brain Dev 2003;25:225–228.

Conversion Disorder

American Psychiatric Association. Task Force on DSM-IV. Diagnostic and Statistical Manual of Mental Disorders: DSM-IV, 4th ed. Washington, DC: American Psychiatric Association, 1994.

Creutzfeldt-Jakob Disease

Budka H, Agguzi A, Brown P, et al. Neuropathological diagnostic criteria for Creutzfeldt-Jakob disease (CJD) and other human spongiform encephalopathies (prion diseases). Brain Pathol 1995;5:459–466.

World Health Organization. Global surveillance, diagnosis and therapy of human transmissible spongiform encephalopathies: Report of a WHO consultation. Geneva, Switzerland, 9–11 February 1998.

World Health Organization. Human transmissable spongiform encephalopathies. Wkly Epidemiol Rec 1998;73:361–365.

Delirium and Intoxications

American Psychiatric Association. Task Force on DSM-IV. Diagnostic and Statistical Manual of Mental Disorders: DSM-IV, 4th ed. Washington, DC: American Psychiatric Association, 1994.

Lerner AJ, Hedera P, Koss E, Stuckey J, Friedland RP. Delirium in Alzheimer disease. Alzheimer Dis Assoc Disord 1997;11:16–20.

World Health Organization. ICD-10, the ICD-10 classification of mental and behavioural disorders: diagnostic criteria for research. World Health Organization, Geneva, 1993.

Dementia With Lewy Bodies

Byrne EJ, Lennox G, Godwin-Austen RB, et al. Dementia associated with cortical Lewy bodies. Proposed diagnostic criteria. Dementia 1991;2:283, 284.

Hohl U, Tiraboschi P, Hansen LA, et al. Diagnostic accuracy of dementia with Lewy bodies. Arch Neurol 2000;57:347–351.

Holmes C, Cairns N, Lantos P, Mann A. Validity of current clinical criteria for Alzheimer's disease, vascular dementia and dementia with Lewy bodies. Br J Psychiatry 1999;174:45–50.

Hulette C, Mirra S, Wilkinson W, et al. The consortium to establish a registry for Alzheimer's disease (CERAD). Part IX. A prospective clinicopathologic study of Parkinson's features in Alzheimer's disease. Neurology 1995;45:1991–1995.

Knopman DS, Boeve BF, Petersen RC. Essentials of the proper diagnoses of mild cognitive impairment, dementia and major subtypes of dementia. Mayo Clin Proc 2003;78:1290–1308.

Litvan I, Bhatia KP, Burn DJ, et al. SIC Task Force appraisal of clinical diagnostic criteria for Parkinsonian disorders. Mov Disord 2003;18:467–486.

Litvan I, MacIntyre A, Goetz CG, et al. Accuracy of the clinical diagnosis of Lewy body disease. Parkinson disease, and dementia with Lewy bodies: a clinicopathologic study. Arch Neurol 1998;55:969–978.

Lopez OL, Becker JT, Kaufer DI, et al. Research evaluation and prospective diagnosis of dementia with Lewy bodies. Arch Neurol 2002;59:43–46.

Lopez OL, Litvan I, Catt KE, et al. Accuracy of four clinical diagnostic criteria for the diagnosis of neurodegenerative dementias. Neurology 1999;53:1292–1299.

Luis CA, Barker WW, Gajaraj K, et al. Sensitivity and specificity of three clinical criteria for dementia with Lewy bodies in an autopsy-verified sample. Int J Geriatr Psychiatry 1999;14:526–533.

McKieth IG, Galasko D, Kosaka K, et al. Consensus guidelines for the clinical and pathological diagnosis of dementia with Lewy bodies (DLB): report of the consortium on DLB international workshop. Neurology 1996;47:1113–1124.

McKieth IG, Ballard CG, Perry RH, et al. Prospective validation of consensus criteria for the diagnosis of dementia with Lewy bodies. Neurology 2000;54:1050–1058.

McKieth IG, Perry RH, Fairbairn AF, et al. Operational criteria for senile dementia of Lewy body type (SDLT). Psychol Med 1992;22:911–922.

Mega MS, Masterman DL, Benson DF, et al. Dementia with Lewy bodies: reliability and validity of clinical and pathologic criteria. Neurology 1996;47:1403–1409.

Veghese J, Crystal HA, Dickson DW, Lipton RB. Validity of clinical criteria for the diagnosis of dementia with Lewy bodies. Neurology 1999;53:1974–1982.

Walker MP, Ayre GA, Cummings JL, et al. Quantifying fluctuation in dementia with Lewy bodies, Alzheimer's disease, and vascular dementia. Neurology 2000;54:1616–1625.

Frontotemporal Dementia

Cairns NJ, Lee V M-Y, Trojanowski JQ. The cytoskeleton in neurodegenerative diseases. J Pathol 2004;204:438–449.

Knopman DS, Boeve BF, Petersen RC. Essentials of the proper diagnoses of mild cognitive impairment, dementia and major subtypes of dementia. Mayo Clin Proc 2003;78:1290–1308.

Knopman DS, DeKosky ST, Cummings JL, et al. Practice parameter: diagnosis of dementia (an evidence-based review). Neurology 2001;56:1143–1153.

Lopez OL, Litvan I, Catt KE, et al. Accuracy of four clinical diagnostic criteria for the diagnosis of neurodegenerative dementias. Neurology 1999;53:1292–1299.

Mckhann GH, Albert MS, Grossman M, Miller B, Dickson D, Trojanowski JQ. Clinical and pathological diagnosis of frontotemporal dementia: report of the work group on frontotemporal dementia and Pick's disease. Arch Neurol 2001;58:1803–1809.

Neary D, Snowden JS, Gustafson L, et al. Frontotemporal lobar degeneration: a consensus on clinical diagnostic criteria. Neurology 1998;51:1546–1554.

Mild Cognitive Impairment

Berg L. Clinical dementia rating (CDR). Psychopharmacol Bull 1988;24:637–639.

Busse A, Bischkopf J, Riedel-Heller SG, Angermeyer MC. Mild cognitive impairment: prevalence and incidence according to different diagnostic criteria. Results of the Liepzig longitudinal study of the aged (LEILA75+). Br J Psychiatry 2003;183:449–454.

Morris JC, Storandt M, Miller JP, et al. Mild cognitive impairment represents early-stage Alzheimer disease. Arch Neurol 2001;58:397–405.

Peterson RC. Aging, mild cognitive impairment and Alzheimer's disease. Neurol Clin 2000;18:799–805.

Petersen RC, Smith GE, Waring SC, Ivnik RJ, Tangalos EG, Kokmen E. Mild cognitive impairment: clinical characterization and outcome. Arch Neurol 1999;56:303–308.

Munchausen Syndrome by Proxy

Rosenberg DA: Munchausen's syndrome by proxy: medical diagnostic criteria. Child Abuse Negl 2003;27:421–430.

Normal Pressure Hydrocephalus

Adams RD, Fisher CM, Hakim S, Ojemann RG, Sweet WH. Symptomatic occult hydrocephalus with "normal" cerebrospinal-fluid pressure: A treatable syndrome. N Engl J Med 1965;273:117–126.

Hakim S, Adams RD. The special clinical problem of symptomatic hydrocephalus with normal cerebrospinal fluid pressure: Observations on cerebrospinal fluid dynamics. J Neurol Sci 1965;2:307–327.

Marmarou, A, Bergsneider, M Relkin, N Klinge, P; Black, Peter McL. Development of guidelines for idiopathic normal-pressure hydrocephalus: introduction. Guidelines for the diagnosis and management of idiopathic normal-pressure hydrocephalus. Neurosurgery 2005;57:S2-1–S2-3.

Relkin N, Marmarou A, Klinge P, Bergsneider M, Black PM. Diagnosing idiopathic normal-pressure hydrocephalus. Guidelines for the diagnosis and management of idiopathic normal-pressure hydrocephalus. Neurosurgery 57:2005; S2-4–S2-16.

Obsessive-Compulsive Disorder

American Psychiatric Association. Task Force on DSM-IV. Diagnostic and Statistical Manual of Mental Disorders: DSM-IV, 4th ed. Washington, DC: American Psychiatric Association, 1994.

Olfactory Reference Syndrome

Lochner C, Stein DJ. Olfactory reference syndrome: diagnostic criteria and differential diagnosis. Postgrad Med J 2003;49:328–331.

Primary Progressive Aphasia

Mesulam MM. Primary progressive aphasia. Ann Neurol 2001;49:425–432.

American Psychiatric Association. Task Force on DSM-IV. Diagnostic and Statistical Manual of Mental Disorders: DSM-IV, 4th ed. Washington, DC: American Psychiatric Association, 1994.

Mesulam MM. Primary progressive aphasia—differentiation from Alzheimer's disease. Ann Neurol 1987;22:533, 534.

Weintraub S, Rubin NP, Mesulam MM. Primary progressive aphasia. Longitudinal course, neuropsychological profile, and language features. Arch Neurol 1990;47:1329–1335.

Transient Global Amnesia

Caplan LR. Transient global amnesia. In: Vinken PJ, Bruyn GW, Klawans HL, eds. Handbook of Clinical Neurology, vol 1. Amsterdam: Elsevier Science, 1985;205–218.

Hodges JR, Warlow CP. Syndromes of transient amnesia: towards a classification. A study of 153 cases. J Neurol Neurosurg Psychiatr 1990;53:834–843.

Lampl Y, Sadeh M, Lorberboym M. Transient global amnesia—not always a benign process. Acta Neurol Scand 2004;110:75–79.

Sedlaczek O, Hirsch JG, Grips E, et al. Detection of delayed focal MR changes in the lateral hippocampus in transient global amnesia. Neurology 2004;62:2165–2170.

Tong DC, Grossman M. What causes transient global amnesia? New insights from DWI. Neurology 2004;62:2154, 2155.

4
Demyelinating Disorders

MULTIPLE SCLEROSIS

Perhaps no neurological condition better illustrates the evolution of diagnostic criteria over time or has better known criteria than multiple sclerosis (MS).

The criteria have evolved with technological advances in neuroimaging and diagnostic testing, so-called paraclinical data, as well as increased knowledge about the natural history of MS. However, despite the apparent increasing rate of diagnostic acumen and technical sophistication, we have had revisions 18 years, respectively, after each set of published criteria—Schumacher, 1965; Poser, 1983; and McDonald, 2001.

Because of the increased reliance on magnetic resonance imaging (MRI) in the McDonald criteria, and the changes in terminology, many studies have looked at both the sensitivity and specificity of MRI in predicting MS after a single event, and comparisons with the Poser criteria. In light of the development of new therapies for MS and the realization that axonal loss may occur with demyelination, even with a clinically isolated syndrome, there has been increased emphasis on early diagnosis by whatever criteria the clinician chooses.

Tintore et al. examined individuals with a clinically isolated syndrome (that is, patients with a single episode) and MRI findings suggestive of MS. At a 1-year follow-up, 11% had clinically definite MS by Poser criteria and 37% by McDonald criteria. Eighty percent of those who fulfilled the McDonald criteria had a second event over the follow-up period (mean: 49 months). In another study, Fangerau et al. found that all patients with definite MS by Poser criteria met criteria by McDonald criteria. However, many of the patients labeled as *laboratory-supported MS* by Poser criteria would be classified as *possible MS* because of the inability to meet the additional data or second attack criteria.

The MRI itself has been investigated in terms of interrater reliability. Even within this narrower field, there exist several criteria for what constitutes a positive MRI scan (for current criteria, *see* Tables 4 and 5). In general, there was poor agreement for the total number of lesions, and better agreement for the presence of a lesion. Interestingly, lesion location influenced agreement rates, and using a dichotomous lesion vs no lesion on T2-weighted images produced good agreement.

NEUROMYELITIS OPTICA

Also known as Devic's disease, neuromyelitis optica (NMO) has been considered a syndrome in its own right or a variant of MS. It has generally been considered a rare disease, but it is unclear if this is because of true rarity vs poor ascertainment methods, or whether its incidence varies by population. It has been estimated to cause about 5% of demyelinating disorders in Japan and India.

All of the criteria listed in Table 6 agree that NMO must present with optic neuritis and myelitis, but the relative timing is not always specified. The addition of neuroimaging criteria, especially the

From: *Current Clinical Neurology: Diagnostic Criteria in Neurology*
Edited by: A. J. Lerner © Humana Press Inc., Totowa, NJ

Table 1
Schumacher Criteria for the Diagnosis of Multiple Sclerosis

1. Neurological examination reveals objective abnormalities of central nervous system (CNS) function.
2. History indicates involvement of two or more parts of the CNS.
3. CNS disease predominately reflects white matter involvement.
4. Involvement of CNS follows one of two patterns:
    a. Two or more episodes, each lasting at least 24 hours and at least 1 month apart.
    b. Slow or stepwise progression of signs and symptoms over at least 6 months.
5. Patient aged 10–50 years old at onset.
6. Signs and symptoms cannot be better explained by other disease process.

Adapted from Schumacher FA, Beeve GW, Kibler RF, et al. Problems of experimental trials of multiple sclerosis. Ann NY Acad Sci 1965;122:552–568.

Table 2
Poser Criteria for the Diagnosis of Multiple Sclerosis

Clinically definite multiple sclerosis (MS)
- Two attacks and clinical evidence of two separate lesions.
- Two attacks, clinical evidence of one, and paraclinical evidence[a] of another separate lesion.

Laboratory-supported definite MS
- Two attacks, either clinical or paraclinical evidence of one lesion, and cerebrospinal fluid (CSF) immunological abnormalities.
- One attack, clinical evidence of two separate lesions, and CSF abnormalities.
- One attack, clinical evidence of one, and paraclinical evidence of another separate lesion, and CSF abnormalities.

Clinically probable MS
- Two attacks and clinical evidence of one lesion.
- One attack and clinical evidence of two separate lesions.
- One attack, clinical evidence of one lesion, and paraclinical evidence of another separate lesion.

Laboratory-supported probable MS
- Two attacks and CSF abnormalities.

[a]Paraclinical evidence includes the results of magnetic resonance imaging, evoked potentials, or other diagnostic tests of central nervous system dysfunction.

(Adapted with permission from Poser CM, Paty DW, Scheinberg L, et al. New diagnostic criteria for multiple sclerosis: guidelines for research protocols Ann Neurol 1983;13:227–231, and from John Wiley and Sons.)

requirement that the spinal lesion span several vertebral levels, has helped in excluding cases of MS that clinically present as NMO. The differential diagnosis must also include individuals with a history of isolated optic neuritis who later develop a myelopathy. Care must be taken to ascertain that mass lesions, cervical spondylosis, or other pathological entities have been excluded. Conversely, there may be individuals with incomplete syndromes, such as recurrent optic neuritis or recurrent "transverse myelitis," without other extensive disease who should be considered at-risk for developing NMO. This is important, because the clinical course of NMO is often more virulent than typical MS. The current standard therapy for attack prevention combines oral corticosteroids with immunosuppressive agents, such as azathioprine. Early initiation of therapy is recommended to prevent attack-related disability.

TRANSVERSE MYELITIS

An inflammatory disease of the spinal cord, transverse myelitis is a rare but often devastating syndrome. Its incidence is about one to four individuals per million per year. It may be associated with

Table 3
McDonald Criteria for the Diagnosis of Multiple Sclerosis

Clinical presentation	Additional data needed for MS diagnosis
Two or more attacks, objective clinical evidence of two or more lesions	None[a]
Two or more attacks, objective clinical evidence of one lesion	Dissemination in space, demonstrated by: • MRI, *or* • Two or more MRI-detected lesions consistent with MS plus positive CSF, *or* • Further clinical attack, implicating a different site
One attack; objective clinical evidence of two or more lesions	• Dissemination in time (demonstrated by MRI), *or* • Second clinical attack
One attack; objective clinical evidence of one lesion (monosymptomatic presentation, clinically isolated syndrome)	Dissemination in space, demonstrated by: • MRI, *or* • Two or more MRI-detected lesions consistent with MS plus positive CSF, *and* Dissemination in time, demonstrated by: • MRI, *or* • Second clinical attack
Insidious neurological progression suggestive of MS	Positive CSF, *and* Dissemination in space, demonstrated by: • Nine or more T2 lesions in brain, *or* • Two or more lesions in spinal cord, *or* • Four to eight brain lesions plus one spinal cord lesion, *or* • Abnormal VEP associated with four to eight brain lesions, *or* • Abnormal VEP with fewer than four brain lesions plus one spinal cord lesion; *and* Dissemination in time, demonstrated by: • MRI, *or* • Continued progression for 1 year

[a]Caution urged if all tests are negative.

MS, multiple sclerosis; MRI, magnetic resonance imaging; CSF, cerebrospinal fluid (oligoclonal bands or raised immunoglobulin G index); VEP, visually evoked potential.

(Adapted with permission from McDonald WI, Compton A, Edan G, et al. Recommended diagnostic criteria for multiple sclerosis: guidelines from the International Panel on the diagnosis of multiple sclerosis. Ann Neurol 2001; 50:121–127, and from John Wiley and Sons.)

Table 4
Guidelines for Magnetic Resonance Imaging Criteria or Brain Abnormality

Three of the four following guidelines:
1. One gadolinium-enhancing lesion or nine T2-hyperintense lesions if there is no gadolinium-enhancing lesions.
2. At least one infratentorial lesion.
3. At least one juxtacortical lesion.
4. At least three periventricular lesions.

Note: One spinal cord lesion can be substituted for one brain lesion.

(Adapted with permission from McDonald WI, Compton A, Edan G, et al. Recommended diagnostic criteria for multiple sclerosis: guidelines from the International Panel on the diagnosis of multiple sclerosis. Ann Neurol 2001;50:121–127.)

numerous viral, bacterial, parasitic (e.g., schistosomiasis), or autoimmune collagen vascular diseases. Transverse myelitis may be the presenting symptom of MS, and is an integral part of NMO.

Table 5
Magnetic Imaging Criteria for Dissemination of Lesions in Time

1. If a first scan occurs 3 months or more after the onset of the clinical event, the presence of a gadolinium-enhancing lesion is sufficient to demonstrate dissemination in time, provided that it is not at the site implicated in the original clinical event. If there is no enhancing lesion at this time, a follow-up scan is required. The timing of this scan is not crucial, but 3 months is recommended. A new T2- or gadolinium-enhancing lesion at this time fulfills the criterion for dissemination in time.

2. If the first scan is performed less than 3 months after the onset of the clinical event, a second scan done 3 months or more after the clinical event showing a new gadolinium-enhancing lesion provides sufficient evidence for dissemination in time. However, if no enhancing lesion is seen at the second scan, a further scan not less than 3 months after the first scan that shows a new T2 lesion or an enhancing lesion will suffice.

Adapted from McDonald WI, Compton A, Edan G, et al. Recommended diagnostic criteria for multiple sclerosis: guidelines from the International Panel on the diagnosis of multiple sclerosis. Ann Neurol 2001;50:121–127.

Table 6
Comparison of the Definitions of Neuromyelitis Optica

Gault and Devic (Lyon, France)
  Retrobulbar neuritis or papillitis accompanied by acute myelitis and occasionally other neurological symptoms or signs not restricted to the spinal cord or optic nerves.
Shibasaki et al. (Kyushu University, Japan)
  Acute bilateral visual impairment (optic neuritis) and transverse myelitis occurring successively within an interval of 4 weeks that follows a monophasic course.
O'Riordan and colleagues (Queen Square, England)
  1. Complete transverse myelitis: an acutely developing and severe paraparesis or tetraparesis affecting motor and sensory pathways with or without sphincteric involvement, evolving over 1–14 days, with a sensory level and in the absence of cord compression.
  2. Acute unilateral or bilateral optic neuropathy.
  3. No clinical involvement beyond the spinal cord or optic nerves.
  4. The disease can be monophasic or multiphasic.
Mandler and colleagues (University of New Mexico)
  1. Clinical: Acute involvement of spinal cord and optic nerves, either coincidental or separated by months or years, independent of its subsequent progression but without the development of brainstem, cerebellar, or cortical features at any time in the disease course.
  2. Imaging: Normal-appearing brain MRI, enlargement and cavitation on spinal cord MRI.
  3. CSF: Decreased serum/CSF albumin ratio with normal CNS daily IgG synthesis and usually absence of oligoclonal bands.
  4. Pathology: Spinal cord necrosis and cavitation with thickened vessel walls and absence of inflammatory infiltrates; demyelination of optic nerves with or without cavitation; no demyelinating lesions in the brain, brainstem, or cerebellum.
Wingerchuk and colleagues (Mayo Clinic)
  Diagnosis requires all absolute criterion and one major supportive criterion or two minor supportive criteria.
Absolute criteria:
  1. Optic neuritis.
  2. Acute myelitis.
  3. No evidence of clinical disease outside of the optic nerve or spinal cord.
Major supportive criteria:
  1. Negative brain MRI at onset (does not meet criteria for multiple sclerosis).
  2. Spinal cord MRI with signal abnormality extending over three or more vertebral segments.
  3. CSF pleocytosis of >50 WBC/mm^3 or >5 PMNs/mm.^{3}
Minor supportive criteria:
  1. Bilateral optic neuritis.
  2. Severe optic neuritis with fixed visual acuity worse than 20/200 in at least one eye.
  3. Severe, fixed, attack-related weakness (MRC ≤2) in one or more limbs.

(Continued)

Table 6 *(Continued)*

de Seze and colleagues (CHRU de Lille, France)
  1. An acutely developing myelopathy affecting motor and sensory pathways with or without sphincter dysfunction, evolving in less than 1 month.
  2. An acute unilateral or bilateral optic neuritis.
  3. No clinical neurological involvement beyond the spinal cord or optic nerves.
  4. Monophasic or polyphasic course.

MRI, magnetic resonance imaging; CSF, cerebrospinal fluid; CNS, central nervous system; IgG, immunoglobulin G; MRC, Medical Research Council; WBC, white blood cell; PMN, polymorphonuclear neutrophil.
(Adapted from Cree BA, Goodin DS, Hauser SL. Neuromyelitis optica. Semin Neurol 2002;22:105–122.)

Table 7
Diagnostic Criteria for Idiopathic Acute Transverse Myelitis

Inclusion criteria	*Exclusion criteria*
• Development of sensory, motor, or autonomic dysfunction attributable to the spinal cord.	• History of previous radiation to the spine within the last 10 years.
• Bilateral signs and/or symptoms (though not necessarily symmetric).	• Clear arterial distribution clinical deficit consistent with thrombosis of the anterior spinal artery.
• Clearly defined sensory level.	
• Exclusion of extra-axial compressive etiology by neuroimaging (MRI or myelography; CT of spine not adequate).	• Abnormal flow voids on the surface of the spinal cord consistent with AVM.
• Inflammation within the spinal cord demonstrated by CSF pleocytosis or elevated IgG index or gadolinium enhancement. If none of the inflammatory criteria are met at symptom onset, repeat MRI and lumbar puncture evaluation between 2 and 7 days following symptom onset meet criteria.	• Serological or clinical evidence of connective tissue disease (sarcoidosis, Behcet's disease, Sjögren's syndrome, SLE, mixed connective tissue disorder, and so on).[a]
	• CNS manifestations of syphilis, Lyme disease, HIV, HTLV-1, mycoplasma, other viral infection (e.g., HSV-1, HSV-2, VZV, EBV, CMV, HHV-6, enteroviruses).[a]
• Progression to nadir between 4 hours and 21 days following the onset of symptoms (if patient awakens with symptoms, symptoms must become more pronounced from point of awakening).	• Brain MRI abnormalities suggestive of MS.[a]
	• History of clinically apparent optic neuritis.[a]

[a]Do not exclude disease-associated acute transverse myelitis.
MRI, magnetic resonance imaging, CT, computed tomography; AVM, arteriovenous malformation; CSF, cerebrospinal fluid; IgG index, immunoglobulin G index; SLE, systemic lupus erythematosus; HTLV-1, human T-cell lymphotropic virus-1; HSV, herpes simplex virus, VZV, varicella zoster virus; EBV, Epstein Barr virus; CMV, cytomegalovirus; HHV, human herpes virus.
(Adapted with permission from Transverse myelitis consortium working group. Proposed diagnostic criteria and nosology of transverse myelitis. Neurology 2002;59:499–505.)

SOURCES

Multiple Sclerosis

Barkhof F, Filippi M, Miller DH, Ader HJ. Interobserver agreement for diagnostic MRI criteria in suspected multiple sclerosis. Neuroradiology 1999;41:347–350.

Dalton CM, Chard DT, Davies GR, et al. Early development of multiple sclerosis is associated with progressive grey matter atrophy in patients presenting with clinically isolated syndromes. Brain 2004;127(Part 5):1101–1107.

Fangerau T, Schimrigk S, Haupts M, et. al. Diagnosis of multiple sclerosis: comparison of the Poser criteria and the new McDonald criteria. Acta Neurol Scand 2004;109:385–389.

McDonald WI, Compton A, Edan G, et al. Recommended diagnostic criteria for multiple sclerosis: guidelines from the International Panel on the diagnosis of multiple sclerosis. Ann Neurol 2001;50:121–127.

Poser CM, Paty DW, Scheinberg L, et al. New diagnostic criteria for multiple sclerosis: guidelines for research protocols. Ann Neurol 1983;13:227–231.

Schumacher FA, Beeve GW, Kibler RF, et al. Problems of experimental trials of multiple sclerosis. Ann NY Acad Sci 1965;122:552–568.

Thompson AJ, Montalban X, Barkhof F, et al. Diagnostic criteria for primary progressive multiple sclerosis: a position paper. Ann Neurol 2000;47:831–835.

Tintore M, Rovira A, Rio J, et al. New diagnostic criteria for multiple sclerosis: application in first demyelinating episode. Neurology 2003;60:27–30.

Neuromyelitis Optica

Cree BA, Goodin DS, Hauser SL. Neuromyelitis optica. Semin Neurol 2002;22:105–122.

de Seze J, Stojkovic T, Ferriby D, et al. Devic's neuromyelitis optica: clinical, laboratory, MRI and outcome profile. J Neurol Sci 2002;197:57–61.

Devic E. Myelite aigue dorse-lombaire avec névrite optique, autopsie. Congrés français de méd [in French]. Premiére Session, Lyon 1895;1:434–439.

Devic E. Myélite subaiguë compliquée de névrite optique [in French]. Bull Med (Paris) 1894;8:1033–1034.

Gault F. De la neuromyélite optique aiguë [in French]. PhD thesis, Lyons, France: 1894.

Mandler RN, Davis LE, Jeffery DR, Kornfeld M. Devic's neuromyelitis optica: a clinicopathological study of 8 patients. Ann Neurol 1993;34:162–168.

O'Riordan JI, Gallagher HL, Thompson AJ, et al. Clinical, CSF, and MRI findings in Devic's neuromyelitis optica. J Neurol Neurosurg Psychiatr 1996;60:382–387.

Shibasaki H, McDonald WI, Kuroiwa Y. Racial modification of clinical picture of multiple sclerosis: comparison between British and Japanese patients. J Neurol Sci 1981;49:253–271.

Wingerchuk DM, Hogancamp WF, O'Brien PC, Weinshenker BG. The clinical course of neuromyelitis optica (Devic's syndrome). Neurology 1999;53:1107–1114.

Transverse Myelitis

Berman M, Feldman S, Alter M, Zilber N, Kahana E. Acute transverse myelitis: incidence and etiologic considerations. Neurology 1981;31:966–971.

Jeffery DR, Mandler RN, Davis LE. Transverse myelitis. Retrospective analysis of 33 cases, with differentiation of cases associated with multiple sclerosis and parainfectious events. Arch Neurol 1993;50:532–535.

Ropper AH, Poskanzer DC. The prognosis of acute and subacute transverse myelopathy based on early signs and symptoms. Ann Neurol 1979:4:51–59.

Transverse myelitis consortium working group. Proposed diagnostic criteria and nosology of transverse myelitis. Neurology 2002;59:499–505.

5
Disorders of Consciousness and Brain Death

BRAIN DEATH IN ADULTS

There is no universal consensus regarding the diagnosis of brain death using standardized criteria (*see* the excellent review of this by Wijdicks, 2002). The most widely known are the original Harvard criteria from 1968. The lack of widely accepted criteria operationally means that physicians are subject to local guidelines in specific cases. Other sets of guidelines for determining brain death include the Ad Hoc Committee on Death of the Minnesota Medical Association (1976), the Conference of the Medical Royal Colleges (1976), the United States Collaborative Study of Cerebral Death (1977), and the President's Commission for the Study of Ethical Problems in Medicine and Biomedical and Behavioral Research (1981). Differences among their criteria include (1) the regions of brain that must lose all function, (2) the extent and characteristics of areflexia, (3) the duration of the clinical observation, and (4) the role and category of confirmatory tests.

In the United States, the criteria for brain death usually follow The Uniform Determination of Death Act, which are (1) irreversible cessation of circulatory and respiratory functions or (2) irreversible cessation of all functions of the entire brain, including the brain stem, as well as the neocortex.

It also states that a determination of death must be made in accordance with "accepted medical standards." The Act does not define these medical standards; rather, it leaves them open for refinement as medical technology advances.

In Virginia, there is a requirement for a specialist in neurology, neurosurgery, or electroencephalography to declare a patient brain-dead. Kentucky requires two licensed physicians to make the determination of brain death. Alaska and Georgia allow for determination of brain death to be made by registered nurses. In Florida, a requirement for two physicians includes "one physician shall be the treating physician, and the other physician shall be a board-eligible or board-certified neurologist, neurosurgeon, internist, pediatrician, surgeon, or anesthesiologist." In New Jersey and New York, brain death cannot be declared against the patient's religious beliefs. Table 1 contains current brain death criteria recommended by the American Academy of Neurology.

BRAIN DEATH IN CHILDREN

For children, the recommendations of the 1987 Task Force of the American Academy of Pediatrics depend on age, as detailed in Table 2. The guidelines rightly emphasize caution because there have been case reports of good outcomes in children after near-drowning, and so on, who would transiently have met some or all of the diagnostic criteria. There have also been case reports of children with Guillain-Barré syndrome, who present without reflexes or voluntary respirations, but whose true clinical state is revealed by electroencephalography. The guidelines were formulated before some newer technologies, such as transcranial Doppler ultrasonography or radionuclide scanning, were widely used for demonstrating absence of cerebral blood flow.

From: *Current Clinical Neurology: Diagnostic Criteria in Neurology*
Edited by: A. J. Lerner © Humana Press Inc., Totowa, NJ

Table 1
Determining Brain Death in Adults (American Academy of Neurology)

I. Diagnostic criteria for clinical diagnosis of brain death
   A. Prerequisites. Brain death is the absence of clinical brain function when the proximate cause is known and demonstrably irreversible.
      1. Clinical or neuroimaging evidence of an acute central nervous system catastrophe that is compatible with the clinical diagnosis of brain death.
      2. Exclusion of complicating medical conditions that may confound clinical assessment (no severe electrolyte, acid–base, or endocrine disturbance).
      3. No drug intoxication or poisoning.
      4. Core temperature ≥32°C (90°F).
   B. The three cardinal findings in brain death are coma or unresponsiveness, absence of brainstem reflexes, and apnea.
      1. Coma or unresponsiveness—no cerebral motor response to pain in all extremities (nail-bed pressure and supraorbital pressure).
      2. Absence of brainstem reflexes.
         a. Pupils
            i. No response to bright light.
            ii. Size: midposition (4 mm) to dilated (9 mm).
         b. Ocular movement
            i. No oculocephalic reflex (testing only when no fracture or instability of the cervical spine is apparent).
            ii. No deviation of the eyes to irrigation in each ear with 50 mL of cold water (allow 1 minute after injection and at least 5 minutes between testing on each side).
         c. Facial sensation and facial motor response
            i. No corneal reflex to touch with a throat swab.
            ii. No jaw reflex.
            iii. No grimacing to deep pressure on nail bed, supraorbital ridge, or temporomandibular joint.
         d. Pharyngeal and tracheal reflexes
            i. No response after stimulation of the posterior pharynx with tongue blade.
            ii. No cough response to bronchial suctioning.
      3. Apnea—testing performed as follows:
         a. Prerequisites
            i. Core temperature ≥36.5°C or 97°F.
            ii. Systolic blood pressure ≥90 mmHg.
            iii. Euvolemia. *Option:* positive fluid balance in the previous 6 hours.
            iv. Normal PCO_2. *Option:* arterial PCO_2 ≥40 mmHg.
            v. Normal PO_2. *Option:* preoxygenation to obtain arterial PO_2 ≥200 mmHg.
         b. Connect a pulse oximeter and disconnect the ventilator.
         c. Deliver 100% O_2, 6 L/minute, into the trachea. *Option:* place a cannula at the level of the carina.
         d. Look closely for respiratory movements (abdominal or chest excursions that produce adequate tidal volumes).
         e. Measure arterial PO_2, PCO_2, and pH after approx 8 minutes and reconnect the ventilator.
         f. If respiratory movements are absent and arterial PCO_2 is ≥60 mmHg (*option:* 20-mmHg increase in PCO_2 over a baseline normal PCO_2), the apnea test result is positive (i.e., it supports the diagnosis of brain death).
         g. If respiratory movements are observed, the apnea test result is negative (i.e., it does not support the clinical diagnosis of brain death), and the test should be repeated.
         h. Connect the ventilator if, during testing, the systolic blood pressure equals 90 mmHg or the pulse oximeter indicates significant oxygen desaturation and cardiac arrhythmias are present; immediately draw an arterial blood sample and analyze arterial blood gas. If PCO_2 is equal to 60 mmHg or PCO_2 increase is equal to 20 mmHg over baseline normal PCO_2, the apnea test result is positive (it supports the clinical diagnosis of brain death); if PCO_2 is <60 mmHg or PCO_2 increase is <20 mmHg over baseline normal PCO_2, the result is indeterminate, and an additional confirmatory test can be considered.

(Continued)

Table 1 *(Continued)*

II. Pitfalls in the diagnosis of brain death

The following conditions may interfere with the clinical diagnosis of brain death, so that the diagnosis cannot be made with certainty on clinical grounds alone. Confirmatory tests are recommended.

   A. Severe facial trauma.
   B. Preexisting pupillary abnormalities.
   C. Toxic levels of any sedative drugs, aminoglycosides, tricyclic antidepressants, anticholinergics, antiepileptic drugs, chemotherapeutic agents, or neuromuscular blocking agents.
   D. Sleep apnea or severe pulmonary disease resulting in chronic retention of CO_2.

III. Clinical observations compatible with the diagnosis of brain death

These manifestations are occasionally seen and should not be misinterpreted as evidence for brainstem function.

   A. Spontaneous movements of limbs other than pathological flexion or extension response.
   B. Respiratory-like movements (shoulder elevation and adduction, back arching, intercostal expansion without significant tidal volumes).
   C. Sweating, blushing, tachycardia.
   D. Normal blood pressure without pharmacological support or sudden increases in blood pressure.
   E. Absence of diabetes insipidus.
   F. Deep tendon reflexes superficial abdominal reflexes, triple flexion response.
   G. Babinski reflex.

IV. Confirmatory laboratory tests (options)

Brain death is a clinical diagnosis. A repeat clinical evaluation 6 hours later is recommended, but this interval is arbitrary. A confirmatory test is not mandatory, but is desirable in patients in whom specific components of clinical testing cannot be reliably performed or evaluated. It should be emphasized that any of the suggested confirmatory tests may produce similar results in patients with catastrophic brain damage who do not (yet) fulfill the clinical criteria of brain death. The following confirmatory test findings are listed in the order of the most sensitive test first. Consensus criteria are identified by individual tests.

   A. Conventional angiography. No intracerebral filling at the level of the carotid bifurcation or circle of Willis. The external carotid circulation is patent, and filling of the superior longitudinal sinus may be delayed.
   B. Electroencephalography (EEG). No electrical activity during at least 30 minutes of recording that adheres to the minimal technical criteria for EEG recording in suspected brain death as adopted by the American Electroencephalographic Society, including 16-channel EEG instruments.
   C. Transcranial Doppler ultrasonography.
      1. Ten percent of patients may not have temporal insonation windows. Therefore, the initial absence of Doppler signals cannot be interpreted as consistent with brain death.
      2. Small systolic peaks in early systole without diastolic flow or reverberating flow, indicating very high vascular resistance associated with greatly increased intracranial pressure.
   D. Technetium-99m hexamethylpropyleneamineoxime brain scan. No uptake of isotope in brain parenchyma ("hollow skull phenomenon").
   E. Somatosensory-evoked potentials. Bilateral absence of N20-P22 response with median nerve stimulation. The recordings should adhere to the minimal technical criteria for somatosensory evoked potential recording in suspected brain death as adopted by the American Electroencephalographic Society.

V. Medical record documentation (standard)

   A. Etiology and irreversibility of condition.
   B. Absence of brainstem reflexes.
   C. Absence of motor response to pain.
   D. Absence of respiration with PCO_2 equal to 60 mmHg.
   E. Justification for confirmatory test and result of confirmatory test; antiepileptic drugs, chemotherapeutic agents, or neuromuscular blocking agents.
   F. Repeat neurological examination. Option: the interval is arbitrary, but a 6-hour period is reasonable.

Note on confirmatory tests:

Although confirmatory tests are optional in the United States, they are mandated in some other countries in specific circumstances.

Adapted with permission from The Quality Standards Subcommittee of the American Academy of Neurology. Practice parameters for determining brain death in adults [summary statement]. Neurology 1995;45:1012–1014.)

Guidelines of the Task Force for the Determination of Brain Death in Children

Clinical History and Examination

The critical initial assessment is the clinical history and examination. The most important factor is determination of the proximate cause of coma to ensure absence of remediable or reversible conditions. Most difficulties with the determination of death based on neurological criteria have resulted from overlooking this basic fact. Especially important are detection of toxic and metabolic disorders, sedative–hypnotic drugs, paralytic agents, hypothermia, hypotension, and surgically remediable conditions. The physical examination is necessary to determine the failure of brain function.

Physical Examination Criteria

1. Coma and apnea must coexist. The patient must exhibit complete loss of consciousness, vocalization, and volitional activity.
2. Absence of brainstem function as defined by:
   a. Midposition or fully dilated pupils which do not respond to light. Drugs may influence and invalidate pupillary assessment.
   b. Absence of spontaneous eye movements and those induced by occulocephalic and caloric (oculovestibular) testing.
   c. Absence of movement of bulbar musculature including facial and oropharyngeal muscles. The corneal, gag, cough, suckling, and rooting reflexes are absent.
   d. Respiratory movements are absent with the patient off the respirator. Apnea testing using standardized methods can be performed, but is done after other criteria are met.
3. The patient must not be significantly hypothermic or hypotensive for age.
4. Flaccid tone and absence of spontaneous or induced movements, excluding spinal cord events, such as reflex withdrawal or spinal myoclonus, should exist.
5. The examination should remain consistent with brain death throughout the observation and testing period.

Observation Periods According to Age (Table 2)

Table 2
Age-Dependent Observation Period for Determination of Brain Death in Children

Age	Hours between two examinations	Recommended number of EEGs
7 days–2 months	48	2
2 months–1 year	24	2
>1 year	12	Not needed

Seven days–2 months—Two examinations and electroencephalograms (EEGs) separated by at least 48 hours. Two months to 1 year—Two examinations and EEGs separated by at least 24 hours. A repeat examination and EEG are not necessary if a concomitant radionuclude angiographic study demonstrates no visualization of cerebral arteries.
Observation period
  If hypoxic encephalopathy present, observation for 24 hours is recommended. This may be reduced if an EEG shows electrocerebral silence or a radionuclide study is negative for cerebral blood flow.

Adapted with permission from American Academy of Pediatrics Task Force on Brain Death in Children. Report of special Task Force. Guidelines for the determination of brain death in children. Pediatrics 1987;80:298–300.

Laboratory Testing

ELECTROENCEPHALOGRAPHY

Electroencephalography to document electrocerebral silence should, if performed, be done over a 30-minute period using standardized techniques for brain death determinations. In small children, it may not be possible to meet the standard requirement for 10-cm electrode separation. The interelectrode distance should be decreased in proportion to the patient's head size. Drug concentrations should be insufficient to suppress electroencephalographic activity.

Table 3
The Minimally Conscious State

Definition of the minimally conscious state (MCS).
   The MCS is a condition of severely altered consciousness in which minimal but definite behavioral evidence of self or environmental awareness is demonstrated.
Diagnostic criteria for the MCS.
   1.   MCS is distinguished from the vegetative state by the presence of behaviors associated with conscious awareness. In MCS, cognitively mediated behavior occurs inconsistently, but is reproducible or sustained long enough to be differentiated from reflexive behavior. The reproducibility of such evidence is affected by the consistency and complexity of the behavioral response. Extended assessment may be required to determine whether a simple response (e.g., a finger movement or eye blink) that is observed infrequently is occurring in response to a specific environmental event (e.g., command to move fingers or blink eyes) or on a coincidental basis. In contrast, a few observations of a complex response (e.g., intelligible verbalization) may be sufficient to determine the presence of consciousness.
   2.   To make the diagnosis of MCS, limited but clearly discernible evidence of self- or environmental awareness must be demonstrated on a reproducible or sustained basis by one or more of the following behaviors:
       a.   Following simple commands.
       b.   Gestural or verbal yes/no responses (regardless of accuracy).
       c.   Intelligible verbalization.
       d.   Purposeful behavior, including movements or affective behaviors that occur in contingent relation to relevant environmental stimuli and are not because of reflexive activity.
            i.   Examples include:
                 • Appropriate smiling or crying in response to the linguistic or visual content of emotional but not to neutral topics or stimuli.
                 • Vocalizations or gestures that occur in direct response to the linguistic content of questions—reaching for objects that demonstrate a clear relationship between object location and direction of reach.
                 • Touching or holding objects in a manner that accommodates the size and shape of the object—pursuit eye movement or sustained fixation that occurs in direct response to moving or salient stimuli.
   3.   Although it is not uncommon for individuals in MCS to demonstrate more than one of the above criteria, in some patients the evidence is limited to only one behavior that is indicative of consciousness. Clinical judgments concerning a patient's level of consciousness depend on inferences drawn from observed behavior. Thus, sensory deficits, motor dysfunction, or diminished drive may result in underestimation of cognitive capacity.
Proposed criteria for emergence from MCS.
Recovery from MCS to higher states of consciousness occurs along a continuum in which the upper boundary is necessarily arbitrary. Consequently, the diagnostic criteria for emergence from MCS are based on broad classes of functionally useful behaviors that are typically observed as such patients recover.
Emergence from MCS is characterized by reliable and consistent demonstration of one or both of the following.
   1.   Functional interactive communication.
   2.   Functional use of two different objects.
   3.   Functional interactive communication occurring through:
       a.   Verbalization.
       b.   Writing.
       c.   Yes/no signals.
       d.   Use of augmentative communication devices.
       e.   Functional use of objects requires demonstration of behavioral evidence of object discrimination.
To facilitate consistent reporting of findings among clinicians and investigators working with patients in MCS, the following parameters for demonstrating response reliability and consistency should be used:
Functional communication: accurate yes/no responses to six of six basic situational orientation questions on two consecutive evaluations. Situational orientation questions include items, such as "Are you sitting down?" and "Am I pointing to the ceiling?"
Functional object use: generally appropriate use of at least two different objects on two consecutive evaluations. This criterion may be satisfied by behaviors such as bringing a comb to the head or a pencil to a sheet of paper.

(Continued)

Table 3 *(Continued)*

It is necessary to exclude aphasia, agnosia, apraxia, or sensorimotor impairment as the basis for nonresponsiveness, as opposed to diminished level of consciousness. As noted previously, the criteria for emergence from MCS may underestimate the level of consciousness in some patients. For example, patients with some forms of akinetic mutism demonstrate limited behavioral initiation but are capable of occasional complex cognitively mediated behavior. When there is evidence to suggest that the assessment of level of consciousness is confounded by diminished behavioral initiation, further diagnostic investigation is indicated. Until these diagnostic ambiguities can be resolved by future research, the above definitions should be applied to all patients whose behavior fails to substantiate higher levels of consciousness. It is likely that studies investigating the neurological substrate underlying subgroups of MCS patients will, in the future, allow the development of diagnostic criteria that are more reliably tied to the level of consciousness.

Recommendations for behavioral assessment of neurocognitive responsiveness.

Differential diagnosis among states of impaired consciousness is often difficult. The following steps should be taken to detect conscious awareness and to establish an accurate diagnosis:

- Adequate stimulation should be administered to ensure that arousal level is maximized.
- Factors adversely affecting arousal should be addressed (e.g., sedating medications and occurrence of seizures).
- Attempts to elicit behavioral responses through verbal instruction should not involve behaviors that frequently occur on a reflexive basis.
- Command-following trials should incorporate motor behaviors that are within the patient's capability.
- A variety of different behavioral responses should be investigated using a broad range of eliciting stimuli.
- Examination procedures should be conducted in a distraction-free environment.
- Serial reassessment incorporating systematic observation and reliable measurement strategies should be used to confirm the validity of the initial assessment. Specialized tools and procedures designed for quantitative assessment may be useful.
- Observations of family members, caregivers, and professional staff participating in daily care should be considered in designing assessment procedures.

Special care must be taken when evaluating infants and children younger than 3 years of age who have sustained severe brain injury. In this age group, assessment of cognitive function is constrained by immature language and motor development. This limits the degree to which command following, verbal expression, and purposeful movement can be relied on to determine whether the diagnostic criteria for MCS have been met.

Adapted with permission from Giacino JT, Ashwal S, Childs N, et al. The minimally conscious state. Definition and diagnostic criteria. Neurology 2002;58:349–353.)

Table 4
The Vegetative State

Definitions

The *vegetative state* is a clinical condition of complete unawareness of the self and the environment accompanied by sleep–wake cycles with either complete or partial preservation of hypothalamic and brainstem autonomic functions.

Diagnostic criteria

The vegetative state can be diagnosed using the following criteria.

Patients in a vegetative state show:

- No evidence of awareness of self or environment and an inability to interact with others.
- No evidence of sustained, reproducible, purposeful, or voluntary behavioral responses to visual, auditory, tactile, or noxious stimuli.
- No evidence of language comprehension or expression.
- Intermittent wakefulness manifested by the presence of sleep–wake cycles.
- Sufficiently preserved hypothalamic and brainstem autonomic functions to permit survival with medical and nursing care.
- Bowel and bladder incontinence.
- Variably preserved cranial nerve (pupillary, oculocephalic, corneal, vestibulo-ocular, gag) and spinal reflexes.

Table 4 *(Continued)*

The *persistent vegetative state* (PVS) can be defined as a vegetative state present at 1 month after acute traumatic or nontraumatic brain injury, and present for at least 1 month in degenerative/metabolic disorders or developmental malformations.

The *permanent vegetative state* means an irreversible state, a definition, as with all clinical diagnoses in medicine, based on probabilities, not absolutes. A patient in PVS becomes permanently vegetative when the diagnosis of irreversibility can be established with a high degree of clinical certainty, i.e., when the chance of regaining consciousness is exceedingly rare.

Diagnosis of PVS. PVS can be diagnosed on clinical grounds with a high degree of medical certainty in most adult and pediatric patients after careful, repeated neurological examinations. The diagnosis of PVS should be established by a physician who, by reason of training and experience, is competent in neurological function, assessment, and diagnosis. Reliable criteria do not exist for making a diagnosis of PVS in infants younger than 3 months, except in patients with anencephaly. Other diagnostic studies may support the diagnosis of PVS, but none adds to diagnostic specificity with certainty.

Categories and clinical course of PVS. There are three major categories of diseases in adults and children that result in PVS. The clinical course and outcome of PVS patients depends on the specific etiology:

A. Acute traumatic and nontraumatic brain injury. PVS usually evolves within 1 month of injury from a state of eyes-closed coma to a state of wakefulness without awareness with sleep–wake cycles and preserved brainstem functions.

B. Degenerative and metabolic disorders of the brain. Many degenerative and metabolic nervous system disorders in adults and children inevitably progress toward an irreversible vegetative state. Patients who are severely impaired but retain some degree of awareness may lapse briefly into a vegetative state from the effects of medication, infection, superimposed illnesses, or decreased fluid and nutritional intake. Such a temporary encephalopathy must be corrected before establishing that the patient is in PVS. If the vegetative state persists for several months, recovery of consciousness is unlikely.

C. Severe developmental malformations of the nervous system. The developmental vegetative state is a form of PVS that affects some infants and children with severe congenital malformations of the nervous system. These children do not acquire awareness of the self or the environment. This diagnosis can be made at birth only in infants with anencephaly.

For children with other severe malformations who appear vegetative at birth, observation for 3–6 months is recommended to determine whether these infants acquire awareness. The majority of such infants who are vegetative at birth remain vegetative; those who acquire awareness usually recover only to a severe disability.

Recommendations. Diagnostic standard and management guidelines for adults and children in PVS include the following:

Diagnostic standard for establishing a persistent vegetative state. The vegetative state is diagnosable. It is defined as being persistent at 1 month. Based on class II evidence and consensus that reflect a high degree of clinical certainty, the following is a standard concerning PVS:

A. PVS can be judged to be permanent 12 months after traumatic injury in adults and children. Special attention to signs of awareness should be devoted to children during the first year after traumatic injury.

B. PVS can be judged to be permanent for nontraumatic injury in adults and children after 3 months. The chance for recovery after these periods is exceedingly low, and recovery is almost always to a severe disability.

Adapted with permission from Practice parameters: assessment and management of patients in the persistent vegetative state [summary statement]. The Quality Standards Subcommittee of the American Academy of Neurology. Neurology 1995;45:1015–1018.)

ANGIOGRAPHY

A cerebral radionuclude angiogram confirms cerebral death by demonstrating the lack of visualization of the cerebral circulation. A technically satisfactory study demonstrates arrest of carotid circulation at the base of the skull, and absence of intracranial arterial circulation can be considered confirmatory of brain death, although there may be some visualization of the intracranial venous sinuses. Contrast angiography can document lack of effective blood flow to the brain.

Table 5
Comparison of Clinical Features Associated With Coma, Vegetative State, Minimally Conscious State, and Locked-In Syndrome

Condition	Consciousness	Sleep–Wake	Motor function	Auditory function	Visual function	Communication	Emotion
Coma	None	Absent	Reflex and postural responses only	None	None	None	None
Vegetative state	None	Present	Postures or withdraws to noxious stimuli; Occasional nonpurposeful movement	Startle; Brief orienting to sound	Startle; Brief visual fixation	None	None; Reflexive crying or smiling
Minimally conscious state	Partial	Present	Localizes noxious stimuli; Reaches for objects; Holds or touches objects in a manner that accommodates size and shape; Automatic movements (e.g., scratching)	Localizes sound location; Inconsistent command following	Sustained visual fixation; Sustained visual pursuit	Contingent vocalization; Inconsistent but intelligible verbalization or gesture	Contingent smiling or crying
Locked-in syndrome	Full	Present	Quadriplegic	Preserved	Preserved	Aphonic/dysarthric; Vertical eye movement and blinking usually intact	Preserved

Adapted with permission from Giacino JT, Ashwal S, Childs N, et al. The minimally conscious state: definition and diagnostic criteria. Neurology 2002;58:349–353.

MINIMALLY CONSCIOUS STATE

See Table 3.

VEGETATIVE STATE

The American Academy of Neurology addressed the terminology and prognosis of individuals diagnosed with a vegetative state. The basics of the diagnosis include lack of consistent response to external stimuli in any modality. The term *persistent vegetative state* may be used when the duration is more than 1 month. *Permanency of vegetative status* involves a degree of prognostication, and should be based on both extensive review of history and careful physical examination. Individuals who fail to meet strict criteria for the vegetative state may meet criteria for the minimally conscious state (*see* Tables 4 and 5).

SOURCES

Brain Death in Adults

An appraisal of the criteria of cerebral death. A summary statement. A collaborative study. JAMA 1977;237:982–986.

Conference of Medical Royal Colleges and their Faculties in the United Kingdom: Diagnosis of brain death. Br Med J 1976;2:1187–1188.

Conrad GR, Sinha. Scintigraphy as a confirmatory test of brain death. Semin Nucl Med 2003;33:31–323.

Cranford RE. Minnesota Medical Association criteria. Brain death: concept and criteria, I. Minn Med 1978;61:561–563.

Cranford RE. Minnesota Medical Association criteria. Brain death: concept and criteria, II. Minn Med 1978;61:600–603.

Plum F, Posner JB. The diagnosis of stupor and coma, 3rd ed. Contemporary Neurology Series, vol. 19. Philadelphia: Davis, 1980.

President's Commission for the Study of Ethical Problems in Medicine and Biomedical and Behavioral Research. Guidelines for the determination of death. JAMA 1981;246:2184–2186.

Quality Standards Subcommittee of the American Academy of Neurology, The. Practice parameters for determining brain death in adults (summary statement). Neurology 1995;45:1012–1014.

Report of the Ad Hoc Committee of the Harvard Medical School to Examine the Definition of Brain Death: a definition of irreversible coma. JAMA 1968;205:337–340.

Wijdicks EF. Determining brain death in adults. Neurology 1995;45:1003–1011.

Wijdicks EF. The diagnosis of brain death. N Engl J Med 2001;344:1215–1221.

Wijdicks EF. Brain death worldwide: accepted fact but no global consensus in diagnostic criteria. Neurology 2002;58:20–25.

Brain Death in Children

Alvarez LA, Moshe SL, Belman AL: EEG and brain death determination in children. Neurology 1988;38:227–230.

American Academy of Pediatrics Task Force on Brain Death in Children. Report of special Task Force. Guidelines for the determination of brain death in children. Pediatrics 1987;80:298–300.

American Electroencephalographic Society; Guidelines in EEG and evoked potential. J Clin Neurophysiol 1986;3(Suppl 1):12–17.

Ashwal S, Schneider S. Failure of electroencephalography to diagnose brain death in comatose children. Ann Neurol 1979;6 (6): 512–517.

Blend MJ, Pavel DG, Hughes JR. Normal cerebral radionuclide angiogram in a child with electrocerebral silence. Neuropediatrics 1986;17:168–170.

Grattan-Smith PJ, Butt W. Suppression of brainstem reflexes in barbiturate coma. Arch Dis Child 1993;69:151, 152.

Green JB, Lauber A. Return of EEG activity after electrocerebral silence: two case reports. J Neurol Neurosurg Psychiatry 1972;35:103–107.

Hassan T, Mumford C. Guillain-Barre syndrome mistaken for brain stem death. Postgrad Med J 1991;67:280, 281.

Holzman BH, Curless RG, Sfakianakis GN. Radionuclide cerebral perfusion scintigraphy in determination of brain death in children. Neurology 1983;33:1027–1031.

Kohrman MH, Spivack BS. Brain death in infants: sensitivity and specificity of current criteria. Pediatr Neurol 1990;6:47–50.

Langendorf FG, Mallin JF, Masdeu JC. Fulminant Guillain-Barre syndrome simulating brain death. Electroencephalogr Clin Neurophysiol 1986;64:74.

Medlock MD, Hanigan WC, Cruse RP. Dissociation of cerebral blood flow, glucose metabolism, and electrical activity in pediatric brain death. Case report. J Neurosurg 1993;79:752–755.

Schwartz JA, Baxter J, Brill DR. Diagnosis of brain death in children by radionuclide cerebral imaging. Pediatrics 1984;73: 14–18.

Silverman D, Saunders MG, Schwab RS. Cerebral death and the electroencephalogram. Report of the ad hoc committee of the American Electroencephalographic Society on EEG Criteria for determination of cerebral death. JAMA 1969;209: 1505–1510.

Task Force for the Determination of Brain Death in Children: Guidelines for the determination of brain death in children. Task Force for the Determination of Brain Death in Children. Arch Neurol 1987;44:587, 588.

Minimally Conscious State

Giacino JT, Ashwal S, Childs N, et al. The minimally conscious state. Definition and diagnostic criteria. Neurology 2002;58:349–353.

Vegetative State

Practice parameters: assessment and management of patients in the persistent vegetative state (summary statement). The Quality Standards Subcommittee of the American Academy of Neurology. Neurology 199545:1015–1018.

6

Epilepsy

AICARDI-GOUTIERES SYNDROME

Aicardi-Goutieres syndrome was first described in 1984 in a series of eight patients. The clinical picture is of infants with familial progressive encephalopathy, basal ganglia calcification, and chronic cerebrospinal fluid pleocytosis (Table 1). It is a very rare syndrome, suspected to be familial with autosomal-recessive inheritance, and occurrence in siblings has been reported. A majority of reported cases have elevated serum levels of α-interferon, which is of unclear pathogenic significance.

EARLY MYOCLONIC ENCEPHALOPATHY

Criteria for this syndrome have been developed by the International League Against Epilepsy (ILAE). However, this epileptic syndrome is nonspecific with regard to origin, and not all patients fulfill all of the ILAE criteria. In particular, there may be clinical overlap with the syndrome of early infantile epileptic encephalopathy, which is recognized by the ILAE as distinct from early myoclonic epilepsy (Table 2).

IDIOPATHIC LOCALIZATION-RELATED EPILEPSIES

This group, known by the acronym ILRE, includes the so-called benign partial epilepsies in infancy and childhood. Entities originally falling into this category included benign childhood epilepsy with centrotemporal spikes, childhood epilepsy with occipital paroxysms, and primary reading epilepsy. Some authors would now include benign partial epilepsies of infancy, and Panayiotopoulos-type early-onset benign childhood occipital epilepsy (also called benign childhood epilepsy with occipital paroxysms) (Table 3).

LENNOX-GASTAUT SYNDROME

Originally described in the 1930s, Lennox-Gastaut syndrome is a childhood-onset epileptic syndrome almost always associated with developmental delay or congenital anomalies (Table 4).

MESIAL TEMPORAL LOBE EPILEPSY

Mesial temporal lobe epilepsy (MTLE) may occur with or without accompanying pathological lesions. One of the more common forms occurs in conjunction with hippocampal sclerosis. Diagnostic criteria for hippocampal sclerosis have been defined based on pathological examination, primarily from surgical specimens; autopsy material is relatively rare. The primary feature is that of neuronal cell loss and gliosis with relative sparing of transitional cortex in the mid-hippocampus. Hippocampal sclerosis may be an isolated finding, without the individual having concomitant mesial temporal lobe epilepsy.

From: *Current Clinical Neurology: Diagnostic Criteria in Neurology*
Edited by: A. J. Lerner © Humana Press Inc., Totowa, NJ

Table 1
Diagnostic Criteria for Aicardi-Goutieres Syndrome

1. Progressive encephalopathy with infantile onset (under 1 year of age).
2. Basal ganglia calcification.
3. Chronic cerebrospinal fluid pleocytosis.
4. Negative toxoplasmosis, rubella, cytomegalovirus, herpes simplex serology.
5. Exclusion of other toxic or metabolic disorders, such as lymphocytic choriomeningitis.

Table 2
Diagnostic Criteria for Early Myoclonic Encephalopathy

1. Electroencephalogram with suppression–burst pattern.
2. Occurrence of erratic, fragmentary myoclonus of early onset in association with other types of seizures.
3. The seizures are resistant to conventional antiepileptic therapy.
4. No known obstetric complications or perinatal insults.

Adapted with permission from Wang PJ, Lee WT, Hwu WL, et al. The controversy regarding diagnostic criteria for early myoclonic encephalopathy. Brain Dev 1998;20:530–535.

Table 3
Diagnostic Criteria for Idiopathic Localization-Related Epilepsies

Clinical features
1. Normal neurological examination.
2. Normal neuroimaging.
3. Family history of benign type epilepsy.
4. Brief stereotypes seizures.
5. Frequent nocturnal occurrences.
6. Easy to control epilepsy except with ethosuximide.
7. Remission before adolescence.

Electroencephalogram features
1. Normal background activity.
2. Spikes with a characteristic morphology and location.
3. Sleep activation.
4. Occasional generalized paroxysms.

Adapted with permission from Negoro T. Diagnosis and treatment of idiopathic focal epilepsies (benign partial epilepsies) in infancy and childhood. Epilepsia 2005;46:S3–S38, and from Blackwell Publishing.

Table 4
Diagnostic Criteria for Lennox-Gastaut Syndrome

1. Multiple seizure types including atypical absence and seizures resulting in falls (axial tonic, massive myoclonic, and atonic seizures).
2. Electroencephalogram demonstrating slow spike and wave (<2.5 Hz) and bursts of fast rhythms at 10–12 Hz during sleep.
3. Static encephalopathy and learning disabilities, most often associated with profound mental retardation
   Other seizure types usually are present, including generalized tonic–clonic seizures and partial seizures.

No electroclinical feature *per se* distinguishes MTLE with or without hippocampal sclerosis, although the presence of olfactory–gustatory auras is felt to be more common in patients with MTLE secondary to a neoplasm (Table 5). MTLE also needs to be distinguished from neocortical temporal lobe epilepsy, with which it shares some broad features. History of febrile seizures, abdominal auras, contralateral dystonic posturing, and ipsilateral mesial temporal spike waves on electroencephalogram suggest MTLE. In Pfander's multiple logistic regression model, this combination yielded diagnostic accuracy of 73%, and positive and negative predictive values of 81 and 70%, respectively.

Table 5
Status of Various Criteria in the Diagnosis of Mesial Temporal Lobe Epilepsy With Hippocampal Sclerosis

	Distinguishes			Essential	
Characteristic	Does not	May	Does	Yes	No
History of initial precipitating incident		+			+
Family history		+			+
Latent period		+			+
Silent period		+			+
Seizure onset between 6 and 14 years	+				+
Predominantly unilateral HS on magnetic resonance imaging			+		+
Hypometabolism on positron-emission tomography	+				+
Characteristic seizure semiology	+			+[a]	
Characteristic interictal and ictal EEG	+				+
Memory disturbance	+				+
Pharmacoresistance	+				+
Good surgical outcome	+				+
Progressive course		+			+

[a]Except in young children.

HS, hippocampal sclerosis; EEG, electroencephalogram.

Exclusionary criteria would include seizures that begin with primary visual, auditory or focal somatosensory auras, focal, or violent bilateral motor behaviors, and extratemporal EEG spikes. Evidence of diffuse brain damage on neuroimaging, EEG, and/or neurocognitive testing, and focal neurological findings other than memory deficit, are also inconsistent with a diagnosis of mesial temporal lobe epilepsy with HS, although some of these patients may have dual pathology.

Table 6
Guidelines to Assist in the Identification of Sudden Unexpected Death in Epilepsy

- The victim had epilepsy, defined as recurrent unprovoked seizures.
- The victim died unexpectedly while in a reasonable state of health.
- The death occurred suddenly, where known.
- The death occurred during normal activities and benign circumstances.
- An obvious medical cause of death was not found.
- The death was not the direct cause of the seizure or status epilepticus.

Adapted with permission from Langan Y, Sander JWAS. Sudden unexpected death in patients with epilepsy. Definition, epidemiology and therapeutic implications. CNS Drugs 2000:13:337–349, and from ADIS International.

SUDDEN UNEXPECTED DEATH IN EPILEPSY

There are no universal guidelines in determining this diagnosis, which is by definition always made retrospectively (Table 6).

One proposed diagnosis is sudden unexpected, nontraumatic, and nondrowning death in an individual with epilepsy with or without evidence for a seizure and excluding documented status epilepticus, where postmortem examination does not reveal a cause for death.

Common findings include pulmonary edema, bitten tongue, and incontinence. The relationship of sudden unexpected death in this population to suffocation is unknown.

SOURCES

Aicardi-Goutieres Syndrome

Goutieres F, Aicardi J, Barth PG, Lebon P. Aicardi-Goutieres syndrome: an update and results of interferon-alpha studies. Ann Neurol 1998;44:900–907.
Koul R, Chacko A, Joshi S, Sankhla D. Aicardi-Goutieres syndrome in siblings. J Child Neurol 2001;16:759–761.

Early Myoclonic Encephalopathy

Aicardi J. Early myoclonic encephalopathy. In: Roger J, Dravet C, Bureau M, Dreifuss FE, Wolf P, eds. Epileptic Syndromes of Infancy and Adolescence. London: John Libbey, 1985:12–22.

Commission on Classification and Terminology of the International League Against Epilepsy. Proposal for revised classification of epilepsies and epileptic syndromes. Epilepsia 1989;30:389–399.

Lombroso CT. Early myoclonic encephalopathy, early infantile epileptic encephalopathy, and benign and severe infantile myoclonic epilepsies: a critical review and personal contributions. J Clin Neurophysiology 1990;7:380–408.

Wang PJ, Lee WT, Hwu WL, et al. The controversy regarding diagnostic criteria for early myoclonic encephalopathy. Brain Dev 1998;20:530–535.

Idiopathic Localization-Related Epilepsies

Negoro T. Diagnosis and treatment of idiopathic focal epilepsies (benign partial epilepsies) in infancy and childhood. Epilepsia 2005;46(Suppl 3):S3–S38.

Lennox-Gastaut Syndrome

Lennox WG, Davis JP. Clinical correlates of the fast and the slow spike-wave electroencephalogram. Pediatrics 1950;5:626–644.

Medial Temporal Lobe Epilepsy

ILAE commission report. Mesial temporal lobe epilepsy with hippocampal sclerosis. Epilepsia 2004;45:695–714.

Pfander M, Arnold S, Henkel A, et al. Clinical features and EEG findings differentiating mesial from neocortical temporal lobe epilepsy. Epileptic Disord 2002;4:189–195.

Sudden Unexpected Death in Epilepsy

Langan Y, Sander JWAS. Sudden unexpected death in patients with epilepsy. Definition, epidemiology and therapeutic implications. CNS Drugs 2000;13:337–349.

Nashef F. Sudden unexpected death in epilepsy: terminology and definitions. Epilepsia 1997;38:S6–S8.

7

Genetic Syndromes

ADENYLOSUCCINATE LYASE DEFICIENCY

A disorder of purine synthesis, adenylosuccinate lyase deficiency is a rare condition, with only about 40 published cases. It presents in early life with mental retardation and seizures. Although no specific diagnostic criteria have been proposed for the clinical syndrome, Table 1 summarizes clinical findings in 20 patients and may be useful as a guide in suspecting the diagnosis.

ALEXANDER'S DISEASE

Alexander's disease is a rare genetic disease, presenting primarily in childhood. The genetic basis of Alexander's disease involves mutations in the glial fibrillar acidic protein (*GFAP*) gene. Individuals with Alexander's disease may present as infants, children, or rarely, as adults. Infants and children typically present with seizures, megalencephaly, developmental delay, and spasticity. Particularly in older patients, there may be bulbar or pseudobulbar symptoms, and spasticity, especially of the legs. The disease is progressive, with most patients dying within 10 years of onset.

Until recently, the diagnosis has been pathological, with demonstration of Rosenthal fibers on brain biopsy. Genetic testing combined with clinical course and neuroimaging may be sufficient for diagnosis. Other similar clinical syndromes may be seen with mutations in other genes, and differential diagnosis is that of other leukoencephalopathies.

In the study presented in Table 2, patients were included if they fulfilled the following minimum criteria: (1) magnetic resonance imaging findings of white matter changes with preferential involvement of the frontal regions of the brain; (2) normal karyotype; (3) normal metabolic screening; and (4) no family history of any leukoencephalopathy.

ANGELMAN SYNDROME

These criteria are applicable for the three major types of Angelman syndrome: molecular deletions involving the critical region (deletion-positive), uniparental disomy, and nondeletion/nonuniparental disomy.

Angelman syndrome is currently clinically diagnosed and can be confirmed by laboratory testing in about 80% of cases. Individuals whose developmental history conforms to that described in Table 3, and who have all of the clinical findings of groups A and B in Table 4 should have a chromosome study, as well as molecular analysis by fluorescence *in situ* hybridization, polymorphism analysis, or methylation testing to look for alterations in chromosome region 15q11–q13. A positive genetic test (Table 5) may confirm the diagnosis, but a normal result does not exclude the diagnosis. In individuals with fewer clinical findings, a positive genetic test is presumptive evidence for Angelman syndrome. The judgment of the clinician is crucial when genetic testing is negative and clinical findings suggest the syndromic diagnosis. For individuals with no deletion or uniparental disomy, the clinician should be reasonably certain that the clinical findings in Tables 3 and 4 are present if the diagnosis of Angelman syndrome is still considered.

From: *Current Clinical Neurology: Diagnostic Criteria in Neurology*
Edited by: A. J. Lerner © Humana Press Inc., Totowa, NJ

Table 1
Clinical Findings in 20 Patients With Adenylosuccinate Lyase Deficiency

Author	Sex	Seizure onset	EEG	Psychomotor retardation	Autistic features	Others	CT/MRI	S-Ado/ SAICAR, md/mL	Outcome
Jaeken et al., 1984	F	—	Normal	Yes	No eye contact	Axial hypotonia, growth retardation	Cerebellar hypoplasia	—	Severe mental retardation
	M	7 years	Generalized abnormalities	Yes	No eye contact, no language	Axial hypotonia, growth retardation, muscular wasting	Cerebellar hypoplasia, cortical atrophy	—	Seizure controlled by CBZ
	F	2 years	Diffuse slowing	Yes	No eye contact, no language	Growth retardation, muscular wasting	Cerebellar hypoplasia	—	Seizure controlled by CBZ
Jaeken et al., 1988	M	NR	Abnormal	Yes	—	Unvoluntary movements of extremities, peripheral hypertonicity	—	—	Died (13 years)
	F	NR	Abnormal	Yes	No eye contact	—	Cerebellar hypoplasia	—	Mild mental retardation
	F	1 week	Hypsarrhythmia	Yes	No eye contact, stereotypies	Peripheral hypertonicity	Cortical/ cerebellar atrophy	—	Severe mental retardation, intractable epilepsy
	M	—	Normal	Yes	No eye contact, stereotypies	Strabismus, growth retardation	Normal	—	Severe mental retardation
	F	NR	Diffuse slowing	Yes	No eye contact, hypoacusia	Growth retardation	Cerebral atrophy	4–5	Mild mental retardation, intractable epilepsy

Reference	Sex	Age	EEG	Seizures	Behavior	Neurologic	MRI/CT	Ratio	Outcome
Jaeken et al., 1992	F	5 years	Generalized abnormalities	Yes	Aggressivity, stereotypies	—	Slight cerebral atrophy	1.77	Mild mental retardation
Salerno and Crifo 1994	F	7 months	Focal/generalized abnormalities	Yes	No language, stereotypies	Ataxia, strabismus, muscular wasting, hyperactivity, Apraxia, growth retardation	—	1.2	Severe mental retardation, intractable epilepsy
Sebesta et al., 1997	M	NR	Abnormal	Yes	—	Hypotonia, hyperactivity	Abnormal	—	Mild mental retardation
	F	NR	Abnormal	Yes	—	Hypotonia, hyperactivity	Abnormal	—	Mild mental retardation
	F	1 month	Abnormal	Yes	—	—	Abnormal	—	Severe mental retardation
	F	NR	Abnormal	Yes	—	—	Abnormal	—	Died (15 years)
	M	1 month	Abnormal	Yes	—	—	Abnormal	—	Severe mental retardation
Maaswinkel-Mooij et al., 1997	F	9 weeks	Hypsarrhythmia	Yes	—	Axial hypotonia, peripheral hypertonia	Lack of myelinization	1.02	Severe mental retardation, intractable epilepsy
Valik et al., 1997	F	—	Normal	Yes	—	Muscular hypotonia, fasciculations, strabismus	Increased T2 signal in semiovale center	2.5–2.6	Severe mental retardation
van den Bergh et al., 1998	M	2 days	Burst suppression	Yes	—	Axial hypotonia	—	—	Died (7 months)
Kohler et al., 1999	M	3 weeks	Focal abnormalities	Yes	No eye contact, stereotypies	Muscular hypotonia	Slight cerebral atrophy	0.9	Severe mental retardation, seizure-free
	M	3 days	Status epilepticus, burst suppression	Yes	—	—	Lack of myelinization	1.5	Died (6 months)

EEG, electroencephalography; CT, computerized tomography; MRI, magnetic resonance imaging; S-Ado, succinyladenosine; SAICA-R, succinylaminoimidazole carboxamide ribotide; NR, nonreferred; CBZ, carbamazepine.

(Adapted with permission from Ciardo F, Costantino S, Curatolo P. Neurologic aspects of adenylosuccinate lyase deficiency. J Child Neurol 2001;16:301–308, and from BC Decker.)

Table 2
Clinical and Molecular Findings in Patients With Alexander Disease

Patient no./sex	Mutation: exon/base change/amino acid change	Initial presentation	Age at onset[a]/current age	↑HC[b]	Current status — Bulbar and/or pseudobulbar signs	Current status — Seizures	Current status — Spasticity	Current status — Dementia or cognitive deficits	Other findings
Infancy onset									
1/F	Exon 1 249C→G R79G[c]	Seizures	3 months/ 3 years	−	Dysphagia, frequent vomiting, or frequent choking episodes	+	+	+	Linear growth failure, truncal hypotonia, no language development
2/M	Exon 1 249C→T R79C[d]	Seizures	6 months/ 5 years	+	Strabismus	+	−	+	Hypothyroidism
3/M[e]	Exon 1 250G→A R79H[d]	Seizures	18 months/ 9 years	+	Dysphagia, frequent vomiting, or frequent choking episodes; dysarthria or slurred speech	+	−	+	Born 3 weeks after term; linear sebaceous nevi on scalp
4/M[f]	Exon 1 250G→A R79H[d]	Seizures	7 months/ 2 years	+	−	+	+	−	
5/M	Exon 4 729C→T R239C[d]	Delayed motor development	9 months/ 4 years	+	Dysarthria or slurred speech	−	+	−	
6/M	Exon 4 738T→G Y242D[c]	Failure to thrive; hypotonia	12 months/ 5 years	+	Strabismus	−	−	+	
7/F	Exon 6 1131G→A E373K[c]	Seizures	2 months/ 5 months	+	−	+	−	N/A	Born 10 days after term; noncongenital truncal and appendicular hypotonia; poor weight gain, fussiness

86

Juvenile onset

8/M	Exon 1 232T→G M73R	Strabismus	+	9 years/ 15 years	+	Dysphagia, frequent vomiting, or frequent choking episodes; dysarthria or slurred speech; strabismus	+	+	+	Stellate nevi
9/M	Exon 1 276C→T R88C[d]	Excessive sleepiness, frequent vomiting	−	7 years/ 9 years	−	Dysphagia, frequent vomiting, or frequent choking episodes; dysarthria or slurred speech; strabismus	−	−	+	Linear growth failure
10[e]/M	Exon 1 276C→T R88C[d]	MRI changes observed during evaluation for short stature	+	N/A[a]/4 years	−	—	−	−	−	Linear growth failure
11/F	Exon 8 1260C→T R416W[d]	Intractable vomiting	−	5 years/ 7 years	−	Dysphagia, frequent vomiting, or frequent choking episodes	−	−	−	Prone to episodes of syncope after hyperventilation
12[g]/M	Exon 8 1260C→T R416W[d]	MRI changes observed after accidental eye injury	−	N/A[a]/11 years	−	—	−	−	−	Clumsiness and poor coordination (nonprogressive)
13[h]/F	—	Seizures	+	2 months/ 10 years[b]	+	—	+	−	+	Frontal and parietal white matter changes

[a] No age at onset is reported for Patients 10 and 12; evaluation for leukodystrophy was initiated only after incidental findings of white matter changes were discovered by MRI performed as part of examination for other conditions.

[b] Increased head circumference (↑HC) (megaencephaly) is positive (+) when the occipitofrontal circumference is >95th percentile for age. Patient 1 had HC trending at 2nd percentile, although her height and weight were <10th percentile as well; no language development is noted at current age (3 years).

[c] Parents' DNA tested negative for the mutation.

[d] These mutations have previously been described: R79C, R79H, R88C, R239C, R416W.

[e] Patient 3 was also homozygous for a 879G→A nucleotide change that results in a D295N amino acid change. This nucleotide change has previously been observed in 3% of healthy control subjects. In addition, this patient was also heterozygous for a silent 872G→A nucleotide change previously found in 9% of control subjects. Patients 10 and 13 were likewise heterozygous for these two nucleotide changes. Both of these nucleotide changes are found in exon 5.

[f] Patient 4 was also heterozygous for a silent 110T→C nucleotide change in exon 1.

[g] Patient 12 also carried a 154C→T nucleotide change in exon 1 that is predicted to result in a P47L amino acid change. This nucleotide change has previously been described in another patient with Alexander disease who a so had the 729C→T mutation.

[h] Patient 13 recently died in a drowning accident.

N/A, not applicable; MRI, magnetic resonance imaging.

(Reprinted with permission from Gorospe JR, Naidu S, Johnson AB, et al. Molecular findings in symptomatic and pre-symptomatic Alexander disease patients Neurology 2002;58:1494–1500.)

Table 3
Angelman Syndrome: Developmental History and Laboratory Findings

1. Normal prenatal and birth history with normal head circumference.
2. Absence of major birth defects.
3. Developmental delay evident by 6–12 months of age.
4. Delayed but forward progression of development (no loss of skills).
5. Normal metabolic, hematological, and chemical laboratory profiles.
6. Structurally normal brain using magnetic resonance imaging or computerized tomography (may have mild cortical atrophy or dysmyelination).

These findings are useful as inclusion criteria, but deviations should not exclude diagnosis.
(Adapted with permission from Williams CA, Angelman H, Clayton-Smith J, et al. Angelman syndrome: consensus for diagnostic criteria. Angelman Syndrome Foundation. Am J Med Genet. 1995;27;56:237—238, and from John Wiley and Sons.)

Table 4
Angelman Syndrome: Clinical Characteristics

A. **Consistent (100%)**
   1. Developmental delay, functionally severe.
   2. Speech impairment, none or minimal use of words; receptive and nonverbal communication skills higher than verbal ones.
   3. Movement or balance disorder, usually ataxia of gait and/or tremulous movement of limbs.
   4. Behavioral uniqueness: any combination of frequent laughter/smiling; apparent happy demeanor; easily excitable personality, often with hand flapping movements; hypermotoric behavior; short attention span.

B. **Frequent (more than 80%)**
   1. Delayed, disproportionate growth in head circumference, usually resulting in microcephaly (absolute or relative) by age 2.
   2. Seizures, onset usually younger than 3 years of age.
   3. Abnormal electroencephalography, characteristic pattern with large amplitude slow spike waves (usually 2 to 3 per second), facilitated by eye closure.

C. **Associated (20–80%)**
   1. Flat occiput.
   2. Occipital groove.
   3. Protruding tongue.
   4. Tongue thrusting; suck/swallowing disorders.
   5. Feeding problems during infancy.
   6. Prognathia.
   7. Wide mouth, widely spaced teeth.
   8. Frequent drooling.
   9. Excessive chewing/mouthing behaviors.
   10. Strabismus.
   11. Hypopigmented skin, light hair and eye color (compared with family), seen only in deletion cases.
   12. Hyperactive lower limb deep tendon reflexes.
   13. Uplifted, flexed arm position especially during ambulation.
   14. Increased sensitivity to heat.
   15. Sleep disturbance.
   16. Attraction to/fascination with water.

Adapted with permission from Williams CA, Angelman H, Clayton-Smith J, et al. Angelman syndrome: consensus for diagnostic criteria. Angelman Syndrome Foundation. Am J Med Genet 1995;56:237–238, and from John Wiley and Sons.)

In about 20% of individuals whose clinical presentation is characteristic of Angelman syndrome, genetic laboratory studies of chromosome 15 will be normal. These individuals are the "nondeletion/nondisomy type." It is in the families of these individuals where familial recurrence is a possibility, whether methylation patterns are normal or abnormal. Although affected nondeletion/nondisomy siblings have

Table 5
Angelman Syndrome: Genetic Testing Abnormalities

1. High-resolution Giemsa (G)-banded chromosome study showing deletion of chromosome region 15q11–q13. Because of the possibility of false-positive and negative results from this study, G-banding should not be used as a stand-alone test but should be confirmed by fluorescence *in situ* hybridization (FISH), polymorphism, or methylation analysis.
2. Abnormal FISH indicating a deletion of cloned 15q11–q13 DNA sequences that are included in the Angelman syndrome deletion overlap region. Use of a pericentromeric FISH probe enhances ability to detect subtle translocation.
3. DNA polymorphism analysis showing absence of maternal alleles at 15q11–q13 loci, which may result either from maternal deletion or from paternal uniparental disomy
4. Characteristic DNA methylation pattern (i.e., paternal imprint only) of 15q11–q13 cloned DNA sequences using methylation-sensitive restriction endonucleases
5. An abnormal methylation pattern in individuals without 15q11–q13 deletion is not a stand-alone test for uniparental disomy.

Number of tests necessary and order of testing may vary. Chromosome study is necessary in all suspected cases to rule out chromosome rearrangements or other chromosome disorders.

(Adapted with permission from Williams CA, Angelman H, Clayton-Smith J, et al. Angelman syndrome: consensus for diagnostic criteria. Angelman Syndrome Foundation. Am J Med Genet 1995;56:237–238, and from John Wiley and Sons.)

been shown to share molecular haplotypes of the maternal 15 chromosome, there is currently no diagnostic test applicable to these individuals. Diagnosis in these situations remains clinical, although that may change as new testing and additional insight into the molecular cause of Angelman syndrome evolves.

The clinical diagnosis of Angelman syndrome usually is not suspected during the first year of life, but becomes a more frequent diagnostic consideration between 1 and 4 years of age. Angelman syndrome can be diagnosed in the first year (6–12 months) if the diagnosis is given due consideration. An abnormal electroencephalography may be the first sign for diagnostic evaluation. During infancy, other clinical disorders can mimic the features of Angelman syndrome. These include Rett's syndrome, nonspecific cerebral palsy, Lennox-Gastaut syndrome, static encephalopathy with mental retardation, infantile autism, and α-thalassemia X-linked mental retardation syndrome.

CHARGE SYNDROME

Originally described in the early 1980s, CHARGE is the acronym for *c*oloboma, *h*eart disease, *a*tresia choanae, *r*etarded growth and retarded development and/or central nervous system anomalies, *g*enital hypoplasia, and *e*ar anomalies and/or deafness. CHARGE is clinically diagnosed, so the frequency and certainty will depend on who is doing the evaluation. With the establishment of specific etiology or etiologies for CHARGE, the diagnostic criteria will likely improve. Most cases of CHARGE syndrome appear to be new mutations; the loci for many has been mapped to chromosome 8q12. The incidence is about 1:10,000 births, but high infantile mortality rates likely obscure the true incidence of this syndrome.

The original diagnostic criteria proposed by Pagon in 1981 included four of the six CHARGE features. It has also been suggested that at least one of the abnormalities be coloboma of the iris or choanal atresia. However, several features not included in the acronym are specific to CHARGE and rare in other conditions. Other criteria included (heart disease, retarded growth and retarded development, genital hypoplasia) are less specific to CHARGE and are frequently seen in other conditions. Many individuals have also been found with "partial," "atypical," or "incomplete" CHARGE.

Blake et al. proposed more detailed criteria in 1998, including major, minor, and other congenital anomalies found in this pleomorphic syndrome (Tables 6–8). Verloes has proposed modifications to this, based on examination of the specific embryological defects, and avoiding secondary and gender-dependent abnormalities (Table 9).

Several syndromes have clinical findings similar to CHARGE and should be considered in the differential diagnosis. These include the following:

Table 6
1998 Revised Clinical Diagnostic Criteria for CHARGE Syndrome: Major Characteristics of CHARGE, Very Common in CHARGE, and Relatively Rare in Other Conditions

Finding	Includes	Frequency
Coloboma of the eye	Coloboma of the iris, retina, choroid, disc (not including colobomas of the eyelid); microphthalmos or cryptophthalmos	80–90%
Choanal atresia or stenosis	Unilateral/bilateral; bony or membranous. Atresia or stenosis	50–60%
Cranial nerve dysfunction or anomaly	I Anosmia	Frequent
	VII Facial palsy (unilateral or bilateral)	40%
	IX/X Swallowing difficulties	70–90%
Characteristic CHARGE ear	Short, wide ear with little or no lobe; "snipped-off" helix; prominent antihelix that is discontinuous with tragus; triangular concha; decreased cartilage; often sticks out; usually asymmetric	Frequent
	Middle ear: ossicular malformations seen on MRI	Frequent
	Malformed inner ear (Mondini defect) with deformed cochlea and vestibule seen on MRI	80–90%

MRI, magnetic resonance imaging.

(Adapted with permission from Blake KD, Davenport SLH, Hall B, et al. CHARGE Association—an update and review for the primary pediatrician. Clin Pediatr 1998;37:159–173.)

Table 7
Minor Characteristics of CHARGE: Significant Features That May Be More Difficult to Diagnose or Less Specific to CHARGE

Finding	Includes	Frequency
Distinctive face	Square face with broad prominent forehead, arched eyebrows, large eyes, occasional ptosis, prominent nasal bridge with square root, thick nostrils, prominent nasal columella, flat midface, small mouth, occasional small chin, larger chin with age. Facial asymmetry even without facial palsy.	70–80%
Characteristic CHARGE hand	Small or unusual thumb; broad palm with hockey-stick palmar crease; short fingers.	>50%
Orofacial cleft	Cleft palate; submucous cleft palate; cleft lip with or without cleft palate.	20–30%
Congenital heart defects	All types, especially conotruncal types (aortic arch anomalies, atrioventricular canal, tetralogy of Fallot).	60–70%
Genital (hypogonadotropic hypogonadism)	Males: micropenis; cryptorchidism. Females: hypoplastic labia.	70–80%
	Both: lack of pubertal development.	? 50%
Postnatal growth deficiency	Growth hormone deficiency.	? (*not* rare)
	Other short stature.	70%

Definite CHARGE: three or more major characteristics or two major and three minor characteristics
Probable/possible CHARGE: one major characteristic and several minor or other characteristics

(Adapted with permission from Blake KD, Davenport SLH, Hall B, et al. CHARGE Association—an update and review for the primary pediatrician. Clin Pediatr 1998;37:159–173.)

- DiGeorge syndrome.
- VATER syndrome (*v*ertebrae problems, *a*nal anomalies, *t*rachea, *e*sophagus, *r*adius [lower arm bone] and/or *r*enal problems).
- *Velocardiofacial* (VCF) syndrome and other similar conditions.
- *PAX2* mutation (coloboma, hearing loss, and renal abnormalities).
- Retinoic acid embryopathy.

Table 8
Other Characteristics Associated With CHARGE Syndrome

Finding	Includes	Frequency
Anomalies of trachea and/or esophagus	Tracheoesophageal fistula, esophageal atresia. Tracheomalacia.	15–20% Frequent
Chronic otitis and sinusitis	Chronic serious otitis in early years; chronic recurrent sinusitis.	85%
Sloping shoulders	Because of underdeveloped shoulder muscles or absent/hypoplastic pectoral muscles.	Frequent
Limb/skeletal	Absent thumb, polydactyly.	Rare?
Central nervous system anomalies	No consistent anomalies. Seizures are rare.	Occasional
Thymic or parathyroid hypoplasia	DiGeorge sequence *without* chromosome 22 deletion.	Rare
Urinary tract and/or renal anomalies	Small, absent, horseshoe or ectopic kidney; hydronephrosis or reflux; ureteral anomalies.	40%
Nipple anomalies	Extra or misplaced nipples; hypoplasia.	Occasional
Omphalocele	Umbilical hernia or omphalocele.	15%
Developmental delay	Delayed milestones; mental retardation.	>90%

Adapted with permission from Blake KD, Davenport SLH, Hall B, et al. CHARGE Association—an update and review for the primary pediatrician. Clin Pediatr 1998;37:159–173.

Table 9
Major and Minor Signs of CHARGE Syndrome

I.   The major signs ("the three Cs")
  A.   Coloboma (iris or choroids, with or without microphthalmia).
  B.   Atresia of chanae.
  C.   Hypoplastic semicircular canals.
II. Minor signs
  A.   Rhomboencephalic dysfunction (brainstem dysfunction, cranial VII–XII palsies and neurosensory deafness).
  B.   Hypothalamo-hypophyseal dysfunction including growth hormone and gonadotropin deficiencies.
  C.   Abnormal middle or external ear.
  D.   Malformation of mediastinal organs (heart, esophagus).
  E.   Mental retardation.

Typical CHARGE
Three major signs.
Two of three major signs and two of five minor signs.
Partial/incomplete CHARGE
Two of three major signs and one of five minor signs.
Atypical CHARGE
Two of three major signs alone.
One of three major signs and three of five minor signs.

Adapted with permission from Verloes A. Update diagnostic criteria for CHARGE syndrome: a proposal. Am J Med Genet 2005;133:306–308.

CHILDHOOD ATAXIA WITH CENTRAL NERVOUS SYSTEM HYPOMYELINATION/VANISHING WHITE MATTER

Clinical Diagnosis

The diagnosis of childhood ataxia with central nervous system hypomyelination/leukoencephalopathy with vanishing white matter can be made with confidence in patients with typical clinical findings, characteristic abnormalities on cranial magnetic resonance imaging (Figs. 1–3), and identifiable mutations in one of the five causative genes.

Table 10
Diagnostic Criteria in Childhood Ataxia With Central Nervous System Hypomyelination/Vanishing White Matter Syndrome

I.   Clinical findings
- Initial motor and mental development is normal or mildly delayed.
- Neurological deterioration has a chronic progressive or subacute course. Episodes of subacute deterioration may follow minor infection or minor head trauma and may lead to lethargy or coma.
- Clinical examination usually shows a combination of truncal and appendicular ataxia, pyramidal syndrome, and spasticity with increased tendon reflexes. The peripheral nervous system is usually not involved.
- Optic atrophy may develop.
- Epilepsy may occur, but is not the predominant sign of the disease.
- Mental abilities may be affected but not to the same degree as motor functions.

II. Magnetic resonance imaging (MRI) criteria present in all patients regardless of age of onset.
- The cerebral hemispheric white matter is symmetrically and diffusely abnormal.
- The abnormal white matter has signal intensity close to or the same as cerebrospinal fluid (CSF) on T1-weighted (Fig. 1) and T2-weighted (Fig. 2) images.
- On T1-weighted and fluid-attenuated inversion recovery (FLAIR) images (Fig. 3), a fine meshwork of remaining tissue strands is visible within the areas of CSF-like white matter, with a typical radiating appearance on sagittal and coronal images and a dot-like pattern in the centrum semiovale on the transverse images.

These MRI abnormalities are present even in asymptomatic children. Over time, increasing amounts of white matter vanish and are replaced with CSF, and cystic breakdown of the white matter is seen on proton density or FLAIR. Cerebellar atrophy varies from mild to severe and primarily involves the vermis.

Cranial computer tomography scan shows diffuse and symmetric hypodensity of the hemispheric white matter. Computer tomography is primarily used to rule out the presence of brain calcifications.

Testing
Routine laboratory tests, including cerebrospinal fluid analysis, are normal.

Neuropathological examination
The findings in general are a "cavitating orthochromatic leukodystrophy with rarity of myelin breakdown and relative sparing of axons." Cerebral and cerebellar myelin is markedly diminished, whereas the spinal cord is relatively spared. Vacuolation and cavitation of the white matter are diffuse. The hallmark is the presence of oligodendrocytes with "foamy" cytoplasm and markedly hypotrophic and sometimes atypical astrocytes.

Genes
Mutations in the five genes *(EIF2B1, EIF2B2, EIF2B3, EIF2B4,* and *EIF2B5)* encoding the five subunits of the eucaryotic translation initiation factor EIF2B are known to be associated with central nervous system hypomyelination/vanishing white matter syndrome.

Adapted with permission from Schiffman R, Fogli A, van der Knaap M, Boespflug-Tanguy O. Childhood ataxia with central nervous system hypomyelination/vanishing white matter. GeneReviews, February 2003. Available online at http://www.geneclinics.org/servlet/access?id=8888891&key=Ztnfp2fvDYe5R&gry=INSERTGRY&fcn=y&fw=xLNP& filename=/profiles/cach/index.html.

COWDEN SYNDROME

Cowden syndrome is a genetic syndrome of multiple hamartomas. Current nosology includes Lhermitte-Duclos disease, a condition of cerebellar dysplastic gangliocytomas with other findings characteristic of Cowden syndrome. Lhermitte-Duclos disease can be thought of as the neurological variant of Cowden syndrome. Also included is a syndrome of macrocephaly, multiple lipomas, and hemangiomata (Bannayan-Riley-Ruvalcaba syndrome). The phosphatase and tensin homolog deleted on chromosome ten *(PTEN)* gene causing Cowden syndrome is located on chromosome 10q23.31. *PTEN* is a widely expressed, dual-specificity phosphatase, which has actions as a tumor suppressor. The exact mechanism of *PTEN* action is unclear, but it may act to arrest the cell cycle and be a mediator of apoptosis.

The current criteria (published in 2000) supplant the 1995 criteria, which are similar but not as inclusive. The International Cowden Consortium maintains surveillance of emerging data and knowledge to revise and update the criteria as needed.

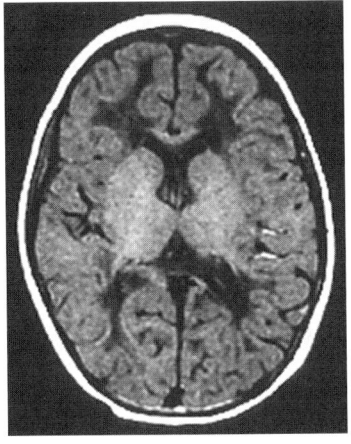 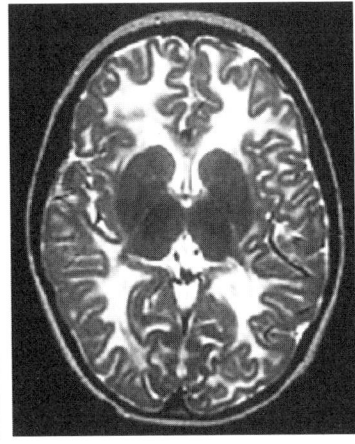 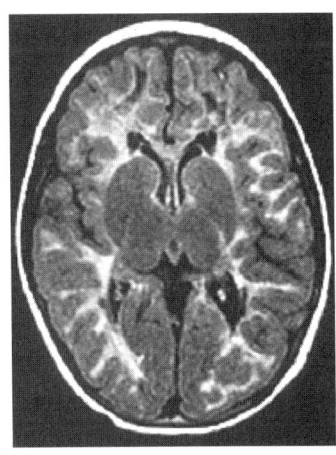

Fig. 1. T1-weighted MRI image.   Fig. 2. T2-weighted MRI image.   Fig. 3. FLAIR image.

FRAGILE X SYNDROME

Fragile X syndrome is the most common genetic cause for mental retardation and the most common known cause for autism.

Table 11
International Cowden Consortium Operational Criteria as of 2000 for the Diagnosis of Cowden's Syndrome

Pathognomonic criteria
1. Mucocutaneous lesions
    a. Trichilemmomas, facial.
    b. Acral keratoses.
    c. Papillomatous papules.
    d. Mucosal lesions.

Major criteria
1. Breast carcinoma.
2. Thyroid carcinoma (nonmedullary), especially follicular thyroid carcinoma.
3. Macrocephaly (megalencephaly) (≥95th percentile).
4. Lhermitte-Duclos disease (LDD).
5. Endometrial carcinoma.

Minor criteria
1. Other thyroid lesions (e.g., adenoma or multinodular goiter).
2. Mental retardation.
3. Gastointestinal hamartomas.
4. Fibrocystic disease of the breast.
5. Lipomas.
6. Fibromas.
7. Genitourinary tumors (e.g., renal cell carcinoma, uterine fibroids) or malformation.

Operational diagnosis in a person
1. Mucocutaneous lesions alone if:
    a. There are six or more facial papules, of which three or more must be trichilemmoma, or
    b. Cutaneous facial papules and oral mucosal papillomatosis, or
    c. Oral mucosal papillomatosis and acral keratoses, or
    d. Palmoplantar keratoses, six or more.
2. Two major criteria, but one must include macrocephaly or Lhermitte-Duclos disease.
3. One major and three minor criteria.
4. Four minor criteria.

(Continued)

Table 11 *(Continued)*

Operational diagnosis in a family where one person is diagnostic for Cowden's syndrome
1. The pathognomonic criterion.
2. Any one major criterion with or without minor criteria.
3. Two minor criteria.

Adapted with permission from Eng C. Will the real Cowden syndrome please stand up: revised diagnostic criteria. J Med Genet 2000;37:828–830.

Table 12
Diagnostic Criteria Scoring for Fragile X Syndrome

	Not present (0 points)	Borderline or present in the past (1 point)	Definitely present (2 points)
Mental retardation			
Hyperactivity			
Short attention span			
Tacitly defensive[a]			
Hand flapping			
Hand biting			
Poor eye contact			
Perseverative speech[b]			
Hyperextensible metacarpophalangeal joints[c]			
Large or prominent ears			
Large testicles			
Simian crease[d] or Sydney line[e]			
Family history of mental retardation			
Total score			

[a]Having a negative response to touch.
[b]Continued repetition of words or phrases.
[c]Double-jointed.
[d]Single horizontal crease on the palm instead of the usual two creases.
[e]Horizontal crease that goes from edge to edge across the palm.
(Adapted with permission from Hagerman RJ, Amiri K, Cronister A. Fragile X checklist. Am J Med Genet 1991;38:283–287, and from John Wiley and Sons.)

As the name implies, the disorder is associated with mutations in the fragile X mental retardation-1 (*FMR1*) gene, located on chromosome Xq27.3, coding for the mRNA-binding fragile X mental retardation protein (FMRP). FMRP is active in many tissues, including brain. FMR1 contains a polymorphic CGG repeat that can be categorized into four classes based on the size of the repeat: common (6–40 repeats), intermediate (41–60 repeats), premutation (61–200 repeats), and full mutation (>200–230 repeats). The presence of the full mutation accounts for clinical disease, and the permutation is the carrier form. Estimates of the prevalence of fragile X syndrome have varied from 1 in 2500 to 1 in 6000 males. Females may also suffer from fragile X syndrome. Based on studies of male prevalence of the full mutation, 1 in 8000 females to 1 in 9000 females in the general population may be affected by the fragile X syndrome. It is estimated that perhaps only 20% of individuals with fragile X are correctly diagnosed. The diagnosis can be suspected on clinical grounds, and directly tested for in cytogenetics laboratories. Table 12 contains the fragile X syndrome scoring system. Hagerman, Amiri, and Cronister found that 45% of males with a score of 16 or higher and 60% of those with a score of 19 or higher on the fragile X checklist had fragile X syndrome. Females are generally less severely affected, presumably because of X inactivation.

In 1994, a working group for the American College of Medical Genetics published guidelines for fragile X testing. These included testing any person with unexplained mental retardation, developmental delay, or autism, especially if physical or behavioral characteristics commonly associated with the

Table 13
Diagnostic Criteria for Fraser Syndrome

Major criteria
1. Cryptophthalmos.
2. Syndactyly.
3. Abnormal genitalia.
4. Sibling with Fraser syndrome.

Minor criteria
1. Congenital malformation of nose.
2. Congenital malformation of ears.
3. Congenital malformation of larynx.
4. Cleft lip and/or palate.
5. Skeletal defects.
6. Umbilical hernia.
7. Renal malformation.
8. Mental retardation.

Reprinted with permission from Slavotinek AM, Tifft CJ. Fraser syndrome and cryptophthalmos: review of the diagnostic criteria and evidence for phenotypic modules in complex malformation syndromes. J Med Genet 2002;39:623–633, and from BMJ Publishing Group.)

Table 14
Diagnostic Criteria for Friedreich's Ataxia

QCSFA	Harding	Filla et al.
Onset ≤20 years	Onset ≤25 years	Onset ≤20 years
Progressive ataxia	Progressive ataxia	Progressive ataxia
Lower limb areflexia	Lower limb areflexia	Lower limb areflexia
Decreased vibration sense	Dysarthria after 5 years	One of the following:
		Dysarthria
Weakness	Babinski sign	Babinski sign
Dysarthria	Small/absent SAPs[a]	LVH

[a]Small or absent sensory action potentials (SAPs) in upper limbs, with motor nerve conduction velocity >40 m/s.
QCSFA, Quebec Cooperative Study on Friedreich's Ataxia; LVH, left ventricular hypertrophy.
Filla et al. propose a category of "possible FA" to include ignoring age of onset and requiring lower limb areflexia and dysarthria, Babinski sign, or repolarization abnormalities on electrocardiography. Alternatively, repolarization abnormalities on electrocardiogram in patients with retained lower limb reflexes.
"Probable FA" would fulfill the QCSFA or Harding criteria.
"Definite FA:" molecularly confirmed.
(Adapted with permission from Filla A, De Michele G, Coppola G, et al. Accuracy of clinical diagnostic criteria for Friedreich's ataxia. Mov Dis 2000;15:1255–1258, and from John Wiley and Sons.)

fragile X syndrome are evident. The working group also recommended carrier testing based on family history of unexplained mental retardation. In some countries (Finland and Israel), labs testing pregnant women have developed. Among male carriers of the premutation, a late-life neurological disorder consisting of tremor and ataxia has been described.

FRASER SYNDROME

Fraser syndrome is a rare constellation of signs of a multisystem congenital malformations described in Table 13. Slavotinek and Tifft have reviewed the known cases, and found that cryptophthalmos, syndactyly, and ambiguous genitalia are the most common signs.

FRIEDREICH'S ATAXIA

Friedreich's ataxia is the most common hereditary ataxia. It is a childhood-onset disorder, and one of its clinical hallmarks is absence of deep tendon reflexes. Direct genetic testing is now available, but the basic clinical criteria continue to be important for screening patients with further biochemical and genetic studies (Table 14).

Table 15
The Curacao Criteria for Hereditary Hemorrhagic Telangiectasia Syndrome

Criteria

1. Epistaxis (spontaneous, recurrent nose bleeds).
2. Telangiectases (multiple, at characteristic sites):
   a. Lips.
   b. Oral cavity.
   c. Fingers.
   d. Nose.
3. Visceral lesions, such as:
   a. Gastrointestinal telangiectasia (with or without bleeding).
   b. Pulmonary arteriovenous malformation (AVM).
   c. Hepatic AVM.
   d. Cerebral AVMs.
   e. Spinal AVM.
4. Family history (a first-degree relative with hemorrhagic telangiectasia syndrome [HHT] according to the following criteria):
   a. The HHT diagnosis is *definite* if three criteria are present,
   b. *Possible* or *suspected* if two criteria are present, and
   c. *Unlikely* if fewer than two criteria are present.

All offspring of an individual with HHT are at risk of having the disease, because HHT may not manifest until late in life. If there is any concern regarding the presence of physical signs, an experienced physician should be consulted. Coagulation disorders should be excluded. The presence of visceral abnormalities in children should prompt a particularly careful check of other family members. These criteria are likely to be further refined as molecular diagnostic tests become available in the next few years.

(Adapted with permission from Shovlin CL, Guttmacher AE, Buscarini E, et al. Diagnostic criteria for hereditary hemorrhagic telangiectasia [Rendu-Osler-Weber syndrome]. Am J Med Gen 2000;91:66, 67, and from John Wiley and Sons.)

The discovery of expanded GAA repeats in the Friedreich's ataxia gene on chromosome 9q has enlarged the clinical phenotype of Friedreich's ataxia. Several sets of clinical criteria have been proposed. Filla et al. compared the criteria, splitting cases into "possible," "probable," and "definite." Positive predictive values ranged from 88 to 98%, depending on criteria and level of clinical determination.

HEREDITARY HEMORRHAGIC TELANGIECTASIA (OSLER-WEBER-RENDU SYNDROME)

Hereditary hemorrhagic telangiectasia syndrome is an autosomal-dominant disorder, presenting classically as anemia with epistaxis or gastrointestinal bleeding and demonstration of cutaneous or visceral telangiectasias. Neurological symptoms may be the result of cerebral hemorrhages or strokes associated with pulmonary arteriovenous malformations and strokes with paradoxical embolism. Arteriovenous malformations may also occur in the spinal cord.

Genes responsible for hereditary hemorrhagic telangiectasia are present on chromosomes 9 and 12. However, the main basis of diagnosis is to suspect the condition in a symptomatic individual with a positive family history of bleeding disorder (Table 15).

MACHADO-JOSEPH DISEASE

Machado-Joseph disease is an autosomal-dominant disorder now described worldwide, but described originally in families residing in the Azore Islands. The symptoms are frequently pleomorphic within extended kindred (Table 16).

Molecular analysis indicates that Machado-Joseph disease is identical to spinocerebellar ataxia type 3, and is associated with an expansion of CAG trinucleotide repeats on chromosome 14q. It may be that the majority of the families reported worldwide may stem from a single mutation with a founder effect.

Table 16
Diagnostic Criteria for Machado-Joseph Disease

1. Autosomal-dominant inheritance.
2. Cerebellar ataxia with pyramidal signs.
3. Dystonic or akinetic-rigid syndrome.
4. Peripheral amyotrophy with motor neuron features and areflexia.
5. Other neurological abnormalities
   • Progressive external ophthalmoplegia.

Adapted with permission from Lima L, Coutinho P. Clinical criteria for diagnosis of Machado-Joseph disease: report of a non-Azorean Portuguese family. Neurology 1980;30:319–322.)

MITOCHONDRIAL DISORDERS

Mitochondrial disorders may present at any age, and consist of a growing number of recognized disorders of fatty acid metabolism, pyruvate metabolism, and respiratory chain abnormalities. The genes responsible for a given syndrome may be either nuclear genes expressed in mitochondria or genes of the mitochondrial DNA.

Diagnostic criteria exist on both a biochemical and clinical basis, and incorporate genetic information. Wolf and Smeitink provided a matrix for correlating the general criteria (Table 17, with the likelihood of mitochondrial disease based on biochemical criteria [Table 18]. Table 19 forms a matrix assessing the probability of a mitochondrial disease using general and biochemical criteria.)

Table 17
Mitochondrial Disease Criteria: General Criteria

A. **Muscular presentation**
   Muscular signs and symptoms (maximum 2 points):
   1. Progressive external ophthalmoplegia (2 points).
   2. Ptosis, facies myopathica (1 point).
   3. Exercise intolerance (a symptom characterized by abnormal, premature fatigue/weakness/muscle aches or cramps after normal play or activities of daily living) (1 point).
   4. Reduced muscle power (as evident by formal testing revealing weakness, if possible, or signs, such as Gower's sign, or absent or bad head control or delayed motor milestones—the latter only if mental development is normal or much advanced in comparison to motor development) or muscular hypotonia (in the newborn period and up to a developmental age of 6 months, with head lag in traction test, poor head control, "slipping through" sign, frog-like posture when awake and with limply hanging head and limbs in ventral suspension) (1 point).
   5. Episodes of acute rhabdomyolysis (acute episodes with severe muscle pain, muscle weakness, excessive elevation of creatinine kinase, or detection of myoglobin in urine) (1 point).
   6. Abnormal electromylogram (mild myopathic changes: early recruitment or reduction in amplitude and duration of motor unit action potentials with an increase in the number of polyphasic potentials).
   7. Any other involvement—central nervous system (CNS) (maximum 1 point) or multisystem (maximum 2 points).

B. **CNS presentation**
   CNS signs and symptoms (maximum 2 points, 1 point each)
   1. Delayed or absent psychomotor development (significant delay in two or more developmental domains: gross/fine motor skills, cognition, speech/language, personal/social or activities of daily living, as revealed by developmental screening tests), or mental retardation (IQ <70).
   2. Loss of acquired skills.
   3. Stroke-like episodes (transient hemianopia, hemiplegia, etc.).
   4. Migraine.
   5. Frank seizures or abnormal electroencephalogram (slowing of background activity, generalized epileptiform activity, or focal slow wave or seizure activity).
   6. Myoclonus or myoclonic epilepsy.

(Continued)

Table 17 *(Continued)*

7. Cortical blindness (loss of vision and optokinetic nystagmus in a patient with otherwise normal ocular examination and intact pupillary light responses).

8. Signs and symptoms of pyramidal tract involvement (increased muscle tone, opisthotonus, increased tendon reflexes, extensor plantar response, etc.).

9. Signs and symptoms of extrapyramidal involvement (athetosis, dystonia, involuntary movements).

10. Signs and symptoms of brainstem involvement (autonomic disturbance as central apneas, central hypoventilation, sinus bradycardia or tachycardia; swallowing difficulties, nystagmus, strabismus; abnormal or absent waves III–V in brainstem auditory evoked response).

11. Signs and symptoms of cerebellar involvement (ataxia, intention tremor, dysdiadochokinesis, etc.).

12. Any other involvement—muscle (maximum 1 point) or multisystem (maximum 2 points).

C. **Multisystemic involvement**

   Multisystemic involvement (maximum 3 points, 1 point each system)

Hematology

1. Sideroblastic anemia.
2. Pancytopenia.

Gastrointestinal tract

1. Acute or chronic hepatic dysfunction (elevated liver enzymes, decreased synthesis of liver proteins, decreased excretion of bilirubin, hypoglycemia).

2. Failure to thrive (no adequate weight gain, weight below third percentile/–2 standard deviation or crossing of percentiles).

3. Exocrine pancreatic dysfunction (>7% fat excretion).

4. Intestinal pseudo-obstruction (characterized by constipation, colicky pain, and vomiting, but without organic obstruction).

5. Otherwise unexplained chronic diarrhea (>3 weeks).

Endocrine

1. Short stature (>2 standard deviation below mean or < third percentile).
2. Delayed puberty.
3. Diabetes mellitus type I or type II or impaired glucose tolerance.
4. Hypoparathyroidism.
5. Central diabetes insipidus.

Heart

1. Cardiomyopathy (hypertrophic or dilatative) in the absence of a vitium cordis or hypertension.
2. Conduction block (atrioventricular-block I to III, bundle branch blocks, preexcitation syndromes).

Kidney

1. Proximal tubular dysfunction (complete or partial Fanconi syndrome).
2. Focal segmental glomerulosclerosis (biopsy).

Eyes

1. Cataract.
2. Retinopathy (impairment or loss of retinal function as seen in electroretinogram).
3. Optic atrophy.

Ears

1. Sensorineural hearing loss.

Nerve

1. Peripheral neuropathy.

General

1. Exacerbation of listed symptoms or signs with minor illness.
2. Sudden unexplained neonatal or infantile death in family history.
3. Any other involvement—muscle (maximum 1 point) or CNS (maximum 1 point): maximum 1 point.

   Metabolic and other investigations (maximum 4 points)

1. Elevated lactate (blood) more than 2000 µmol/L on at least three occasions (spontaneous, postprandial or postglucose tolerance test) (2 points).

2. Elevated lignin/phosphorus ratio higher than 18 (only if lactate is elevated) (1 point).

3. Elevated alanine (blood) higher than 450 µmol/L (2 points).

Table 17 *(Continued)*

4. Elevated cerebrospinal fluid (CSF) lactate (>1800 μmol/L, score only if blood lactate is normal) (2 points).
5. Elevated CSF protein (1 point).
6. Elevated CSF alanine (2 points).
7. Urine: elevated excretion of lactate or tricarboxylic acid cycle intermediates (2 points).
8. Elevated excretion of ethylmalonic acid or 3-methylglutaconic acid or dicarbonic acids (adipic, suberic, and sebacic acid) (1 point).
   Other
1. Abnormal ^{31}P-magnetic resonance spectroscopy in muscle—abnormally elevated inorganic phosphate and reduced phosphocreatine/inorganic phosphate ratio as compared to normal controls (2 points).
2. Magnetic resonance imaging: Leigh syndrome (T2-hyperintense lesions in putamina, globi pallidi, caudate nuclei) (2 points).
3. Magnetic resonance imaging: stroke-like picture (not confined to a vascular territory) or leukodystrophy or cerebral or cerebellar atrophy (maximum 1 point).
4. ^{1}H-magnetic resonance spectroscopy brain: clearly discernible lactate peak (1 point).
   Morphology (maximum 4 points)
1. Ragged red fibers or ragged blue fibers (if any in a pediatric patient, score 2 points; if more than 2%, score 4 points).
2. Cytochrome oxidase-negative fibers (if any in a pediatric patient, score 2 points: if more than 2%, score 4 points).
3. Strongly reduced overall cytochrome oxidase staining (CAVE technical problems) (4 points).
4. Abnormal (reduced or patchy) succinate dehydrogenase staining (1 point).
5. Strongly succinate dehydrogenase-reactive blood vessels (2 points).
6. Electron microscopy: abnormal mitochondria (2 points at maximum):
   a. Subsarcolemmal or intermyofibrillar aggregates of mitochondria (1 point).
   b. Enlarged or elongated mitochondria (2 points).
   c. Increased cristae with irregular orientation, honeycomb pattern, concentric wheels, or paucity of cristae (in the latter case, vacuolated or empty appearance of mitochondria) (2 points).
   d. Abnormal mitochondrial inclusions (cristalline, globular) (2 points).
   e. Lipid droplets (1 point).

Evaluation:

1 point:	respiratory chain disorder unlikely.
2–4 points:	respiratory chain disorder possible.
5–7 points:	respiratory chain disorder probable.
8–12 points:	respiratory chain disorder definite.

Adapted with permission from data supplement to Wolf NI, Smeitink JA. Mitochondrial disorders: a proposal for consensus diagnostic criteria in infants and children. Neurology 200212;59:1402–1405. Also available via www.neurology.org.

Table 18
Biochemical Criteria of the Mitochondrial Diagnostic Criteria Taking Into Account
^{14}C-Oxidation Rates, Adenosine Triphosphate Plus Phosphocreatine Production,
and Single-Enzyme Measurements (Single Enzymes = Complexes I–V)

Scoring	*^{14}C oxidation rates*		*ATP plus PCr production*		*Single enzymes*
Unlikely	Normal	and	Normal	and	Normal
Possible	Decreased	or	Decreased	or	Decreased
Probable	Decreased	and	Decreased	and	Normal
Definite	Decreased	and	Decreased	and	Decreased

ATP, adenosine triphosphate; PCr, phosphocreatine; decreased; lower than the lowest control value.
(Adapted with permission from Wolf NI, Smeitink JA. Mitochondrial disorders: a proposal for consensus diagnostic criteria in infants and children. Neurology 2002;59:1402–1405.)

In Tables 20 and 21, a revision of general diagnostic criteria for respiratory chain disorders published in 2002 is presented. These extend a prior, separate set of diagnostic criteria based on the presence of major and minor characteristics, and were validated in a large concurrent study.

Table 19
Combination of Biochemical and General Criteria and Final Patient Assignment of Mitochondrial Disorders

Biochemical criteria	General criteria			
	Unlikely	*Possible*	*Probable*	*Definite*
Unlikely	Unlikely	Possible	Possible	Probable
Possible	Possible	Possible	Probable	Probable
Probable	Possible	Probable	Probable	Definite
Definite	Probable	Probable	Definite	Definite

Adapted with permission from Wolf NI, Smeitink JA. Mitochondrial disorders: a proposal for consensus diagnostic criteria in infants and children. Neurology 2002;59:1402–1405.

Table 20
Major Diagnostic Criteria of Respiratory Chain Disorders

Clinical
Clinically complete respiratory chain (RC) encephalomyopathy[a] *or a mitochondrial cytopathy defined as fulfilling all three of the following conditions:*
  1. *Unexplained combination of multisystemic symptoms that is essentially pathognomonic for a RC disorder. Symptoms must include at least three of the organ system presentations described elsewhere, namely neurological, muscular, cardiac, renal, nutritional, hepatic, endocrine, hematological, otological, ophthalmological, dermatological, or dysmorphic.*
  2. *A progressive clinical course with episodes of exacerbation (e.g., following intercurrent illnesses) or a family history that is strongly indicative of a mitochondrial DNA mutation (at least one maternal relative other than the proband whose presentation predicts a probable or definite RC disorder).*
  3. *Other possible metabolic or nonmetabolic disorders have been excluded by appropriate testing, which may include metabolite, enzyme, or mutation analyses, imaging, electrophysiological studies, and histology.*

Histology
  >2% Ragged red fibers in skeletal muscle.
Enzymology[b]
  >2% Cytochrome oxidase-negative fibers if <50 years of age.
  >5% Cytochrome oxidase-negative fibers if >50 years of age.
  <20% Activity of any RC complex in a tissue.
  <30% Activity of any RC complex in a cell line.
  <30% Activity of the same RC complex activity in at least two tissues.
Functional
Fibroblast adenosine triphosphate synthesis rates more than 3 standard deviations below mean.
Molecular
Identification of a nuclear or mtDNA mutation of undisputed pathogenicity.

[a]Presentations include Leigh's disease, Alpers' disease, lethal infantile mitochondrial disease, Pearson's syndrome, Kearns-Sayre syndrome, mitochondrial encephalomyopathy, lactic acidosis, and stroke-like episodes, myoclonic epilepsy with ragged-red fibers, neuropathy, ataxia, and retinitis pigmentosa, mitochondrial neuro-gastrointestinal encephalomyopathy, and Leber's hereditary optic neuropathy.
[b]Enzyme activities represent percentage of normal control mean relative to an appropriate reference enzyme such as citrate synthase or RC complex II.
Modifications to the original adult diagnostic criteria (Walker UA, Collins S, Byrne E. Respiratory chain encephalomyopathies: a diagnostic classification. Eur Neurol 1996;36:260–267) that were developed in this study are shown in italics.
(Adapted with permission from Bernier FP, Boneh A, Dennett X, Chow CW, Cleary MA, Thorburn DR. Diagnostic criteria for respiratory chain disorders in adults and children. Neurology 2002;59:1406–1411.)

NEUROFIBROMATOSIS TYPE I

Inherited as an autosomal-dominant disorder with frequent new mutations (up to 50%), neurofibromatosis type I is caused by mutation in the neurofibromin gene located on chromosome 17q11.2. It is a relatively frequent disease with population estimates of 1 in 3400. A frequency of 1 in 390 has been found in young Israeli adults in a survey of military recruits (Table 22).

Table 21
Minor Diagnostic Criteria of Respiratory Chain Disorders

Clinical

Symptoms compatible with a respiratory chain (RC) defect[a]

Histology

1 to 2% Ragged red fibers if aged 30–50 years.

Any ragged red fibers if younger than 30 years of age.

More than 2% subsarcolemmal mitochondrial accumulations in a patient younger than 16 years of age.

Widespread electron microscopic abnormalities in any tissue.

Enzymology

Antibody-based demonstration of a defect in RC complex expression.

20–30% Activity of any RC complex in a tissue.

30–40% Activity of any RC complex in a cell line.

30–40% Activity of the same RC complex activity in at least two tissues.

Functional

Fibroblast adenosine triphosphate synthesis rates 2 to 3 standard deviations below mean.

Fibroblasts unable to grow on media with glucose replaced by galactose.

Molecular

Identification of a nuclear or mitochondrial DNA mutation of probable pathogenicity.

Metabolic

One or more metabolic indicators of impaired RC function.

---

[a]In addition to the symptoms listed elsewhere, we regarded pediatric features such as stillbirth associated with a paucity of intrauterine movement, neonatal death or collapse, movement disorder, severe failure to thrive, neonatal hypotonia, and neonatal hypertonia as minor clinical criteria. The adult criteria required muscle or neurologic involvement, but these do not have to be present in the modified general criteria.

Modifications to the original adult diagnostic criteria (Walker UA, Collins S, Byrne E. Respiratory chain encephalomyopathies: a diagnostic classification. Eur Neurol 1996;36:260–267) that were developed in this study are shown in italics.

(Adapted with permission from Bernier FP, Boneh A, Dennett X, Chow CW, Cleary MA, Thorburn DR. Diagnostic criteria for respiratory chain disorders in adults and children. Neurology 2002;59:1406–1411.)

Table 22
Diagnostic Criteria for Neurofibromatosis Type 1

Two or more filled criteria are diagnostic.

1. Six or more café au lait spots, larger than 5 mm in diameter in prepubertal, and larger than 15 mm in diameter in postpubertal individuals.
2. Two or more neurofibromas of any type or one plexiform neurofibroma.
3. Axillary and/or inguinal freckling.
4. Optic nerve glioma.
5. Osseous lesions, such as dysplasia of the sphenoid wing, thinning of long bone cortex, with or without pseudoarthrosis.
6. First-degree relative (parent, sibling, or offspring) with neurofibromatosis type 1, according to above criteria.

Adapted from the National Institute of Neurological Disorders and Stroke. Available at http://www.ninds.nih.gov/disorders/neurofibromatosis/detail_neurofibromatosis.htm.

NEUROFIBROMATOSIS TYPE 2

Table 23
Diagnostic Criteria for Neurofibromatosis Type 2

1987 National Institute of Health criteria

A. Bilateral vestibular schwannomas.
B. First-degree family relative with neurofibromatosis type 2 (NF2) *and* unilateral vestibular schwannoma *or* any two of the following: meningioma, schwannoma, glioma, neurofibroma, or juvenile posterior subcapsular lenticular opacity.

(Continued)

Table 23 *(Continued)*

1991 National Institute of Health criteria

A. Bilateral vestibular schwannomas.

B. First-degree family relative with NF2 *and* unilateral vestibular schwannoma *or* any one of the following: meningioma, schwannoma, glioma, neurofibroma, or juvenile posterior subcapsular lens opacity.

Manchester criteria[a]

A. Bilateral vestibular schwannomas.

B. First-degree family relative with NF2 *and* unilateral vestibular schwannoma *or* any two of the following: meningioma, schwannoma, glioma, neurofibroma, or posterior subcapsular lenticular opacities.

C. Unilateral vestibular schwannoma *and* any two of the following: meningioma, schwannoma, glioma, neurofibroma, or posterior subcapsular lenticular opacities.

D. Multiple meningiomas (two or more) *and* unilateral vestibular schwannoma *or* any two of the following: schwannoma, glioma, neurofibroma, or cataract.

National Neurofibromatosis Foundation criteria

A. *Confirmed or definite NF2*

   1. Bilateral vestibular schwannomas.

   2. First-degree family relative with NF2 *and* unilateral vestibular schwannoma at less than 30 years of age *or* any two of the following: meningioma, schwannoma, glioma, or juvenile lens opacity (posterior subcapsular cataract or cortical cataract).

B. *Presumptive or probable NF2*

   1. Unilateral vestibular schwannoma at less than 30 years of age *and* at least one of the following: meningioma, schwannoma, glioma, or juvenile lens opacity (posterior subcapsular cataract or cortical cataract).

   2. Multiple meningiomas (two or more) *and* unilateral vestibular schwannoma at less than 30 years of age *or* at least one of the following: schwannoma, glioma, or juvenile lens opacity (posterior subcapsular cataract or cortical cataract).

---

[a]In the Manchester criteria, "any two of" refers to two individual tumors or cataract, whereas in the other sets of criteria, it refers to two tumor types or cataract.

(Adapted with permission from Baser ME, Friedman JM, Wallace AJ, Ramsden RT, Joe H, Evans DGR. Evaluation of clinical diagnostic criteria for neurofibromatosis 2. Neurology 2002;59:1759–1765.)

Table 24
Diagnostic Criteria for PEHO Syndrome

Clinical criteria

1. Infantile—usually neonatal—hypotonia.

2. Convulsions, seizure onset at 2–52 weeks of life, myoclonic jerking and infantile spasms, and/or hypsarrhythmia.

3. Early arrest of mental development, absence of motor milestones (no head support or ability to sit unsupported), no speech, and later, profound psychomotor retardation.

4. Poor or absent visual fixation from the first months of life with atrophy of the optic disks by 2 years of age, normal electroretinogram, extinguished visual evoked potentials.

5. Progressive brain atrophy, as shown by computed tomography or magnetic resonance imaging, particularly of the cerebellum and brain stem; milder supratentorial atrophy.

Additional features present in most patients

1. Subcutaneous peripheral and facial edema.

2. Microcephaly developing at 12 months.

3. Dysmorphic features (narrow forehead, epicanthal folds, short nose, open mouth, small chin, midfacial hypoplasia, protruding lower parts of auricles, and tapering fingers).

Reprinted with permission from Riikonen R. The PEHO syndrome. Brain Dev 2001;23:765–769, and from Elsevier.)

PEHO SYNDROME

A disorder of multiple abnormalities in development, PEHO syndrome consists of *p*rogressive *e*ncephalopathy, with *e*dema, *h*ypsarrhythmia, and *o*ptic atrophy. First described in 1991, the clinical criteria have been developed empirically, and the full extent and variants of the syndrome are unknown (Table 24).

PRADER-WILLI SYNDROME

The criteria for a diagnosis of Prader-Willi syndrome (PWS) are based on a phenotypic scoring system, but incorporate genetic data. Because infants and young children have fewer symptoms than older children and adults with PWS, the scoring system differs by age group. The revised 2001 diagnostic criteria are presented in Tables 25 and 26, and have supplanted the similar 1993 system of Holm et al. Table 26 gives guidelines as to when to perform DNA testing for PWS.

RETT'S SYNDROME

Rett's syndrome (RS) has often been classified among the autistic spectrum disorders. (*See* "Autism Spectrum Disorders" section in Chapter 3 for alternative diagnostic criteria.) Great progress has been

Table 25
Diagnostic Criteria for Prader-Willi Syndrome

Major criteria
1. Neonatal and infantile central hypotonia with poor suck, gradually improving with age.
2. Feeding problems in infancy with need for special feeding techniques and poor weight gain/failure to thrive.
3. Excessive or rapid weight gain on weight-for-length chart (excessive is defined as crossing two centile channels) after 12 months but before 6 years of age; central obesity in the absence of intervention.
4. Characteristic facial features with dolichocephaly in infancy, narrow face or bifrontal diameter, almond-shaped eyes, small appearing mouth with thin upper lip, down-turned corners of the mouth (three or more symptoms are required).
5. Hypogonadism—with any of the following, depending on age:
   a. Genital hypoplasia, (male: scrotal hypoplasia, cryptorchidism, small penis and/or testes for age [<5th percentile]; female: absence or severe hypoplasia or labia minora and/or clitoris).
   b. Delayed or incomplete gonadal maturation with delayed pubertal signs in the absence of intervention after 16 years of age (male: small gonads, decreased facial and body hair, lack of voice change; female: amenorrhea/oligomenorrhea after age 16).
6. Global developmental delay in a child <6 years of age; mild-to-moderate mental retardation or learning problems in older children.
7. Hyperphagia/food foraging/obsession with food.
8. Deletion of chromosome 15q11–13 on high resolution (>650 bands) or other cytogenetic molecular abnormality of the Prader-Willi chromosome region, including maternal disomy.

Minor criteria
1. Decreased fetal movement or infantile lethargy or weak cry in infancy, improving with age.
2. Characteristic behavior problems—temper tantrums, violent outbursts, and obsessive-compulsive behavior; tendency to be argumentative, oppositional, rigid, manipulative, possessive, and stubborn; perseverating, stealing, and lying (five or more of these symptoms required).
3. Sleep disturbance and sleep apnea.
4. Short stature for genetic background by age 15 (in the absence of growth hormone intervention).
5. Hypopigmentation—fair skin and hair compared with family.
6. Small hands (<25th percentile) and/or feet (<10th percentile) for height age.
7. Narrow hands with straight ulnar borders.
8. Eye abnormalities (esotropia, myopia).
9. Thick viscous saliva with crusting at corners of the mouth.
10. Speech articulation defects.
11. Skin picking.

Supportive findings
1. High pain threshold.
2. Decreased vomiting.
3. Temperature instability in infancy or altered temperature sensitivity in older children and adults.
4. Scoliosis and/or kyphosis.
5. Early adrenarche.
6. Osteoporosis.

(Continued)

Table 25 (*Continued*)

7. Unusual skill with jigsaw puzzles.
8. Normal neuromuscular studies.

To score, major criteria are weighted at 1 point each, and minor criteria are weighted at 1/2 point each. Supportive findings increase the certainty of diagnosis but are not scored. For children 3 years of age or younger, 5 points are required, 4 of which should come from the major group. For children older than 3 years of age and for adults, a total score of 8 is required and major criteria must comprise 5 or more points of the total score.

Adapted with permission from Gunay-Aygun M, Schwartz S, Heeger S, O'Riordan MA, Cassidy SB. The changing purpose of Prader-Willi syndrome clinical diagnostic criteria and proposed revised criteria. Pediatrics 2001;108:92, and from the American Academy of Pediatrics.

Table 26
Criteria to Prompt DNA Testing for Prader-Willi Syndrome

Age at assessment features sufficient to prompt DNA testing
  A. Birth–2 years
      1. Hypotonia with poor suck.
  B. 2–6 years
      1. Hypotonia with history of poor suck.
      2. Global developmental delay.
  C. 6–12 years
      1. History of hypotonia with poor suck (hypotonia often persists).
      2. Global developmental delay.
      3. Excessive eating (hyperphagia, obsession with food) with central obesity if uncontrolled.
  D. 13 years through adulthood
      1. Cognitive impairment; usually mild mental retardation.
      2. Excessive eating (hyperphagia, obsession with food) with central obesity if uncontrolled.
      3. Hypothalamic hypogonadism and/or typical behavior problems (including temper tantrums and obsessive-compulsive features).

Adapted with permission from Gunay-Aygun M, Schwartz S, Heeger S, O'Riordan MA, Cassidy SB. The changing purpose of Prader-Willi syndrome clinical diagnostic criteria and proposed revised criteria. Pediatrics 2001;108:92, and from the American Academy of Pediatrics.

made in unraveling the molecular and genetic basis of RS, leading to its inclusion here as a genetic disorder. Based on current molecular biological information, RS should be viewed as a neurodevelopmental disorder instead of a degenerative disorder. Mutations in the methyl-CpG-binding protein 2 (*MECP2*) gene are the molecular basis for more than 80% of girls fulfilling criteria for classic RS.

In September 2001, the International Rett's Syndrome Association convened a panel of international experts, with the aim to establish as simple a dataset as possible to assist physicians in making the clinical diagnosis of RS. The meeting resulted in an updated set of diagnostic/clinical criteria based on observations and knowledge gained from understanding the natural history of RS, and from new information based on the discovery of the *MECP2* gene. The new criteria include information on atypical or borderline variants of RS, which is important for increasing physician awareness and for expanded understanding of RS.

It is important to emphasize that at our present level of knowledge, the diagnosis of RS remains a clinical one, and is not made solely based on *MECP2* mutations. RS can occur with or without mutations in *MECP2*, and *MECP2* mutations can occur without the diagnosis of RS. Therefore, consensus on the diagnostic criteria for classic and variant forms of RS is essential, and these criteria must be applied consistently for the accuracy of phenotype–genotype correlation studies (Tables 27 and 28).

Table 27
Diagnostic Criteria for Rett's Syndrome

Necessary criteria
1. Apparently normal prenatal and perinatal history.
2. Psychomotor development largely normal through the first six months or may be delayed from birth.
3. Normal head circumference at birth.
4. Postnatal deceleration of head growth in the majority.
5. Loss of achieved purposeful hand skill between ages 6 months and 2.5 years.
6. Stereotypic hand movements such as hand wringing/squeezing, clapping/tapping, mouthing, and washing/rubbing automatisms.
7. Emerging social withdrawal, communication dysfunction, loss of learned words, and cognitive impairment.
8. Impaired (dyspraxic) or failing locomotion.

Supportive criteria
1. Awake disturbances of breathing (hyperventilation, breath-holding, forced expulsion of air or saliva, air swallowing).
2. Bruxism.
3. Impaired sleep pattern from early infancy.
4. Abnormal muscle tone successively associated with muscle wasting and dystonia.
5. Peripheral vasomotor disturbances.
6. Scoliosis/kyphosis progressing through childhood.
7. Growth retardation.
8. Hypotrophic small and cold feet; small, thin hands.

Exclusion criteria
1. Organomegaly or other signs of storage disease.
2. Retinopathy, optic atrophy, or cataract.
3. Evidence of perinatal or postnatal brain damage.
4. Existence of identifiable metabolic or other progressive neurological disorder.
5. Acquired neurological disorder resulting from severe infections or head trauma.

Adapted with permission from Hagberg B, Hanefeld F, Percy A, Skjeldal O. An update on clinically applicable diagnostic criteria in Rett syndrome. Eur J Pediatr Neurol 2002;6:293–297, and from Elsevier.

Table 28
Revised Delineation of Variant Phenotypes of Rett's Syndrome

Inclusion criteria
1. Meet at least three main criteria.
2. Meet at least five supportive criteria.

Six main criteria
1. Absence or reduction of hand skills.
2. Reduction or loss of babble speech.
3. Monotonous pattern to hand stereotypies.
4. Reduction or loss of communication skills.
5. Deceleraton of head growth from first years of life.
6. Rett's syndrome disease profile: a regression stage followed by a recovery of interaction contrasting with slow neuromotor regression.

Eleven supportive criteria
1. Breathing irregularities.
2. Bloating/air swallowing.
3. Teeth grinding, harsh-sounding type.
4. Abnormal locomotion.
5. Scoliosis/kyphosis.
6. Lower limb amyotrophy.
7. Cold, purplish feet, usually growth-impaired.
8. Sleep disturbances including night screaming outbursts.
9. Laughing/screaming spells.
10. Diminished response to pain.
11. Intense eye contact/eye pointing.

Adapted with permission from Hagberg B, Hanefeld F, Percy A, Skjeldal O. An update on clinically applicable diagnostic criteria in Rett syndrome. Eur J Pediatr Neurol 2002;6:293–297, and from Elsevier.

Table 29
Proposed Diagnostic Criteria for Schwannomatosis

Definite	*Possible*
Age over 30 years, two or more non-intradermal schwannomas, at least one with histological confirmation, no evidence of vestibular tumor on high-quality MRI scan, and no known constitutional *NF2* mutation	Age under 30 years, two or more non-intradermal schwannomas, at least one with histological confirmation, no evidence of vestibular tumor on high-quality MRI scan, and no known constitutional *NF2* mutation
OR	OR
One pathologically confirmed, nonvestibular schwannoma, plus a first-degree relative who meets above criteria.	Age over 45 years, two or more non-intradermal schwannomas, at least one with histological confirmation, no symptoms of 8th nerve dysfunction, and no known constitutional *NF2* mutation
	OR
	Radiographic evidence of a nonvestibular schwannoma and first-degree relative meeting criteria for definite schwannomatosis.

Segmental
Meets criteria for either definite or possible
schwannomatosis, but limited to one limb
or five or fewer contiguous segments
of the spine.

SCHWANNOMATOSIS

Schwannomatosis represents a recently described third form of neurofibromatosis. It may be recognized in individuals with multiple schwannomas who do not manifest typical features, particularly of neurofibromin 2. Most cases are sporadic, but autosomal-dominant transmission has also been documented. A relatively limited segmental form, with schwannomas limited to a single limb, is also recognized (Table 29).

TUBEROUS SCLEROSIS

Tuberous sclerosis is a genetic condition characterized by the formation of tumors in multiple organs, including brain, eye, kidney, skin, lungs, and many others. The syndrome is genetically (and clinically) heterogeneous, with many mutations having been described (Table 30). The tuberous sclerosis 1 gene is located on chromosome 9q, and the tuberous sclerosis 2 gene on chromosome 16p. Genes located on other chromosomes have been detected in some, but not all, studies of familial inheritance.

Table 30
Diagnostic Criteria for Tuberous Sclerosis

Revised diagnostic criteria for tuberous sclerosis complex (TSC)

Major features
1. Facial angiofibromas or forehead plaque.
2. Nontraumatic ungual or periungual fibroma.
3. Hypomelanotic macules (more than three).
4. Shagreen patch (connective tissue nevus).

(Continued)

Table 30 *(Continued)*

5. Multiple retinal nodular hamartomas.
6. Cortical tuber.[a]
7. Subependymal nodule.
8. Subependymal giant cell astrocytoma.
9. Cardiac rhabdomyoma, single or multiple.
10. Lymphangiomyomatosis.[b]
11. Renal angiomyolipoma.[b]

Minor features

1. Multiple randomly distributed pits in dental enamel.
2. Hamartomatous rectal polyps.[c]
3. Bone cysts.[d]
4. Cerebral white matter migration lines.[a,d,e]
5. Gingival fibromas.
6. Nonrenal hamartoma.[c]
7. Retinal achromic patch.
8. "Confetti" skin lesions.
9. Multiple renal cysts.[c]

Definite TSC: either two major features or one major feature with two minor features.
Probable TSC: one major feature and one minor feature.
Possible TSC: either one major feature or two or more minor features.

[a]When cerebral cortical dysplasia and cerebral white matter migration tracts occur together, they should be counted as one rather than two features of TSC.

[b]When both lymphangiomyomatosis and renal angiomyolipomas are present, other features of TSC should be present before a definitive diagnosis is assigned.

[c]Histological confirmation is suggested.

[d]Radiographic confirmation is sufficient.

[e]One panel member recommended three or more radial migration lines constitute a major feature.

(Adapted from Roach ES, Gomez MR, Northrup H. Tuberous sclerosis complex consensus conference: revised clinical diagnostic criteria. J Child Neurol 1998;13:624–628.)

SOURCES

Adenylosuccinate Lyase Deficiency

Ciardo F, Costantino S, Curatolo P. Neurologic aspects of adenylosuccinate lyase deficiency. J Child Neurology 2001; 16:301–308.

Alexander's Disease

Gorospe JR, Naidu S, Johnson AB, et al. Molecular findings in symptomatic and pre-symptomatic Alexander disease patients. Neurology 2002;58:1494–1500.

Angelman Syndrome

Williams CA, Angelman H, Clayton-Smith J, et al. Angelman syndrome: consensus for diagnostic criteria. Angelman Syndrome Foundation. Am J Med Genet 1995;56:237, 238.

CHARGE Syndrome

Blake KD, Davenport SLH, Hall B, et al. CHARGE Association—an update and review for the primary pediatrician. Clin Pediatr 1998;37:159–173.

Oley CA, Baraitser M, Grant DB. A reappraisal of the CHARGE association. J Med Genet 1988;25:147–157.

Pagon PA, Graham JM, Zonana J, Young SL. Congenital heart disease and choanal atresia with multiple anomalies. J Pediatr 1981;99:223–227.

Verloes A. Update diagnostic criteria for CHARGE syndrome: a proposal. Am J Med Genet 2005;133:306–308.

Vissers ELM, van Ravenswaaij CMA, Admiraal R, et al. Mutations in a new member of the chromodomain gene family cause CHARGE syndrome. Nat Genet 2004;36:955–957. Available online at http://www.nature.com/ng/journal/v36/n9/ abs/ng1407.html;jsessionid=DB84F413FB73F3AA716D210E0AAADC1B.

Childhood Ataxia With Central Nervous System Hypomyelination/Vanishing White Matter

Schiffman R, Fogli A, van der Knaap M, Boespflug-Tanguy O. Childhood ataxia with central nervous system hypomyelination/vanishing white matter. GeneReviews, February 2003. Available online at http://www.geneclinics.org/servlet/access?id=8888891&key=Ztnfp2fvDYe5R&gry=INSERTGRY&fcn=y&fw=xLNP&filename=/profiles/cach/index.html.

van der Knaap MS, Leegwater PA, Konst AA, et al. Mutations in each of the five subunits of translationinitiation factor eIF2B can cause leukoencephalopathy with vanishing white matter. Ann Neurol 2002;51:264–270.

Cowden's Syndrome

Abel TW, Baker SJ, Fraser MM, et al. Lhermitte-Duclos disease: a report of 31 cases with immunohistochemical analysis of the PTEN/AKT/mTOR pathway. J Neuropathol Exp Neurol 2005;64:341–349.

Eng C. Will the real Cowden syndrome please stand up: revised diagnostic criteria. J Med Genet 2000;37:828–830.

Vantomme N, Van Calenbergh F, Goffin J, Sciot R, Demaerel P, Plets C. Lhermitte-Duclos disease is a clinical manifestation of Cowdens syndrome. Surg Neurol 2001;56:201–204.

Fragile X Syndrome

Bailey DB, Nelson D. The nature and consequences of fragile X syndrome. Men Retard Dev Disabilities Res Rev 1995;1:238–244.

Brussino A, Gellera C, Saluto A, et al. *FMR1* gene premutation is a frequent genetic cause of late-onset sporadic cerebellar ataxia. Neurology 2005;64:145–147.

Hagerman RJ, Amiri K, Cronister A. Fragile X checklist. Am J Med Genet 1991;38:283–287.

Hagerman RJ, Cronister A. Fragile X syndrome: diagnosis, treatment, and research. Baltimore: Johns Hopkins University Press, 1996:3–88.

Maddalena A, Richards CS, McGinniss MJ, et al. Technical standards and guidelines for fragile X: the first of a series of disease-specific supplements to the standards and guidelines for clinical genetics laboratories of the American College of Medical Genetics. Genet Med 2001;3:200–205.

Mazzocco MMM. Advances in research on the fragile X syndrome. Men Retard Dev Disabilities Res Rev 2000;6:96–106.

Warren ST, Sherman SL. The fragile X syndrome. In: Scriver C, Beaudet A, Sly W, Valle D, eds. The Metabolic Basis of Inherited Disease. New York: McGraw Hill, 2001:1257–1289.

Fraser Syndrome

Slavotinek AM, Tifft CJ. Fraser syndrome and cryptophthalmos: review of the diagnostic criteria and evidence for phenotypic modules in complex malformation syndromes. J Med Genet 2002;39:623–633.

Friedreich's Ataxia

Filla A, De Michele G, Caruso G, et al. Genetic data and natural history of Friedreich's disease: a study of 80 Italian patients. J Neurol 1990;237:345–351.

Filla A, De Michele G, Coppola G, et al. Accuracy of clinical diagnostic criteria for Friedreich's ataxia. Mov Dis 2000:15:1255–1258.

Geoffrey G, Barbeau A, Breton G, et al. Clinical description and roentgenographic evaluation of patients with Friedreich's ataxia. Can J Neurol Sci 1976;3:279–286.

Harding AE. Friedreich's ataxia: a clinical and genetic study of 90 families with an analysis of early diagnostic criteria and intrafamilial clustering of clinical features. Brain 1981;104:589–620.

Hereditary Hemorrhagic Telangiectasia (Osler-Weber-Rendu Syndrome)

Shovlin CL, Guttmacher AE, Buscarini E, et al. Diagnostic criteria for hereditary hemorrhagic telangiectasia (Rendu-Osler-Weber syndrome). Am J Med Gen 2000;91:66, 67.

Machado-Joseph Disease

Coutinho P, Andrade C. Autosomal dominant system degeneration in Portuguese families of the Azores Islands: a new genetic disorder involving cerebellar, pyramidal, extrapyramidal and spinal cord motor functions. Neurology 1978;28:703–709.

Lima L, Coutinho P. Clinical criteria for diagnosis of Machado-Joseph disease: report of a non-Azorean Portuguese family. Neurology 1980;30:319–322.

Mitochondrial Disorders

Bernier FP, Boneh A, Dennett X, Chow CW, Cleary MA, Thorburn DR. Diagnostic criteria for respiratory chain disorders in adults and children. Neurology 2002;59:1406–1411.

De Vivo DC. The expanding clinical spectrum of mitochondrial diseases. Brain Dev 1993;15:1–22.
Walker UA, Collins S, Byrne E. Respiratory chain encephalomyopathies: a diagnostic classification. Eur Neurol 1996;36:260–267.
Wolf NI, Smeitink JA. Mitochondrial disorders: a proposal for consensus diagnostic criteria in infants and children. Neurology 2002;59:1402–1405.

Neurofibromatosis Type 1

Garty BZ, Laor A, Danon YL. Neurofibromatosis type 1 in Israel: survey of young adults. J Med Genet 1994;31:853–857.
Littler M, Morton NE. Segregation analysis of peripheral neurofibromatosis (NF1). J Med Genet 1990;27:307–310.
Stumpf DA, Alksne JF, Annegers JF, et al. Neurofibromatosis. Arch Neurol 1988;45:575–578.

Neurofibromatosis Type 2

Baser ME, Friedman JM, Wallace AJ, Ramsden RT, Joe H, Evans DGR. Evaluation of clinical diagnostic criteria for neurofibromatosis 2. Neurology 2002;59:1759–1765.

PEHO Syndrome

Riikonen R. The PEHO syndrome. Brain Dev 2001;23:765–769.
Somer M. Diagnostic criteria and genetics of the PEHO syndrome. J Med Gen 1993;30:932–936.

Prader-Willi Syndrome

Gunay-Aygun M, Schwartz S, Heeger S, O'Riordan MA, Cassidy SB. The changing purpose of Prader-Willi syndrome clinical diagnostic criteria and proposed revised criteria. Pediatrics 2001;108:E92.
Holm VA, Cassidy SB, Butler MG, et al. Prader-Willi syndrome: consensus diagnostic criteria. Pediatrics 1993;91:398–402.

Rett's Syndrome

American Psychiatric Association. Diagnostic and Statistical Manual of Mental Disorders, 4th rev. ed. Washington, DC: American Psychiatric Association, 1994.
Hagberg B, Hanefeld F, Percy A, Skjeldal O. An update on clinically applicable diagnostic criteria in Rett syndrome. Eur J Pediatr Neurol 2002;6:293–297.
Jan MM, Dooley JM, Gordon KE. Male Rett syndrome variant: application of diagnostic criteria. Pediatr Neurol 1999;20:238–240.

Tuberous Sclerosis

Roach ES, Gomez MR, Northrup H. Tuberous sclerosis complex consensus conference: revised clinical diagnostic criteria. Journal of Child Neurology, 1998;13:624–628.
Roach ES, DiMario FJ, Kandt RS, Northrup H. Tuberous sclerosis consensus conference: recommendations for diagnostic evaluation. J Child Neurol 1998;14:401–407.

CERVICOGENIC HEADACHE

Headaches caused by disorders of the neck has been a controversial subject; some feel that it is, at best, a rare syndrome. The original diagnostic criteria were proposed by Sjaastad in 1990, and are shown in Table 1.

In a comprehensive review by Antonacci et al., the sensitivity and specificity of the original criteria were measured in an Italian clinic population. Their groups (labeled "A," "B," and "C") correspond to individuals with varying symptoms. Group A includes those individuals with the presence of both unilateral headache without side-shift and pain starting in the neck, eventually spreading to oculofrontotemporal areas, where the maximum pain is often located. The neck pain was invariably unilateral at onset, but could eventually spread across the midline during particularly severe and protracted attacks (Table 2).

Table 1
Pooled Form (1–7) of the Diagnostic Criteria for Cervicogenic Headache Proposed by Sjaastad et al., 1990

1. Unilateral headache without side-shift (I).
2. Symptoms and signs of neck involvement
   a. Pain triggered by neck movement and/or sustained awkward position (IIa1) and/or external pressure over the ipsilateral upper, posterior neck or occipital region (IIa2).
   b. Ipsilateral neck, shoulder and arm pain of a rather vague, nonradicular nature (IIb).
   c. Reduced range of motion in the cervical spine (IIc).
3. Pain episodes of varying duration or fluctuating, continuous pain (IV).
4. Moderate, nonexcruciating pain, usually of a nonthrobbing nature (V).
5. Pain starting in the neck, eventually spreading to oculofrontotemporal areas, where the maximum pain is often located (VI).
6. Anesthetic blockades of the major occipital nerve and/or the C2 root or other appropriate blockades on the symptomatic side abolish the pain transiently, provided complete anesthesia is obtained (VII) *or* sustained a whiplash (neck trauma) a relatively short time before the onset (IX).
7. Various attack-related phenomena: autonomic symptoms and signs, nausea, vomiting (Xa-Xb), ipsilateral edema, and flushing mostly in the periocular area; dizziness (XI); photo- and phonophobia (XII); blurred vision on the eye ipsilateral to the pain (XIII).

The number of the original diagnostic criteria is given in parentheses.

Criterion 6 embraces two criteria; these two criteria were "pooled" after the enrolment of the patients because of the lack of pain, in some of them, at the time of interview, and thus, it was impossible to carry out a nerve blockade. So, in this context, the fulfillment of one criterion suffices.

(Adapted with permission from Antonaci F, Ghrimai S, Bono G, et al. Cervicogenic headache: evaluation of the original diagnostic criteria. Cephalalgia 2001;21:573–583, and from Blackwell Publishing.)

From: *Current Clinical Neurology: Diagnostic Criteria in Neurology*
Edited by: A. J. Lerner © Humana Press Inc., Totowa, NJ

Table 2
Sensitivity and Specificity of Diagnostic Criteria in Patients Fulfilling the Cervicogenic Criteria

Diagnostic criteria	Group A	Specificity	Sensitivity
Major symptoms and signs			
I	Unilateral headache	0	1[a]
II-a-1	Pain triggered by neck movements and/or sustained awkward head positioning	0.75	0.44
II-a-2	Pain elicited by external pressure over the GON or the ipsilateral upper, posterior neck region C2–C3	1	0.17
II-b	Ipsilateral neck, shoulder and arm pain of a rather vague, nonradicular nature	0.88	0.65
II-c	Reduced range of motion in the cervical spine	0.38	0.91
Pain characteristics			
IV	Pain episodes of varying duration or fluctuating continuous pain	0.88	0.78
V	Moderate, nonexcruciating pain, usually of a nonthrobbing nature	0.86	0.91
VI	Pain starting in the neck, eventually spreading to oculofrontotemporal areas	0	1[a]
Other important criteria			
VII	Anesthetic blockades of the GON or C2 root	1.0	0.18
IX	Sustained neck trauma a relatively short time before the onset	0.88	0.65
Minor, more rarely occurring, nonobligatory symptoms and signs			
Xa-b	Rarely occurring nausea, vomiting, and XII photo- and phonophobia	0.88	0.48
Xc	Ipsilateral edema and, less frequently, flushing, mostly in the periocular area	0.88	0.09
XI	Dizziness	0.75	0.26
XIII	"Blurred vision" in the eye ipsilateral to the pain	1.0	0.22
XIV	Difficulty on swallowing	0.88	0.09

[a]Inclusion criterion.
GON, greater optic nerve.
(Adapted with permission from Antonaci F, Ghrimai S, Bono G, et al. Cervicogenic headache: evaluation of the original diagnostic criteria. Cephalalgia 2001;21:573–583, and from Blackwell Publishing.)

Table 3
International Headache Society Diagnostic Criteria for Cluster Headache

A.	At least five attacks fulfilling criteria B–D.
B.	Severe or very severe unilateral orbital, supraorbital, and/or temporal pain lasting 15–180 minutes if untreated.[a]
C.	Headache is accompanied by at least one of the following:

    1. Ipsilateral conjunctival injection and/or lacrimation.
    2. Ipsilateral nasal congestion and/or rhinorrhea.
    3. Ipsilateral eyelid edema.
    4. Ipsilateral forehead and facial sweating.
    5. Ipsilateral miosis and/or ptosis.
    6. A sense of restlessness or agitation.

D. Attacks have a frequency from one every other day to eight per day.[b]
E. Not attributed to another disorder.[c]

[a]During part (but less than half) of the time-course of cluster headache, attacks may be less severe and/or of shorter or longer duration.

[b]During part (but less than half) of the time-course of cluster headache, attacks may be less frequent.

[c]History and physical and neurological examinations do not suggest any of the disorders listed in groups 5–12, or history and/or physical and/or neurological examinations do suggest such disorder but it is ruled out by appropriate investigations, or such disorder is present but attacks do not occur for the first time in close temporal relation to the disorder.

(Adapted with permission from Headache Classification Subcommittee of the International Headache Society. The International Classification of Headache Disorders, 2nd ed. Cephalalgia 2004;24:S9–S60, and from Blackwell Publishing.)

Table 4
International Headache Society Diagnostic Criteria for Episodic and Chronic Cluster Headaches

Episodic cluster headache
Description: Cluster headache attacks occurring in periods lasting 7 days to 1 year separated by pain-free periods lasting 1 month or longer.
Diagnostic criteria:
    A. Attacks fulfilling criteria A–E for Cluster headache.
    B. At least two cluster periods lasting 7–365 days and separated by pain-free remission periods of ≥1 month.
Comment: The duration of the remission period has been increase in this second edition to a minimum of 1 month.
Chronic cluster headache
Description: Cluster headache attacks occurring for more than 1 year without remission or with remissions lasting less than 1 month.
Diagnostic criteria:
    A. Attacks fulfilling criteria A–E for 3.1 Cluster headache.
    B. Attacks recur over more than 1 year with remission periods or with remission periods lasting less than 1 month.

Adapted with permission from Headache Classification Subcommittee of the International Headache Society. The International Classification of Headache Disorders, 2nd ed. Cephalalgia 2004;24:S9–S60.

CLUSTER HEADACHE

Cluster headache is a primary headache disorder of unclear etiology. It is more common in males, and is often precipitated by ingestion of alcohol. Not infrequently, the patient awakes from sleep with the onset of the headache. Patients are typically quite agitated during the attack, which tends to be relatively brief compared with the time-course of migraine or tension-type headaches. Cluster headaches may occur on an episodic or chronic basis. Chronic cluster headache may be primary or a stage evolving from episodic cluster headache (Tables 3 and 4).

EXTERNAL COMPRESSION HEADACHE

Table 5
International Headache Society Diagnostic Criteria for External Compression Headache

A. Results from the application of external pressure in the forehead or the scalp.
B. Is felt in the area subjected to pressure.
C. Is a constant pain.
D. Is prevented by avoiding the precipitating cause.
E. Is not associated with organic cranial or intracranial disease.

Adapted with permission from Headache Classification Subcommittee of the International Headache Society. The International Classification of Headache Disorders, 2nd ed. Cephalalgia 2004;24:S9–S60, and from Blackwell Publishing.

Table 6
Diagnostic Criteria for Headache Related to Intrathecal Injections

A. Headache follows intrathecal injection within 4 hours.
B. Headache is diffuse and present also in the recumbent position.
C. Headache clears completely within 14 days. (If it persists, consider post-lumbar puncture.)

Adapted with permission from Headache Classification Subcommittee of the International Headache Society. The International Classification of Headache Disorders, 2nd ed. Cephalalgia 2004;24:S9–S60, and from Blackwell Publishing.

Table 7
Diagnostic Criteria for Presumed Chemical Meningitis From Intrathecal Injection

1. Headache follows intrathecal injection within 5–72 hours.
2. Headache is diffuse and present also in the recumbent position.
3. Cerebrospinal fluid pleocytosis with negative culture.

Adapted with permission from Headache Classification Subcommittee of the International Headache Society. The International Classification of Headache Disorders, 2nd ed. Cephalalgia 2004;24:S9–S60, and from Blackwell Publishing.

HEADACHE RELATED TO INTRATHECAL INJECTIONS

In the International Headache Society (IHS) classification category, headache related to intrathecal injections is a direct effect of the agent with the following diagnostic criteria (Table 6): if the headache is because of presumed chemical meningitis, the IHS criteria specify the criteria listed in Table 7.

From a clinical standpoint, there may be diagnostic confusion of headache because of a low cerebrospinal fluid (CSF) pressure or post-lumbar puncture (LP) headache, as opposed to a "pure" headache related to intrathecal injections. Headaches after intrathecal injections may be seen after many agents, including anesthetics, inadvertent intrathecal injections of blood patches, chemotherapeutic agents, and gadolinium; the headache may be dose-limiting in some cases. The relationship of more remote complications, such as cerebral ischemia or cerebral venous thrombosis to postdural puncture syndromes, is more obscure, although vascular mechanisms may be related to the pathogenesis of post-LP and intrathecal injection headaches. The choice of smaller needles used in the lumbar puncture with injections of cytotoxic chemicals for chemotherapy has been cited as one method to lower the incidence of intrathecal injection headache.

HEMICRANIA CONTINUA AND PAROXYSMAL HEMICRANIAS

Originally described by Sjaastad and Spierings in 1984, hemicrania continua is a primary headache syndrome classified among the "indomethacin-responsive headaches" because of its selective and consistent response to this agent. It shares some features with cluster headache and migraines as well. Other hemicranial headaches share clinical and probably a pathophysiological basis, and are grouped here. The autonomic manifestations of these disorders are a common feature, and should be routinely

Table 8
Diagnostic Criteria for Hemicrania Continua

A. Headache for a total of more than 2 months.
B. Obligatory features
    1. Unilaterality without side shift.[a]
    2. Absolute and protracted indomethacin effect.[b]
    3. Long-lasting, repetitive attacks—hours/days/weeks, with a tendency to a fluctuating chronic pattern over time.[c]
    4. Intensity of pain: mild, moderate or severe (not excruciatingly severe).
C. Other nonobligatory but frequent characteristics of the pain syndrome
    1. Female sex.
D. Negative provisos
    1. Relative shortage of "local" autonomic phenomena.[d]
    2. Relative lack of "migraine" symptoms and signs.[e]
    3. Relative lack of "cervicogenic" symptoms and signs.[f]
    4. Lack of effect of migraine and cluster headache drugs (triptans and ergotamine).

[a]The pain is mostly in the "anterior" area, but not infrequently also in the auricular/occipital area.

[b]Provided the dosage is adequate: 150 mg per day for 3 days. In the doubtful case, the "indotest" should be carried out (*see* Headache 1998;38:122–128). This is particularly important in the remitting cases, because a betterment of pain in reality being because of a remission may falsely be ascribed to indomethacin.

[c]There are two forms of hemicrania continua from a temporal point of view: a remitting and nonremitting (chronic) form. There may be transitions from the one temporal pattern to the other. The continuous pattern may eventually seem to dominate.

[d]Lacrimation, conjunctival injection, rhinorrhea and nasal obstruction; such signs are usually meager and on the symptomatic side, and, if present, they occur mostly during the more severe attack periods.

[e]Nausea, vomiting, photo- and phonophobia, pulsatile character of pain, and accentuation upon mild physical activity.

[f]Reduction of range of motion in the neck; ipsilateral upper extremity discomfort; mechanical precipitation of pain/attacks.

(Adapted with permission from Pareja, JA, Vincent, M, Antonaci, F, Sjaastad, O. Hemicrania continua: diagnostic criteria and nosologic status. Cephalalgia 2001;21:874–877, and from Blackwell Publishing.)

investigated in the history. SUNCT syndrome (*s*hort-lasting *u*nilateral *n*euralgiform headache with *c*onjunctival injection and *t*earing) is a rare but distinct syndrome.

Secondary causes of paroxysmal hemicranias have been reported as results of various causes including collagen vascular diseases, intrinsic brain tumors, gangliocytoma of the sella turcica, and cavernous sinus meningioma.

An alternative set of diagnostic criteria has also been proposed based on the expansion of the clinical syndrome since the original description of diagnostic criteria presented above. These include some cases not responsive to indomethacin and others responsive to other nonsteroidal anti-inflammatories. Hemicrania continua may also exist in an episodic, as well as a chronic, form, suggesting the existence of clinical (if not biological) subtypes (*see* Tables 10 and 11).

IDIOPATHIC INTRACRANIAL HYPERTENSION

Idiopathic intracranial hypertension is defined by increased CSF pressure without mass lesion, hydrocephalus, or abnormal CSF. It is also called pseudotumor cerebri or benign intracranial hypertension.

Described in the late 19th century, a set of diagnostic criteria known as the modified Dandy criteria were formulated by Smith and are shown in Table 12.

POST-LP AND LOW CSF PRESSURE HEADACHE

Whereas diagnosis of post-LP headache may seem to be self-obvious to most neurologists, post-LP headache is a frequent cause of confusion among other specialties. This is especially true because headache is often the indication for LP in the first place. The existence of diagnostic criteria is a step toward delineating the syndrome, and serves as a reference for future research.

Table 9
Diagnostic Criteria for Hemicrania Continua: An Alternative Proposal

A. Headache present for at least 1 month fulfilling criteria B–D.
B. Unilateral headache.
C. Pain has all three of the following:
    1. Continuous but fluctuating severity.
    2. Painful exacerbations of at least moderate severity.
    3. Lack of precipitating mechanisms.
D.
    1. Absolute response to indomethacin or
    2. One of the following autonomic features with severe pain exacerbation:
        a. Conjunctival injection.
        b. Lacrimation.
        c. Nasal congestion.
        d. Rhinorrhea.
        e. Ptosis.
        f. Eyelid edema.
E. At least one of the following:
    1. No suggestion of a disorder, such as trigeminal neuralgia, idiopathic stabbing headache, cough headache, benign exertional headache, headache associated with sexual activity, or hypnic headache.
    2. Such a disorder is suggested but excluded by appropriate investigations.
    3. Such a disorder is present, but first headache attacks do not occur in close temporal relation to the disorder.

Comment: Hemicrania continua is usually continuous (hemicrania continua-chronic), but rare cases of remission have been reported. Also, an episodic pattern with pain-free remissions lasting weeks to months may precede the continuous headache phase in up to a third of patients, and in some cases the pattern may remain episodic (hemicrania continua-episodic). Painful exacerbations may be associated with migraine-related symptoms of photophobia, phonophobia, nausea, vomiting, and even aura.

Adapted with permission from Goadsby PJ, Lipton RB. A review of paroxysmal hemicranias SUNCT syndrome and other short-lasting headache with autonomic features, including new cases. Brain 1997;120:193–209.

Headaches caused by CSF fistulas and low CSF volume and pressure may be difficult to diagnose easily, and finding the source of the CSF leak can be quite challenging, often requiring imaging of the entire neuraxis, and sometimes involving radionuclide tracer studies to localize the leak. They may resolve spontaneously with simple measures, such as bed rest, or sometimes require surgical repair. Subdural hematoma can occur secondary to low CSF pressure.

MEDICATION-OVERUSE HEADACHE

Whereas a cause and effect has not been firmly established, overuse of symptomatic migraine drugs, opioid or butalbital compounds, or analgesics is implicated in the development of chronic daily headaches with either a migraine-like or a mixed migraine-like and tension-type-like presentation.

Whereas overuse is defined in terms of treatment days (not doses) per month, the stipulation "on a regular basis" is significant—i.e., 2 to 3 days per week on an ongoing basis. Taking symptomatic medications on several successive days with long periods without medication use does not seem to be associated with medication-overuse headache. This strategy, in fact, is often used to prevent severe menstrual migraine attacks.

MIGRAINE DISORDERS

One of the most common neurological disorders, migraine criteria have been formulated by the IHS. Common migraine is now referred to as migraine without aura, and migraine with aura corresponds to classic migraine.

Table 10
Diagnostic Criteria for Paroxysmal Hemicranias

Chronic paroxysmal hemicrania
- A. At least 30 attacks fulfilling criteria B–E.
- B. Attacks of severe unilateral orbital, supraorbital, and/or temporal pain always on the same side, lasting 2–45 minutes.
- C. Attack frequency greater than five a day for more than half the time and tearing (periods with lower frequency may occur).
- D. Pain is associated with at least one of the following signs/symptoms on the pain side:
    1. Conjunctival injection.
    2. Lacrimation.
    3. Nasal congestion.
    4. Rhinorrhea.
    5. Ptosis.
    6. Eyelid edema.
- E. At least one of the following:
    1. There is no suggestion of one of the disorders such as trigeminal neuralgia, idiopathic stabbing headache, cough headache, benign exertional headache, headache associated with sexual activity, or hypnic headache.
    2. Such a disorder is suggested but excluded by appropriate investigations.
    3. Such a disorder is present, but the first headache attacks do not occur in close temporal relation to the disorder.

Note: Most cases respond rapidly and absolutely to indomethacin (usually in doses of 150 mg/day or less)

Episodic paroxysmal hemicrania
- A. At least 30 attacks fulfilling criteria B–F.
- B. Attacks of severe unilateral orbital or temporal pain, or both, that is always unilateral and lasts from 1 to 30 minutes.
- C. An attack frequency of three or more a day.
- D. Clear intervals between bouts of attacks that may last months to years.
- E. Pain is associated with at least one of the following signs or symptoms on the painful side:
    1. Conjunctival injection.
    2. Lacrimation.
    3. Nasal congestion.
    4. Rhinorrhea.
    5. Ptosis.
    6. Eyelid edema.
- F. At least one of the following:
    1. There is no suggestion of one of the disorders such as trigeminal neuralgia, idiopathic stabbing headache, cough headache, benign exertional headache, headache associated with sexual activity, or hypnic headache.
    2. Such a disorder is suggested but excluded by investigations..
    3. Such a disorder is present, but the first headache attacks do not occur in close temporal relation to the disorder.

Note: In most cases responds rapidly and absolutely to indomethacin (usually 150 mg/day or less).

Adapted with permission from Goadsby PJ, Lipton RB. A review of paroxysmal hemicranias SUNCT syndrome and other short-lasting headache with autonomic features, including new cases. Brain 1997;120:193–209.

Chronic Migraine Headache

Migraine that occurs frequently enough, or with the use of frequent medications, may transform itself into a chronic daily headache or chronic migraine. The episodic antecedent headaches are almost always migraine without aura.

Basilar-Type Migraine

Basilar-type migraine, or basilar migraine, is also sometimes known as Bickerstaff's migraine, after his original description in 1961. Basilar-type migraine is a form of migraine with aura characterized

Table 11
Diagnostic Criteria for SUNCT Syndrome

SUNCT (*s*hort-lasting *u*nilateral *n*euralgiform headache with *c*onjunctival injection and *t*earing) syndrome is characterized by short-lasting attacks of unilateral pain that are much briefer than those seen in any other trigeminal-autonomic cephalagia and very often accompanied by prominent lacrimation and redness of the ipsilateral eye.

A. At least 20 attacks fulfilling criteria B–D.
B. Attacks of unilateral orbital, supraorbital, or temporal stabbing or pulsating pain lasting 5–240 seconds.
C. Pain is accompanied by ipsilateral conjunctival injection and lacrimation.
D. Attacks occur with a frequency from 3 to 200 per day.
E. Not attributed to another disorder.[a]

[a]History and physical and neurological examinations do not suggest any of the disorders, such as trigeminal neuralgia, idiopathic stabbing headache, cough headache, benign exertional headache, headache associated with sexual activity, or hypnic headache, or history and/or physical and/or neurological examinations do suggest such disorder but it is ruled out by appropriate investigations, or such disorder is present but attacks do not occur for the first time in close temporal relation to the disorder.

(Adapted with permission from Headache Classification Subcommittee of the International Headache Society. The International Classification of Headache Disorders, 2nd ed. Cephalalgia 2004;24:S9–S60, and from Blackwell Publishing.)

Table 12
Modified Dandy Criteria for Idiopathic Intracranial Hypertension

1. Signs and symptoms of increased intracranial pressure (headaches, nausea, vomiting, transient visual obscurations, papilledema).
2. No localizing neurologic signs, with the exception of unilateral or bilateral cranial nerve VI paresis.
3. Cerebrospinal fluid can show increased pressure, but otherwise without cytological or chemical abnormalities.
4. Normal to small symmetric ventricles must be demonstrated by neuroimaging.

Note: the typical patient profile ("typical patient;" *see* Table 13) of a young obese woman is not required by these criteria, although the presence of idiopathic intracranial hypertension in a child, man, or thin or elderly individual would now be classified as being an "atypical case."

The modified Dandy criteria have been clarified by Friedman and Jacobson, in accordance with improved neuroimaging data.

(Adapted with permission from Friedman DI, Jacobson DM. Diagnostic criteria for idiopathic intracranial hypertension. Neurology 2002;59:1492–1495, and from Lippincott, Williams, and Wilkens.)

Table 13
Criteria for Diagnosing Idiopathic Intracranial Hypertension

1. If symptoms present, they may only reflect those of generalized intracranial hypertension or papilledema.
2. If signs present, they may only reflect those of generalized intracranial hypertension or papilledema.
3. Documented elevated intracranial pressure measured in the lateral decubitus position.
4. Normal cerebrospinal fluid composition.
5. No evidence of hydrocephalus, mass, structural, or vascular lesion on magnetic resonance imaging (MRI) or contrast-enhanced computed tomography for typical patients, and MRI or MR venography for all others.
6. No other cause of intracranial hypertension identified.

Adapted with permission from Friedman DI, Jacobson DM. Diagnostic criteria for idiopathic intracranial hypertension. Neurology 2002;59:1492–1495, and from Lippincott, Williams, and Wilkens.

by combinations of vertigo, diplopia, paresthesias, tinnitus, confusion or stupor, disorientation, and slurred speech. The headache is often a severe occipital throbbing type. Alternating hemiplegia has also been attributed to basilar-type migraine, but some authorities feel that the presence of motor weakness suggests a different form of migraine.

Table 14

Diagnostic Criteria According to the International Headache Society for Postdural (Post-Lumbar) Puncture Headache

A. Headache that worsens within 15 minutes after sitting or standing and improves within 15 minutes after lying down, with at least one of the following and fulfilling criteria C and D:
   1. Neck stiffness.
   2. Tinnitus.
   3. Hypacusia.
   4. Photophobia.
   5. Nausea.
B. Dural puncture has been performed.
C. Headache develops within 5 days after dural puncture.
D. Headache resolves either:[a]
   1. Spontaneously within 1 week.
   2. Within 48 hours after effective treatment of the spinal fluid leak (usually by epidural blood patch).

[a]In 95% of cases, this is so. When headache persists, causation is in doubt.

(Adapted with permission from Headache Classification Subcommittee of the International Headache Society. The International Classification of Headache Disorders, 2nd ed. Cephalalgia 2004;24:S9–S60, and from Blackwell Publishing.)

Table 15

Diagnostic Criteria According to the International Headache Society for Cerebrospinal Fluid Fistula Headache

A. Headache that worsens within 15 minutes after sitting or standing, with at least one of the following and fulfilling criteria C and D:
   1. Neck stiffness.
   2. Tinnitus.
   3. Hypacusia.
   4. Photophobia.
   5. Nausea.
B. A known procedure or trauma has caused persistent cerebrospinal fluid (CSF) leakage with at least one of the following:
   1. Evidence of low CSF pressure on magnetic resonance imaging (e.g., pachymeningeal enhancement).
   2. Evidence of CSF leakage on conventional myelography, computer tomography myelography, or cisternography.
   3. CSF opening pressure lower than 60 mm H_2O in sitting position.
C. Headache develops in close temporal relation to CSF leakage.
D. Headache resolves within 7 days of sealing the CSF leak.

Adapted with permission from Headache Classification Subcommittee of the International Headache Society. The International Classification of Headache Disorders, 2nd ed. Cephalalgia 2004;24:S9–S60, and from Blackwell Publishing.

Table 16

Diagnostic Criteria According to the International Headache Society for Headache Attributed to Spontaneous (or Idiopathic) Low Cerebrospinal Fluid Pressure

Diagnostic criteria

A. Diffuse and/or dull headache that worsens within 15 minutes after sitting or standing, with at least one of the following and fulfilling criterion:
   1. Neck stiffness.
   2. Tinnitus.
   3. Hypacusia.
   4. Photophobia.
   5. Nausea.

(Continued)

Table 16 *(Continued)*

Diagnostic criteria

B. At least one of the following:
    1. Evidence of low cerebrospinal fluid (CSF) pressure on magnetic resonance imaging (e.g., pachymeningeal enhancement).
    2. Evidence of CSF leakage on conventional myelography, computed tomography myelography, or cisternography.
    3. CSF opening pressure lower than 60 mm H_2O in sitting position.
C. No history of dural puncture or other cause of CSF fistula.
D. Headache resolves within 72 hours after epidural blood patching.

Adapted with permission from Headache Classification Subcommittee of the International Headache Society. The International Classification of Headache Disorders, 2nd ed. Cephalalgia 2004;24:S9–S60, and from Blackwell Publishing.

Table 17
Diagnostic Criteria According to the International Headache Society for Medication-Overuse Headache

1. Ergotamines or triptans more than 10 days/month on a regular basis for more than 3 months.
2. Opioids or combination analgesics more than 10 days/month on a regular basis for more than 3 months.
3. Simple analgesics more than 15 days/month for more than 3 months.

Adapted with permission from Headache Classification Subcommittee of the International Headache Society. The International Classification of Headache Disorders, 2nd ed. Cephalalgia 2004;24:S9–S60, and from Blackwell Publishing.

Table 18
Diagnostic Criteria According to the International Headache Society for Migraine Without Aura

Episodic attacks lasting 4 to 72 hours
Two of the following symptoms:
1. Unilateral location.
2. Pulsating quality.
3. Aggravation on movement.
4. Moderate to severe intensity.
AND one of the following symptoms during the headache:
1. Nausea and/or vomiting.
2. Photophobia and phonophobia.
At least five attacks fulfilling the above criteria.

Adapted with permission from Headache Classification Subcommittee of the International Headache Society. The International Classification of Headache Disorders, 2nd ed. Cephalalgia 2004;24:S9–S60, and from Blackwell Publishing.

Table 19
Diagnostic Criteria According to the International Headache Society for Migraine With Aura

1. At least two headache attacks by history, consistent with criteria 2–7.
2. No other disease present that might cause headache or neurological/visual changes.
3. Fully reversible visual or sensory or speech symptoms, and no motor weakness.
4. Unilateral headache location.
5. At least one symptom that develops gradually (>5 minutes) or a variety of symptoms occurring in a sequence.
6. Various symptoms lasting between 5 and 60 minutes.
7. Headache also meets criteria for migraine without aura, beginning within 0–60 minutes of aura.

Adapted with permission from Headache Classification Subcommittee of the International Headache Society. The International Classification of Headache Disorders, 2nd ed. Cephalalgia 2004;24:S9–S60, and from Blackwell Publishing.

Table 20
Diagnostic Criteria According to the International Headache Society of Migraine-Related Vestibulopathy

- Episodic vestibular symptoms: vertigo, illusory sense of motion, positional vertigo.
- Migraine according to International Headache Society criteria.
- At least one of the following migrainous symptoms during at least two vertiginous attacks: headache, photophobia, phonophobia, visual, or other auras.
- Other causes of dizziness ruled out by appropriate investigations.
- Self- or family history of migraine.

Adapted with permission from Headache Classification Subcommittee of the International Headache Society. The International Classification of Headache Disorders, 2nd ed. Cephalalgia 2004;24:S9–S60, and from Blackwell Publishing.

Table 21
International Headache Society Diagnostic Criteria for Chronic Migraine Headache

I. **Chronic migraine**: Headache (not attributable to another disorder) on more than 15 days/month for more than 3 months fulfilling the following criteria for migraine:
   At least two of the following:
   a. Unilateral location.
   b. Pulsating quality.
   c. Moderate/severe pain intensity.
   d. Aggravation by routine physical activity.
   At least one of the following:
   a. Nausea and/or vomiting.
   b. Photophobia and phonophobia.
   Not attributable to another disorder.

II. **Probable chronic migraine:** Headache meeting criteria for chronic migraine but in the presence of recent medication overuse (according to the criteria for medication overuse headache).

Adapted with permission from Headache Classification Subcommittee of the International Headache Society. The International Classification of Headache Disorders, 2nd ed. Cephalalgia 2004;24:S9–S60, and from Blackwell Publishing.

In order to help differentiate basilar migraine from familial hemiplegic migraine, Thomsen et al. suggested adding that basilar migraine not be diagnosed when there is motor weakness. Considering the overlap with both migraine headache and the often genetically determined familial hemiplegic migraine (FHM), the etiology of basilar migraine is intriguing.

FAMILIAL HEMIPLEGIC MIGRAINE

FHM is a dominantly inherited form of migraine with aura. The clinical expression of the disorder may be variable within a family, and attacks of vertigo, periodic ataxia, epilepsy, or coma may occur in about 20% of families. Multiple studies have shown that FHM is linked to the *CACNA1A* gene on chromosome 19q13.

Based on a Danish population based study, Thomsen and colleagues proposed the following modifications to the original IHS familial hemiplegic migraine criteria. The same authors also point out that many patients with FHM also fulfill criteria for basilar migraine, and proposed modifications to that syndrome's criteria (*see* "Basilar Migraine" section).

TENSION HEADACHES

Several variants of tension headaches are recognized, including episodic tension and chronic tension headaches. The diagnostic criteria for these primary, benign headaches are from the IHS

Table 22
Diagnostic Criteria According to the International Headache Society for Basilar-Type Migraine

Description: Migraine with aura symptoms clearly originating from the brainstem and/or from both hemispheres simultaneously affected, but no motor weakness.

Diagnostic criteria:

A. At least two attacks fulfilling criteria B–D.
B. Aura consisting of at least two of the following fully reversible symptoms, but no motor weakness:
    1. Dysarthria.
    2. Vertigo.
    3. Tinnitus.
    4. Hypacusia.
    5. Diplopia.
    6. Visual symptoms simultaneously in both temporal and nasal fields of both eyes.
    7. Ataxia.
    8. Decreased level of consciousness.
    9. Simultaneously bilateral paraesthesias.
C. At least one of the following:
    1. At least one aura symptom develops gradually over at least 5 minutes and/or different aura symptoms occur in succession over at least 5 minutes.
    2. Each aura symptom lasts at least 5 and less than 60 minutes.
D. Headache fulfilling criteria B–D for *Migraine without aura* begins during the aura or follows aura within 60 minutes.
E. Not attributed to another disorder.

Adapted with permission from Headache Classification Subcommittee of the International Headache Society. The International Classification of Headache Disorders, 2nd Edition. Cephalalgia 2004;24:S9–S60, and from Blackwell Publishing.

Table 23
Proposed New Diagnostic Criteria for Familial Hemiplegic Migraine

Description: Migraine with aura including motor weakness and where at least one first- or second-degree relative has migraine aura including motor weakness.

Diagnostic criteria

A. At least two attacks fulfilling criteria B–E.
B. Fully reversible symptoms including motor weakness and at least one of the following:
    1. visual, sensory, or speech disturbance.
C. At least two of the following:
    1. At least one aura symptom develops gradually over at least 5 minutes or symptoms occur in succession.
    2. Each aura symptom lasts less than 24 hours.
    3. Some degree of headache is associated with the aura.
D. At least one first- or second-degree relative has migraine aura including motor weakness fulfilling criteria A, B, C, and E.
E. Not attributed to another disorder.

Adapted with permission from Thomsen LL, Eriksen MK, Roemer SF, Andersen I, Oleson J, Russell MB. A population-based study of familial hemiplegic migraine suggests revised diagnostic criteria Brain 2002;125;1379–1391, and from Oxford University Press.

revised diagnostic criteria. They are distinct from migraine primarily by their lack of nausea or vomiting, and the presence of either phono- or photophobia, but not both. From a clinical perspective, patients may have both classes of headaches at different times, and the criteria do not address issues of pathophysiology. The issue of neuroimaging is also not addressed by the criteria, and many secondary headaches, such as cerebral neoplasms, may present with headaches that fulfill the IHS criteria.

Table 24
Diagnostic Criteria for Tension-Type Headaches

I. **Episodic tension-type headaches**
   A. At least 10 previous headache episodes fulfilling criteria B–D. Number of days with such headache less than 180 per year.
   B. Headache lasting from 30 minutes to 7 days.
   C. At least two of the following pain characteristics:
      1. Pressing/tightening (nonpulsating) quality.
      2. Mild or moderate intensity.
      3. Bilateral location.
      4. No aggravation by walking stairs or similar routine physical activity.
   D. Both of the following:
      1. No nausea or vomiting (anorexia may occur).
      2. Photophobia and phonophobia are absent, or one but not the other is present.
II. **Chronic tension-type headache**
   A. Same as tension-type headache, except number of days with such headaches: at least 15 days per month, for at least 6 months.
III. **Chronic daily headache**
   A. Features of tension-type headache.
   B. Occurs at least 6 days per week.

Adapted with permission from Headache Classification Subcommittee of the International Headache Society. The International Classification of Headache Disorders, 2nd ed. Cephalalgia 2004;24:S9–S60, and from Blackwell Publishing.

SOURCES

Cervicogenic Headache

Antonaci F, Ghrimai S, Bono G, et al. Cervicogenic headache: evaluation of the original diagnostic criteria. Cephalalgia 2001;21:573–583.
Sjaastad O, Fredriksen TA, Pfaffenrath V. Cervicogenic headache: diagnostic criteria. Headache 1990;30:725, 726.

Cluster Headache

Geweke LO. Misdiagnosis of cluster headache. Curr Pain Headache Rep 2002;6:76–82.
Lampl C. Childhood-onset cluster headache. Pediatr Neurol 2002;27:138–140.
Nappi G, Micieli G, Cavallini A, Zanferrari C, Sandrini G, Manzoni GC. Accompanying symptoms of cluster attacks: their relevance to the diagnostic criteria. Cephalalgia 1992;12:165–168.
Smetana GW. The diagnostic value of historical features in primary headache syndromes: a comprehensive review. Arch Intern Med 2000;160:2729–2737.
Torelli P, Cologno D, Cademartiri C, Manzoni GC. Application of the International Headache Society classification criteria in 652 cluster headache patients. Cephalalgia 2001;21:145–150.
van Vliet JA, Eekers PJ, Haan J, Ferrari MD; Dutch RUSSH Study Group. Features involved in the diagnostic delay of cluster headache. J Neurol Neurosurg Psychiatry 2003;74:1123–1125.
Wheeler SD, Carrazana EJ. Delayed diagnosis of cluster headache in African-American women. J Natl Med Assoc 2001;93:31–66.

External Compression Headache

Headache Classification Subcommittee of the International Headache Society. The International Classification of Headache Disorders, 2nd Edition. Cephalalgia 2004;24:S9–S60.

Familial Hemiplegic Migraine

Ducros A, Denier C, Joutel A, et al. The clinical spectrum of Familial Hemiplegic Migraine associated with mutations in a neuronal calcium channel. N Engl J Med 2001;345:17–24.
Ducros A, Joutel A, Vahedi K, Cecillon M, Ferreira A, Bernard E, et al. Mapping of a second locus for familial hemiplegic migraine to 1q21–q23 and evidence of further heterogeneity. Ann Neurol 1997;42:885–890.
Joutel A, Bousser MG, Biousse V, Labauge P, Chabriat H, Nibbio A, et al. A gene for familial hemiplegic migraine maps to chromosome 19. Nature Genet 1993;5:40–45.

Ophoff RA, Terwindt GM, Vergouwe MN, et al. Familial hemiplegic migraine and episodic ataxia type-2 are caused by mutations in the Ca^{2+} channel gene *CACNL1A4*. Cell 1996;87:543–552.

Terwindt GM, Ophoff RA, Haan J, Sandkuijl LA, Frants RR, Ferrari MD. Migraine, ataxia and epilepsy: a challenging spectrum of genetically determined calcium channelopathies. Eur J Hum Genet 1998;6:297–307.

Thomsen LL, Eriksen MK, Roemer SF, Andersen I, Oleson J, Russell MB. A population-based study of familial hemiplegic migraine suggests revised diagnostic criteria Brain 2002;125:1379–1391.

Headache Related to Intrathecal Injections

Bomgaars L, Geyer JR, Franklin J, et al. Phase I trial of intrathecal liposomal cytarabine in children with neoplastic meningitis. J Clin Oncol 2004;22:3916–3921.

Huston CW, Slipman CW, Garvin C. Complications and side effects of cervical and lumbosacral selective nerve root injections. Arch Phys Med Rehabil 2005;86:277–283.

Lo SK, Montgomery JN, Blagden S, et al. Reducing incidence of headache after lumbar puncture and intrathecal cytotoxics. Lancet 1999;353:2038, 2039.

Milhaud D, Heroum C, Charif M, Saulnier P, Pages M, Blard JM. Dural puncture and corticotherapy as risks factors for cerebral venous sinus thrombosis. Eur J Neurol. 2000;7:123, 124.

Tali ET, Ercan N, Kaymaz M, Pasaoglu A, Jinkins JR. Intrathecal gadolinium (gadopentetate dimeglumine)-enhanced MR cisternography used to determine potential communication between the cerebrospinal fluid pathways and intracranial arachnoid cysts. Neuroradiology 2004;46:744–754.

Van de Velde M, Corneillie M, Vanacker B, et al. Treatment for postdural puncture headache associated with late postpartum eclampsia. Acta Anaesthesiol Belg 1999;50:99–102.

Hemicrania Continua

Dodick, D. Hemicrania continua: diagnostic criteria and nosologic status. Cephalalgia 2001;21:869–872.

Goadsby PJ, Lipton RB. A review of paroxysmal hemicranias SUNCT syndrome and other short-lasting headache with autonomic features, including new cases. Brain 1997;120:193–209.

Pareja JA, Vincent M, Antonaci F, Sjaastad O. Hemicrania continua: diagnostic criteria and nosologic status. Cephalalgia 2001;21:874–877.

Sjaastad O, Spierings EL. Hemicrania continua: another headache absolutely responsive to indomethacin. Cephalalgia 1984;4:65–70.

Idiopathic Intracranial Hypertension

Friedman DI, Jacobson DM. Diagnostic criteria for idiopathic intracranial hypertension. Neurology 2002;59:1492–1495.

Smith JL. Whence pseudotumor cerebri? J Clin Neuroophthalmol 1985;5:55, 56.

Medication-Overuse Headache

Headache Classification Subcommittee of the International Headache Society. The International Classification of Headache Disorders, 2nd Edition. Cephalalgia 2004;24:S9–S60.

Silberstein S, Olesen J, Bousser MG, et al. The International Classification of Headache Disorders, 2nd Edition (ICHD-II)-revision of criteria for 8.2 Medication-overuse headache. Cephalalgia 2005;25:460–465.

Migraine Disorders

Headache Classification Subcommittee of the International Headache Society. The International Classification of Headache Disorders, 2nd Edition. Cephalalgia 2004;24:S9–S60.

Neuhauser H, Leopold M, von Brevern M, Arnold G, Lempert T. The interrelations of migraine, vertigo, and migrainous vertigo. Neurology 2001;56:436–441.

Basilar-Type Headache

Bickerstaff ER. Basilar artery migraine. Lancet 1961;1:15–17.

Headache Classification Subcommittee of the International Headache Society. The International Classification of Headache Disorders, 2nd Edition. Cephalalgia 2004;24:S9–S60.

Thomsen LL, Eriksen MK, Roemer SF, Andersen I, Oleson J, Russell MB. A population-based study of familial hemiplegic migraine suggests revised diagnostic criteria Brain 2002;125:1379–1391.

Post-Lumbar Puncture Headache

Headache Classification Subcommittee of the International Headache Society. The International Classification of Headache Disorders, 2nd Edition. Cephalalgia 2004;24:S9–S60.

Mokri B. Headaches caused by decreased intracranial pressure: diagnosis and management. Curr Opin Neurol 200316:319–326.

Vilmin ST, Koster R. Post-lumbar puncture headache: clinical features and suggestions for diagnostic criteria. Cephalalgia 1997;17:778–784.

Tension Headache

Lipton RB, Cady RK, Stewart WF, Wilks K, Hal C. Diagnostic lessons from the Spectrum Study. Neurology 2002;58:S27–S31.

Özge A, Bugdayci R, Sasmaz T, et al. The sensitivity and specificity of the case definition criteria in diagnosis of headache: a school-based epidemiological study of 5562 children in Mersin. Cephalalgia 2003;23:138–145.

Rossi LN, Cortinovis I, Menegazzo L, Brunelli G, Bossi A, Macchi M. Classification criteria and distinction between migraine and tension-type headache in children. Dev Med Child Neurol 2001;43:45–51.

Waldie KE, Poulton R. Physical and psychological correlates of primary headache in young adulthood: a 26-year longitudinal study. J Neurol Neurosurg Psychiatry 2002;72:86–92.

Zebenholzer K, Wober C, Kienbacher C, Wober-Bingol C. Migrainous disorder and headache of the tension-type not fulfilling the criteria: a follow-up study in children and adolescents. Cephalalgia 2000;20:611–616.

9

Immune-Based Disorders

ACUTE RHEUMATIC FEVER

The Jones criteria (Table 1) continue to form the core of diagnosing acute rheumatic fever. It is included here because of its association with neurological disorders, such as Sydenham's chorea, and its etiological link with pediatric autoimmune neuropsychiatric disorder associated with streptococcal infections syndrome (*see* Chapter 10).

NEURO-SWEET DISEASE

Sweet's disease is an inflammatory dermatological condition characterized by malaise, fever, leukocytosis, and raised erythematous plaques. It is also known as acute febrile neutrophilic dermatosis. Painful, dull-red plaques are characteristic. Skin biopsies reveal deep dermal infiltration of mature neutrophils, spared epidermis, and absence of vasculitis.

Sweet's disease may involve the nervous system in multiple ways, and these manifestations have been labeled *Neuro-Sweet disease*. Common manifestations include meningoencephalitis, headache, alterations in consciousness, epilepsy, neuropsychiatric disturbances, and movement disorders. Lesions on neuroimaging may be found in multiple brain areas. It needs to be distinguished from other multisystem inflammatory diseases that involve the nervous system, especially Neuro-Behçet's disease. Recently proposed diagnostic criteria are in Table 2.

PARANEOPLASTIC DISORDERS

Paraneoplastic syndromes are a group of disorders defined by their association with cancer. Although of unknown origin, many are associated with specific antineural antibodies, suggesting an immune basis for these disorders.

Although there are well-known syndromes associated with specific antibodies, such as cerebellar degeneration with anti-Yo antibodies, there may be multiple syndromes associated with an antibody, and multiple sites of origin of cancers associated with that antibody as well.

Recognizing these difficulties, an international panel has published diagnostic criteria for paraneoplastic syndromes (Table 3). The classic and nonclassic paraneoplastic syndromes are listed in Table 4.

POLYARTERITIS NODOSA

Neurological symptoms constitute two of the cardinal features in the American College of Rheumatology (ACR) diagnostic criteria for polyarteritis nodosa. Biopsy of an affected nerve or muscle may show polymorphonuclear infiltrate in blood vessels, consistent with this disorder.

From: *Current Clinical Neurology: Diagnostic Criteria in Neurology*
Edited by: A. J. Lerner © Humana Press Inc., Totowa, NJ

Table 1
Jones Diagnostic Criteria for Acute Rheumatic Fever (in Conjunction With Culture or Serological Evidence of Recent Streptococcal Infection)

Major	*Minor*
Carditis	*Clinical*
Polyarthritis	Fever
Eryhthema marginatum	Arthralgia
Subcutaneous nodules	
Chorea	*Laboratory*
	Increased erythrocyte sedimentation rate
	Increased C-reactive protein
	ECG
	Prolonged P–R interval

ECG, electrocardiogram.
(Reprinted with permission from American Heart Association. Jones criteria, updated. JAMA 1992;268:2069.)

Table 2
Criteria for Neuro-Sweet Disease (NSD)

1. Neurological features
   Highly systemic glucocorticoid-responsive or sometimes spontaneously remitting, but frequently recurrent encephalitis or meningitis, usually accompanied with fever higher than 38°C.
2. Dermatological features
   Painful or tender, dull-red erythematous plaques or nodules preferentially occurring on the face, neck, upper limbs, and upper part of the trunk. Predominantly neutrophilic infiltration of the dermis, spared epidermis, and absence of leukocytoclastic vasculitis.
3. Other features
   Absence of cutaneous vasculitis and thrombosis, which are seen in Behçet disease. Absence of typical uveitis, which is seen in Behçet disease.
4. HLA association
   HLA-Cw1- or B54-positive.
   HLA-B51-negative
   Probable NSD: All of 1, 2, and 3.
   Possible NSD: Any neurological manifestations, either 2 or 4, and one item or more of 3.

Any other neurological diseases that can explain the neurological symptoms and signs, except Neuro-Behçet disease, should be excluded before the diagnosis of Neuro-Sweet disease is made.
(Adapted from Hisanaga K, Iwasaki Y, Itoyama Y, Neuro-Sweet Disease Study Group. Neurology 2005;64:1756–1761.)

Table 3
Diagnostic Criteria for Paraneoplastic Syndromes

Definite paraneoplastic syndromes
1. A classic syndrome and cancer that develops within 5 years of the diagnosis of the neurological disorder.
2. A nonclassic syndrome that resolves or significantly improves after cancer treatment without concomitant immunotherapy, provided that the syndrome is not susceptible to spontaneous remission.
3. A nonclassic syndrome with onconeural antibodies (well-characterized or not) and cancer that develops within 5 years of the diagnosis of the neurological disorder.
4. A neurological syndrome (classic or not) with well characterized onconeural antibodies (anti-HU, Yo, CV2, Ri, Ma2, or amphiphysin), and no cancer.

Possible paraneoplastic syndromes
1. A classic syndrome, no onconeural antibodies, no cancer but at high risk to have an underlying tumor.
2. A neurological syndrome (classic or not) with partially characterized onconeural antibodies and no cancer.
3. A nonclassic syndrome, no onconeural antibodies, and cancer present within 2 years of diagnosis.

Adapted with permission from Graus F, Delattre JY, Antoine JC, et al. Recommended diagnostic criteria for paraneoplastic neurological syndromes. J Neurol Neurosurg Psychiatry 2004;5:1135–1140.

Table 4
Classic and Nonclassic Paraneoplastic Neurological Syndromes

Classic syndromes	Nonclassic syndromes
Syndromes of the central nervous system	
Encephalomyelitis	Brainstem encephalitis
Limbic encephalitis	Optic neuritis[b]
Subacute cerebellar degeneration	Cancer-associated retinopathy[b]
Opsoclonus-myoclonus[a]	Melanoma-associated retinopathy[b]
	Stiff person syndrome
	Necrotizing myelopathy[c]
	Motor neuron diseases[c]
Syndromes of the peripheral nervous system	
Subacute sensory neuropathy	Acute sensorimotor neuropathy
Chronic gastrointestinal pseudo-obstruction	Guillain-Barre Syndrome[c]
	Brachial neuritis[c]
	Subacute/chronic sensorimotor neuropathies[a]
	Neuropathy and paraproteinemia
	Neuropathy with vasculitis[c]
	Acute pandysautonomia[c]
Syndromes of the neuromuscular junction and muscle	
Lambert-Eaton myasthenic syndrome[c]	Myasthenia gravis[b]
Dermatomyositis[c]	Acquired neuromyotonia[c]
	Acute necrotizing myopathy[c]

[a]Associated with onconeural antibodies only with certain types of tumor.
[b]Syndromes not included in Table 3 criteria.
[c]Syndromes not associated with known onconeural antibodies.
(Adapted with permission from Graus F, Delattre JY, Antoine JC, et al. Recommended diagnostic criteria for para-neoplastic neurological syndromes. J Neurol Neurosurg Psychiatry 2004;5:1135–1140, and from BMJ Publishing Group.)

Table 5
1990 Criteria for the Classification of Polyarteritis Nodosa

1. Weight loss: Loss of 4 kg or more of body weight since illness began, not because of dieting or other factors.
2. Livedo reticularis: Mottled reticular pattern over the skin or portions of the extremities or torso.
3. Testicular pain or tenderness: Pain or tenderness of the testicles, not because of infection, trauma, or other causes.
4. Myalgias, weakness, or leg tenderness: Diffuse myalgias (excluding shoulder and hip girdle) or weakness of muscles or tenderness of leg muscles.
5. Mononeuropathy or polyneuropathy: Development of mononeuropathy, multiple mononeuropathies, or polyneuropathy.
6. Diastolic blood pressure higher than 90 mmHg: Development of hypertension with diastolic blood pressure higher than 90 mmHg.
7. Elevated blood urea nitrogen or creatinine: Elevation of blood urea nitrogen greater than 40 mg/dL or creatinine greater than 1.5 mg/dL, not because of dehydration or obstruction.
8. Hepatitis B virus: Presence of hepatitis B surface antigen or antibody in serum.
9. Arteriographic abnormality: Arteriogram showing aneurysms or occlusions of the visceral arteries, not because of arteriosclerosis, fibromuscular dysplasia, or other noninflammatory causes.
10. Biopsy of small or medium-sized artery containing polymorphonuclear neutrophils: Histologicalchanges showing the presence of granulocytes or granulocytes and mononuclear leukocytes in the artery wall.

For classification purposes, a patient shall be said to have polyarteritis nodosa if at least 3 of these 10 criteria are present. The presence of any three or more criteria yields a sensitivity of 82.2% and a specificity of 86.6%.
(Adapted with permission from Lightfoot RW Jr, Michel BA, Bloch DA, et al. The American College of Rheumatology 1990 criteria for the classification of polyarteritis nodosa. Arthritis Rheum 1990;33:1088–1093, and from John Wiley and Sons.)

Table 6
Diagnostic Criteria for Polymyalgia Rheumatica

I. Diagnostic criteria from Bird et al.
   A. Bilateral shoulder pain or stiffness.
   B. Bilateral tenderness in upper arms.
   C. Abrupt onset of illness (<2 weeks).
   D. Erythrocyte sedimentation rate greater than 40 mm/hour.
   E. Morning stiffness (>1 hour in duration).
   F. Age: Older than 65 years (72% sensitivity); older than 50 years (100% sensitivity).
   G. Systemic signs: depression and weight loss.
   The presence of any three criteria *or* at least one criterion coexisting with a clinical or pathological abnormality of the temporal artery, suggests probable polymyalgia rheumatica.
II. Diagnostic criteria from Jones and Hazleman
   All of the following:
   A. Shoulder and pelvic girdle muscle pain without weakness.
   B. Morning stiffness.
   C. Symptom duration of more than 2 months unless treated.
   D. Erythrocyte sedimentation rare greater than 30 mm/hour or C-reactive protein level greater than 6 mg/L.
   E. No rheumatoid arthritis, inflammatory arthritis, or malignant neoplasm.
   F. No objective signs of muscle disease.
   G. Prompt and dramatic response to systemic corticosteroid therapy.

Adapted with permission from Epperly TD, Moore KE, Harrover JD. Polymyalgia and temporal arteritis. Am Fam Physician 2000;62:789–796 and from the American Academy of Family Physicians.

POLYMYALGIA RHEUMATICA

The systemic version of temporal arteritis, polymyalgia rheumatica is a disorder affecting mainly older adults, with subacute onset and bilateral symptoms. Like temporal arteritis, there are elevations of systemic inflammatory markers, and the syndrome responds to corticosteroids. Several sets of diagnostic criteria have been proposed including those of Bird et al. (Table 6) and Jones and Hazelman. In a comparison study of diagnostic criteria, the Bird criteria were found to be 99.5% sensitive. Other criteria have been developed in the setting of research studies, and their application in clinical situations is not always known.

RHEUMATOID ARTHRITIS

The criteria for rheumatoid arthritis as a distinct syndrome encompass both clinical and radiographic features. It is included here because of the multiple syndromes ascribed to rheumatoid arthritis that involve directly or indirectly the central nervous system (CNS) and peripheral nervous system (Table 7).

SJÖGREN'S SYNDROME

A systemic autoimmune condition, Sjögren's syndrome may occur in both a primary form—originally described by Sjögren in 1938—or a secondary form, in association with another connective tissue/autoimmune disorder, such as rheumatoid arthritis or systemic lupus erythematosus (SLE). Cardinal symptoms include dry eyes and dry mouth, with characteristic autoantibody profile, or diagnosis by biopsy of a minor salivary gland.

Both primary and secondary forms may involve the central or peripheral nervous systems, and may be the presenting symptom. There may be focal findings secondary to a small-vessel vasculopathy with perivascular lymphocytic infiltrates. It may also present with "global" CNS dysfunction in the form of mood disturbances, sometimes misdiagnosed as "hysterical" or functional in origin. Neuropsychological testing may show deficits in memory and attention. Peripheral manifestations

Table 7
Diagnostic Criteria for Rheumatoid Arthritis

1. Morning stiffness, lasting as least 1 hour.
2. Involvement of 3 or more of 14 possible joints.
   a. Bilateral, proximal interphalangeal, metacarpophalangeal, wrist, elbow, knee ankle, metatarsophalangeal.
      i. Soft-tissue swelling.
      ii. Fluid around joints.
3. Involvement of hand joints.
   a. Wrist, metacarpophalangeal, or proximal interphalangeal joint.
4. Symmetry.
   a. Any hand joint counts as symmetric to other hand.
5. Rheumatoid nodules.
6. Rheumatoid factor.
7. Radiographic changes typical for rheumatoid arthritis.
   a. Bony erosions.
   b. Decalcification adjacent to involved joints.
   c. Osteoarthritic-type changes do not qualify.

Rheumatoid arthritis: At least four of seven criteria met.
Criteria 1–4 must be present for more than 6 weeks.

Adapted with permission from Arnett FC, Edworthy SM, Bloch DA, et al. The American Rheumatism Association 1987 revised criteria for the classification of rheumatoid arthritis. Arthritis Rheum 1988;31:315–324.

include a small-fiber sensory neuropathy, mononeuritis multiplex, trigeminal neuropathy, or sensineural deafness.

A large number of diagnostic criteria have been published over the past years of varying degrees of strictness. The most recent widely used framework is the European-American consensus criteria and is presented in Tables 8 and 9. It builds on the work of Vitali et al., who have published several sets of criteria similar to the current ones, based on large multicenter studies with criteria optimized for sensitivity and specificity using receiver–operator curve characteristics. In addition to the qualitative criteria, there is also a quantitative approach focused on the Schirmer's test and the rose bengal score for ocular evaluation of xerophthalmia, and measures of salivary gland function and minor salivary gland biopsy. Whereas these tests may be the most reliable in diagnosing Sjögren's syndrome, the sensitivity and specificity may vary depending on the age of the patient and whether the individual has primary or secondary Sjögren's syndrome.

It should also be noted that more than one set of histopathological criteria for grading salivary gland biopsies exist.

SYSTEMIC LUPUS ERYTHEMATOSUS

The wide variety of symptoms and the frequent involvement of peripheral and central nervous system, particularly with advanced disease, makes SLE important to neurologists. The ACR has also published case definitions for neuropsychiatric lupus syndromes (NPSLE), which are presented separately. In attempting to make a diagnosis of NPSLE, the patient must fulfill at least three non-neurological criteria for SLE itself.

Neuropsychiatric Systemic Lupus Erythematosus

In 1992, the ACR published a committee report on classification and case definitions of NPSLE. These case definitions were published in an appendix to the main article and are presented here in complete form. The committee recommended a basic demographic form for case-reporting purposes that is not included here. The syndromes can be subdivided into 19 syndromes encompassing both peripheral nervous system manifestations and CNS syndromes. Each of the guidelines is based on criteria with

Table 8
Revised International Classification Criteria for Sjögren's Syndrome

I. Ocular symptoms: A positive response to at least one of the following questions:
    A. Have you had daily, persistent, troublesome dry eyes for more than 3 months?
    B. Do you have a recurrent sensation of sand or gravel in the eyes?
    C. Do you use tear substitutes more than three times a day?

II. Oral symptoms: A positive response to at least one of the following questions:
    A. Have you had a daily feeling of dry mouth for more than 3 months?
    B. Have you had recurrently or persistently swollen salivary glands as an adult?
    C. Do you frequently drink liquids to aid in swallowing dry food?

III. Ocular signs: That is, objective evidence of ocular involvement defined as a positive result for at least one of the following two tests:
    A. Schirmer's I test, performed without anesthesia ($\leq$5 mm in 5 minutes).
    B. Rose bengal score or other ocular dye score ($\geq$4 according to the van Bijsterveld scoring system).

IV. Histopathology: In minor salivary glands (obtained through normal-appearing mucosa), focal lymphocytic sialoadenitis, evaluated by an expert histopathologist, with a focus score $\geq$1, defined as a number of lymphocytic foci (which are adjacent to normal-appearing mucous acini and contain more than 50 lymphocytes) per 4 mm^2 of glandular tissue.

V. Salivary gland involvement: Objective evidence of salivary gland involvement defined by a positive result for at least one of the following diagnostic tests:
    A. Unstimulated, whole salivary flow ($\leq$1.5 mL in 15 minutes).
    B. Parotid sialography showing the presence of diffuse sialectasias (punctate, cavitary, or destructive pattern), without evidence of obstruction in the major ducts.
    C. Salivary scintigraphy showing delayed uptake, reduced concentration, and/or delayed excretion of tracer.

VI. Serology: Presence in the serum of the following autoantibodies:
    A. Antibodies to Ro(SSA) or La(SSB) antigens, or both.

Adapted with permission from Vitali C, Bombardieri S, Jonsson R, et al. Classification criteria for Sjögren's syndrome: a revised version of the European criteria proposed by the American–European Consensus Group. Ann Rheum Dis 2002;61:554–558 and from BMJ Journals.

Table 9
Revised Rules for Classification of Sjögren's Syndrome

For primary Sjögren's syndrome (SS)
In patients without any potentially associated disease, primary SS may be defined as follows:
1. The presence of any four of the six criteria is indicative of primary SS (Table 8), as long as either item IV (Histopathology) or VI (Serology) is positive.
2. The presence of any three of the four objective criteria items (that is, items III, IV, V, or VI).
3. The classification tree procedure represents a valid alternative method for classification, although it should be more properly used in clinical–epidemiological survey.

For secondary SS
In patients with a potentially associated disease (for instance, another well-defined connective tissue disease), the presence of item I or item II plus any two from among items III, IV, and V may be considered as indicative of secondary SS.

Exclusion criteria:
1. Past head and neck radiation treatment.
2. Hepatitis C infection.
3. AIDS.
4. Preexisting lymphoma.
5. Sarcoidosis.
6. Graft-versus-host disease.
7. Use of anticholinergic drugs (since a time shorter than fourfold the half-life of the drug).

Adapted with permission from Vitali C, Bombardieri S, Jonsson R, et al. Classification criteria for Sjögren's syndrome: a revised version of the European criteria proposed by the American–European Consensus Group. Ann Rheum Dis 2002;61:554–558, and from BMJ Journals.

Table 10
The 1982 Revised Criteria for Classification of Systemic Lupus Erythematosus

Criterion	Definition
1. Malar rash	Fixed erythema, flat or raised, over the malar eminences, tending to spare the nasolabial folds.
2. Discoid rash	Erythematous raised patches with adherent keratotic scaling and follicular plugging; atrophic scarring may occur in older lesions.
3. Photosensitivity	Skin rash as a result of unusual reaction to sunlight, by patient history or physician observation.
4. Oral ulcers	Oral or nasopharyngeal ulceration, usually painless, observed by physician.
5. Arthritis	Nonerosive arthritis involving two or more peripheral joints, characterized by tenderness, swelling, or effusion.
6. Serositis	a. Pleuritis—convincing history of pleuritic pain or rubbing heard by a physician or evidence of pleural effusion. *OR* b. Pericarditis—documented by ECG or rub or evidence of pericardial effusion.
7. Renal disorder	a. Persistent proteinuria greater than 0.5 g/day or greater than 3+ if quantitation not performed. *OR* b. Cellular casts—may be red cell, hemoglobin, granular, tubular, or mixed.
8. Neurological disorder	a. Seizures—in the absence of offending drugs or known metabolic derangements, e.g., uremia, ketoacidosis, or electrolyte imbalance. *OR* b. Psychosis—in the absence of offending drugs or known metabolic derangements, e.g., uremia, ketoacidosis, or electrolyte imbalance.
9. Hematological disorder	a. Hemolytic anemia—with reticulocytosis. *OR* b. Leukopenia—less than 4000/mm^3 total on two or more occasions. *OR* c. Lyphopenia—less than 1500/mm^3 on two or more occasions. *OR* d. Thrombocytopenia—less than 100,000/mm^3 in the absence of offending drugs.
10. Immunological disorder	a. Positive LE cell preparation (removed in later revision). *OR* b. Anti-DNA: antibody to native DNA in abnormal titer. *OR* c. Anti-Sm: presence of antibody to Sm nuclear antigen. *OR* d. False-positive serological test for syphilis known to be positive for at least 6 months and confirmed by *Treponema pallidum* immobilization or fluorescent treponemal antibody absorption test.
11. Antinuclear antibody	An abnormal titer of antinuclear antibody by immunofluorescence or an equivalent assay at any point in time and in the absence of drugs known to be associated with "drug-induced lupus" syndrome.

The proposed classification is based on 11 criteria. For the purpose of identifying patients in clinical studies, a person shall be said to have systemic lupus erythematosus if any 4 or more of the 11 criteria are present, serially or simultaneously, during any interval of observation. ECG, electrocardiogram; LE cell, lupus erythematosus cell; Sm nuclear antigen, Smith nuclear antigen.

(Adapted with permission from Tan EM, Cohen AS, Fries JF, et al. The 1982 revised criteria for the classification of systemic lupus erythematosus. Arthritis Rheum 1982;25:1271–1277, and from John Wiley and Sons.)

substantial interrater reliability. In order for an individual to have NPSLE, three or more of the ACR (non-NPSLE) criteria for SLE must be met. Individuals with NPSLE criteria but not the SLE criteria may be said to have "possible" NPSLE. The ACR did not intend for strict classification to replace

Table 11
Case Definitions for Neuropsychiatric Syndromes in Systemic Lupus Erythematosus

1. **Acute confusional state (*see* "Delirium" section in Chapter 3)**
   Disturbance of consciousness or level of arousal characterized by reduced ability to focus, maintain, or shift attention, and accompanied by disturbances of cognition, mood, affect, and/or behavior. The disturbances typically develop over hours to days and tend to fluctuate during the course of the day. They include hypo- and hyperaroused states and encompass the spectrum from delirium to coma.[a]
   Diagnostic criteria:
   Disturbance of consciousness or level of arousal with reduced ability to focus, maintain, or shift attention, and one or more of the following developing over a short period of time (hours to days) and tending to fluctuate during the course of the day:
   a. Acute or subacute change in cognition that may include memory deficit and disorientation.
   b. A change in behavior, mood, or affect (e.g., restlessness, overactivity, reversal of the sleep/wakefulness cycle, irritability, apathy, anxiety, mood lability, etc.).
   Exclusions:[b]
   - Primary mental/neurological disorder not related to systemic lupus erythematosus (SLE).
   - Metabolic disturbances (including glucose, electrolytes, fluid, osmolarity).
   - Substance or drug-induced delirium (including withdrawal).
   - Cerebral infections.
   Associations:
   - Marked psychosocial stress.
   - Corticosteroid use.
   - Thrombotic thrombocytopenic purpura/hemolytic uremic syndrome.
2. **Acute inflammatory demyelinating polyradiculoneuropathy (*see* "Guillain-Barre Syndrome" section of Chapter 12).**
   Diagnostic criteria:
   a. Clinical features
      i. Progressive polyradiculoneuropathy, usually ascending and predominantly motor, which peaks usually within 21 days or less.
      ii. Reflex loss.
      iii. Symmetric, may involve the trunk and may cause respiratory failure.
   b. Cerebrospinal fluid(CSF)
      i. Increased CSF protein without pleocytosis.
   c. Supportive evidence by nerve conduction study including F-wave ascertainment whereby there is one abnormality in three nerves.[c] The abnormalities are:
      i. Conduction block in which the amplitude of compound muscle action potential diminishes with more proximal sites of nerve stimulation.
      ii. F waves may be absent or prolonged.
      iii. Slowing of conduction velocity.
      iv. Prolongation of distal latencies.
   Exclusions:
   - Acute spinal cord disease.
   - Botulism.
   - Poliomyelitis and other infections.
   - Acute myasthenia gravis.
3. **Anxiety disorder**
   Anticipation of danger or misfortune accompanied by apprehension, dysphoria, or tension. Includes generalized anxiety, panic disorder, panic attacks, and obsessive-compulsive disorders.[d]
   Diagnostic criteria:
   Both of the following:
   a. Prominent anxiety, panic disorder, panic attacks, or obsessions or compulsions.
   b. Disturbance causes clinically significant distress or impaired social, occupational, or other important functioning.
   Exclusions:
   - Adjustment disorder with anxiety (e.g., maladaptive response to stress of having SLE).
   - Substance- or drug-induced anxiety.
   - Anxiety occurring exclusively during the course of an acute confusional state, a mood disorder, or psychosis.

(Continued)

Table 11 *(Continued)*

> *Associations:*
> - Metabolic disorders, e.g., hyperthyroidism, pheochromocytoma.
> - Marked psychosocial stress.
> - Corticosteroid use.

4. **Aseptic Meningitis**
   Diagnostic criteria:
   All the following:
   a. Acute or subacute onset of headache with photophobia, neck stiffness, and fever.
   b. Signs of meningeal irritation.
   c. Abnormal CSF.
   Exclusions:
   Central nervous system (CNS) or meningeal inflammation because of:
   a. Infection by bacteria, mycobacteria, viruses, fungi, parasites.
   b. Subarachnoid hemorrhage.
   c. Malignancy (leukemia, lymphoma, or carcinoma) or granulomatous disease (sarcoidosis).
   d. Medications: nonsteroidal anti-inflammatory drugs, intravenous immunoglobulin, azathioprine, etc.

5. **Autonomic disorder**
   Disorder of the autonomic nervous system with orthostatic hypotension, sphincteric erectile/ejaculatory dysfunction, anhidrosis, heat intolerance, constipation.
   Diagnostic criteria:
   Symptoms and abnormal response to provocative tests:
   Test normal range
   a. Blood pressure response to standing: fall in blood pressure more than 30/15 mmHg or vertical tilt (systolic/diastolic).
   b. Heart rate response to standing: increases 11–29 beats/minute.
   c. Heart rate variation with respiration: maximum–minimum heart rate: 15 beats/minute; E:I ratio (ratio of heart rate during expiration and inspiration): 1:2.
   c. Valsalva ratio: 1:4.
   d. Sweat test: Sweating over all body and limbs.
   Exclusions:
   - Autonomic dysfunction with Lambert-Eaton syndrome.
   - Medications: tricyclic antidepressants.
   - Poisons: organophosphates.
   - Shy-Drager syndrome.
   Associations:
   - Diabetic neuropathy and peripheral neuropathy of other causes.
   - Autonomic failure in elderly.

6. **Cerebrovascular disease** *(see* **"Stroke" section of Chapter 2)**
   Diagnostic criteria:
   One of the following and supporting radioimaging study:
   a. Stroke syndrome: acute focal neurological deficit persisting more than 24 hours (or lasting less than 24 hours with computed tomography (CT) or magnetic resonance imaging (MRI) abnormality consistent with physical findings/symptoms.
   b. Transient ischemic attack: acute, focal neurological deficit with clinical resolution within 24 hours (without corresponding lesion on CT or MRI).
   c. Chronic multifocal disease: recurrent or progressive neurological deterioration attributable to cerebrovascular disease.
   d. Subarachnoid and intracranial hemorrhage: bleeding documented by CSF findings, MRI/CT.
   e. Sinus thrombosis: Acute, focal neurological deficit in the presence of increased intracranial pressure.
Note: The finding of unidentified bright objects on MRI without clinical manifestations is not classified at the present time.
   Exclusions:
   - Infection with space occupying lesions in the brain.
   - Intracranial tumor.
   - Trauma.
   - Vascular malformation.
   - Hypoglycemia.

(Continued)

Table 11 *(Continued)*

Associations:
- Diabetes mellitus.
- Dyslipidemia.
- Atherosclerotic vascular disease.
- Atrial fibrillation.
- Valvular heart disease.
- Atrial septal defect.
- Hypercoagulability state.
- Antiphospholipid antibody syndrome.
- Hypertension.
- Smoking.
- Cocaine or amphetamine abuse.

7. **Cognitive Dysfunction**

   Significant deficits in any or all of the following cognitive functions: simple or complex attention, reasoning, executive skills (e.g., planning, organizing, sequencing), memory (e.g., learning and recall), visuospatial processing, language (e.g., verbal fluency), and psychomotor speed. Cognitive dysfunction implies a decline from a higher level of functioning and ranges from mild impairment to severe dementia. It may or may not impede social, educational, or occupational functioning, depending on the function(s) impaired and the severity of impairment. Subjective complaints of cognitive dysfunction are common and may not be objectively verifiable. Neuropsychological testing should be done in suspected cognitive dysfunction, and its interpretation should be done with a neuropsychologist.

   Diagnostic criteria:
   a. Documented impairment in one or more of the following cognitive domains:
      i. Simple attention.
      ii. Complex attention.
      iii. Memory (e.g., learning and recall).
      iv. Visuospatial processing.
      v. Language (e.g., verbal fluency).
      vi. Reasoning/problem solving.
      vii. Psychomotor speed.
      viii. Executive functions (e.g., planning, organizing, and sequencing).
   b. The cognitive deficits represent a significant decline from a former level of functioning (if known).
   c. The cognitive deficits may cause varying degrees of impairment in social, educational, or occupational functioning, depending on the function(s) impaired and the degree of impairment.

   Associations:
   - Substance abuse.
   - Medication (steroids, sedatives).
   - History of learning disabilities.
   - History of head injury.
   - Other primary neurological and psychiatric disorders.
   - Metabolic disturbances, particularly uremia and diabetes.
   - Antiphospholipid antibody syndrome.
   - Coexisting emotional distress, fatigue, and pain.

8. **Demyelinating syndrome (*see* "Multiple Sclerosis," "Neuromyelitis Optica," and "Transverse Myelitis" sections of Chapter 4)**

   Diagnostic criteria:

   Two or more of the following, each occurring at different times, or one of the following occurring on at least two different occasions:
   a. Multiple discrete areas of damage to white matter within CNS, causing one or more limbs to become weak with sensory loss.
   b. Transverse myelopathy.
   c. Optic neuropathy.
   d. Diplopia because of isolated nerve palsies or internuclear ophthalmoplegia.
   e. Brain stem disease with vertigo, vomiting, ataxia, dysarthria, or dysphagia.
   f. Other cranial nerve palsies.

Table 11 *(Continued)*

Exclusions:
- Infections, e.g., tuberculosis, human T-cell lymphotropic virus-I, HIV, cytomegalovirus, *Borrelia*, CNS Whipple's disease, progressive multifocal leukoencephalopathy, syphilis.
- Vitamin B_{12} deficiency.

Associations:
- Structural lesions, e.g., tumor, arteriovenous malformation.
- Familial disorders, e.g., hereditary spastic paraplegia, ataxia, and leukodystrophies.
- Sarcoid, Behçet's disease, other vasculitis.
- Multiple sclerosis.

9. **Headache (*see* specific sections in Chapter 8 for International Headache Society criteria)**
   a. Migraine
      i. Migraine without aura: Idiopathic, recurrent headache manifested by attacks lasting 4–72 hours. Typical characteristics are unilateral location, pulsating quality, moderate-to-severe intensity, aggravation by routine physical activity, and associated with nausea, vomiting, photo- and phonophobia. At least five attacks fulfilling the aforementioned criteria.
      ii. Migraine with aura: Idiopathic, recurrent disorder manifested by attacks of neurological symptoms localizable to cerebral cortex or brain stem, usually gradually developing over 5–20 minutes and lasting less than 60 minutes. Headache, nausea, and/or photophobia usually follow neurologic aura symptoms directly or after an interval of less than 1 hour. Headache usually lasts 4–72 hours, but may be completely absent.
   b. Tension headache (episodic tension-type headache).
      Recurrent episodes of headaches lasting minutes to days. Pain typically pressing/tightening in quality, of mild-to-moderate intensity, bilateral in location, and does not worsen with routine physical activity. Nausea is rare, but photophobia and phonophobia may be present. At least 10 previous headaches fulfilling these criteria
   c. Cluster headache.
      Attacks of severe, strictly unilateral pain, orbital, supraorbital, and/or temporal, usually lasting 15–180 minutes and occurring from at least once every other day up to eight times per day. Associated with one or more of the following: conjunctival injection, lacrimation, nasal congestion, rhinorrhea, forehead and facial sweating, miosis, ptosis, eyelid edema. Attacks occur in series for weeks or months ("cluster" periods), separated by remissions of usually months or years.
   d. Headache from intracranial hypertension (also called pseudotumor cerebri, benign intracranial hypertension; *see* "Idiopathic Intracranial Hypertension" section of Chapter 8).
      All of the following:
      i. Increased intracranial pressure (200 mm H_2O) measured by lumbar puncture.
      ii. Normal neurological findings, except for papilledema and possible nerve VI palsy.
      iii. No mass lesion and no ventricular enlargement on neuroimaging.
      iv. Normal or low protein and normal white cell count in CSF.
      v. No evidence of venous sinus thrombosis.
   e. Intractable headache, nonspecific.

Exclusions:
- Aseptic meningitis (including drug-induced).
- Drug-induced pseudotumor cerebri (oral contraceptives, sulfonamides, trimethoprim, etc.).
- CNS infection.
- Tumors and other structural lesions.
- Low intracranial pressure.
- Trauma.
- Metabolic headache that remits with elimination of cause (carbon monoxide exposure).
- Withdrawal (caffeine, etc.).
- Seizure/postictal state.
- Sepsis.
- Intracranial hemorrhage or vascular occlusion.

10. **Mononeuropathy (single/multiplex)**
    Disturbed function of one or more peripheral nerve(s) resulting in weakness/paralysis or sensory dysfunction because of either conduction block in motor nerve fibers or axonal loss.

(Continued)

Table 11 *(Continued)*

Conduction block is related to demyelination with preservation of axon continuity. Remyelination may be rapid and complete. If axonal interruption takes place, axonal degeneration occurs below the site of interruption and recovery is often slow and incomplete. Sensory symptoms and sensory loss may affect all modalities or be restricted to certain forms of sensation.

Diagnostic criteria:

a. Clinical demonstration of motor/sensory disturbances in the distribution of a peripheral nerve *and/or*

b. Abnormalities on nerve conduction studies or electromyogram (EMG) (i.e., concentric needle examination).

Associations:

• Diabetic neuropathy.

• Local damage from mechanical injury, radiation, malignancy, sarcoid.

• Infection: Lyme disease, HIV, herpes.

• Vasculitis, polyarteritis nodosa, Wegener's granulomatosis, cryoglobulinemia, rheumatoid arthritis, Sjögren's syndrome, etc.

11. **Mood disorders**

Prominent and persistent disturbance in mood characterized by:

• Depressed mood or markedly diminished interest or pleasure in almost all activities *or*

• Elevated, expansive or irritable mood.

Diagnostic criteria:

a. Major depressive-like episode.

One or more major depressive episodes with at least five of the following symptoms, including either i or ii or both, during a 2-week period and nearly every day:

    i. Depressed mood most of the day, by subjective report or observation made by others.

    ii. Markedly diminished interest or pleasure in all, or almost all, activities most of the day, by subjective report or observation made by others.

    iii.

        (1) Significant weight loss without dieting or weight gain (>5% of body weight in 1 month).

        (2) Insomnia or hypersomnia. Psychomotor agitation or retardation (observable by others, not merely subjective feeling of restlessness or being slowed down).

        (3) Fatigue or loss of energy.

        (4) Feelings of worthlessness or excessive or inappropriate guilt (may be delusional).

        (5) Diminished ability to think or concentrate, or indecisiveness.

        (6) Recurrent thoughts of death (not just fear of dying), recurrent suicidal ideation without a specific plan, or a suicide attempt or a specific plan for committing suicide.

b. Mood disorder with depressive features.

All of the following:

    i. Prominent and persistent mood disturbance characterized by predominantly depressed mood or markedly diminished interest or pleasure in all, or almost all, activities.

    ii. Full criteria for major depressive-like episode are not met.

c. Mood disorder with manic features.

    i. Prominent and persistent mood disturbance characterized by predominantly elevated, expansive, or irritable mood.

e. Mood disorder with mixed features.

    i. Prominent and persistent mood disturbance characterized by symptoms of both depression and mania; neither predominates.

For all mood disorders:[e]

Symptoms must cause significant distress or impairment in social, occupational, or other important areas of functioning.

Exclusions:

• Primary mental disorders.

• Substance-induced mood disorder.

• Adjustment disorder with depressed mood.

12. **Movement disorder (chorea)**

Chorea: Irregular, involuntary brief and unpredictable, jerky movements that may involve any portion of the body in random sequence.

(Continued)

Table 11 (*Continued*)

Diagnostic criteria:

Both of the following:

a. Observed abnormal movements.

b. Random, unpredictable sequence of movements.

Exclusions:

- Wilson's disease.
- Huntington's disease (and other hereditary disorders).
- Medications (neuroleptics, oral contraceptives, phenytoin, L-DOPA, calcium channel blockers).
- Illicit drugs.

13. **Myasthenia gravis (*see* "Myasthenia Gravis" section of Chapter 12)**

Neuromuscular transmission disorder characterized by fluctuating weakness and fatigability of bulbar and other voluntary muscles without loss of reflexes or impairment of sensation or other neurological function.

Myasthenia gravis is an autoimmune disorder mediated by antibodies to acetylcholine receptors. It may occur with other diseases of immunological origin.

Diagnostic criteria:

a. Characteristic signs and symptoms include one or more of the following:

   i. Diplopia, ptosis, dysarthria, weakness in chewing, difficulty in swallowing, muscle weakness with preserved deep tendon reflexes, and, less commonly, weakness of neck extension and flexion, and weakness of trunk muscles.

   ii. Increased weakness during exercise and repetitive use with at least partially restored strength after periods of rest.

   iii. Dramatic improvement in strength following administration of anticholinesterase drug (edrophonium and neostigmine).

And one or more of the following:

b. EMG and repetitive stimulation of a peripheral nerve: In myasthenia gravis, repetitive stimulation at a rate of two per second shows characteristic decremental response that is reversed by edrophonium or neostigmine. Single-fiber studies show increased jitter.

c. Antibodies to acetylcholine receptors.

Exclusions:

- Congenital myasthenic syndrome, progressive restricted myopathies, steroid and inflammatory myopathies, motor neuron disease.
- Multiple sclerosis, variants of Guillain-Barre syndrome (e.g., Miller-Fisher syndrome).
- Organophosphate toxicity, botulism, black widow spider venom.
- Eaton-Lambert syndrome.
- Stroke.
- Medications: neuromuscular blocking agents, aminoglycosides, penicillamine, antimalarial drugs, colistin, streptomycin, polymyxin B, tetracycline.
- Hypokalemia; hypophosphatemia.

Associations:

- Pure red cell aplasia.
- Thyroid abnormalities.
- Thymoma.

14. **Myelopathy (*see* "Transverse Myelitis" section of Chapter 4)**

Diagnostic criteria:

Usually rapid onset (hours or days) of one or more of the following:

a. Bilateral weakness of legs with or without arms (paraplegia/quadriplegia); may be asymmetric.

b. Sensory impairment with cord level similar to that of motor weakness, with or without bowel and bladder dysfunction.

Exclusions:

- Mass lesion causing compression of or within spinal cord (e.g., prolapsed disc, tumor, hematoma, or ruptured spinal arteriovenous malformation).
- *Cauda equina* lesion.

Table 11 *(Continued)*

15. **Neuropathy, cranial**
    Diagnostic criteria:
    Syndrome corresponding to specific nerve function:
    a. Olfactory nerve: loss of sense of smell, distortion of smell, and loss of olfactory discrimination.
    b. Optic nerve: decrease or loss of visual acuity, diminished color perception, afferent pupillary defect, and visual field deficits.
    c. Oculomotor nerve: ptosis of the upper eyelid and inability to rotate eye upward, downward, or inward (complete lesion), and/or dilated nonreactive pupil and paralysis of accommodation (interruption of parasympathetic fibers only).
    d. Trochlear nerve: extorsion and weakness of downward movement of affected eye.
    e. Abducens nerve: weakness of eye abduction.
    f. Trigeminal nerve: paroxysm of pain in lips, gums, cheek, or chin initiated by stimuli in trigger zone (trigeminal neuralgia) and sensory loss of the face or weakness of jaw muscles.
    g. Facial nerve: unilateral or bilateral paralysis of facial expression muscles, or impairment of taste, or hyperacusis (painful sensitivity to sounds).
    h. Vestibulo-cochlear nerve: deafness, tinnitus (cochlear), dizziness, and/or vertigo (vestibular).
    i. Glossopharyngeal nerve: swallowing difficulty, deviation of soft palate to normal side, anesthesia of posterior pharynx and/or glossopharyngeal neuralgia (unilateral stabbing pain in root of tongue and throat, triggered by coughing, sneezing, swallowing, and pressure on ear tragus).
    j. Vagus nerve: soft palate droop, loss of the gag reflex, hoarseness, nasal voice, and/or loss of sensation at external auditory meatus.
    k. Accessory nerve: weakness and atrophy of sternocleidomastoid muscle and upper part of trapezius muscle.
    l. Hypoglossal nerve: paralysis of one side of tongue with deviation to the affected side.
    Exclusions:
    • Skull fracture.
    • Tumor: meningioma, carcinomatous meningitis, aneurysm.
    • Infection: herpes zoster, neuroborreliosis, syphilis, mucormycosis.
    • Miller-Fisher syndrome.

16. **Plexopathy**
    Disorder of brachial or lumbosacral plexus producing muscle weakness, sensory deficit, and/or reflex change not corresponding to the territory of single root or nerve.
    Diagnostic criteria:
    All of the following:
    a. Characteristic signs and symptoms:
       i. Brachial plexus: deep pain in shoulder, muscle weakness, sensory deficit and/or reflex impairment of arm, or
       ii. Lumbosacral plexus: deep boring pain in thigh, muscle weakness, sensory deficit, and/or reflex impairment of leg.
    b. Positive EMG finding (concentric needle examination) *and/or* nerve conduction studies for EMG: more than one root or nerve abnormalities with sparing of paraspinal muscles for nerve conduction study: absent or reduced amplitude on motor or sensory nerve conduction.
    c. Normal MRI or CT scan (optional: myelogram) to rule out a higher neurological lesion.
    Exclusions:
    • Damage from injury, compression, tumor, aneurysm, radiation.
    • Cervical rib, thoracic outlet syndrome.
    • Plexus neuritis.
    • Toxic: heroin.
    • Infectious: Lyme disease, leprosy, herpes zoster.

17. **Polyneuropathy (*see* "Guillain-Barre Syndrome" and "Chronic Inflammatory Demyelinating Polyneuropathy" sections of Chapter 12)**
    Acute or chronic disorder of sensory and motor peripheral nerves with variable tempo characterized by symmetry of symptoms and physical findings in a distal distribution.

(Continued)

Table 11 (*Continued*)

Diagnostic criteria:

One or both of the following:

a. Clinical manifestations:
   i. Clinical demonstration of distal sensory and/or motor deficit.
   ii. Symmetry of signs/symptoms, and/or.
b. Confirmation by EMG:
   i. Concentric needle examination demonstrating denervation of muscle, *or*
   ii. Nerve conduction study demonstrating axonal or demyelinating neuropathy.

Exclusions:

- Vitamin deficiencies: B$_{12}$, niacin, thiamine.
- Hypothyroidism.

18. **Psychosis**

Severe disturbance in the perception of reality characterized by delusions and/or hallucinations

Diagnostic criteria:

All of the following:

a. At least one of the following:
   i. Delusions.
   ii. Hallucinations without insight.
b. The disturbance causes clinical distress or impairment in social, occupational, or other relevant areas of functioning.
c. The disturbance does not occur exclusively during the course of a delirium.
d. The disturbance is not better accounted for by another mental disorder (e.g., mania).

Exclusions:

- Primary psychotic disorder unrelated to SLE (e.g., schizophrenia).
- Substance- or drug-induced psychotic disorder (including nonsteriodal anti-inflammatory drugs, antimalarials).
- Psychologically mediated reaction to SLE (brief reactive psychosis with major stressor).

19. **Seizures and seizure disorders**

Abnormal paroxysmal neuronal discharge in the brain causing abnormal function. Isolated seizures are distinguished from the diagnosis of epilepsy. Epilepsy is a chronic disorder characterized by an abnormal tendency for recurrent, unprovoked seizures that are usually stereotypic. Approximately 3% of the population has epilepsy. Typically, provoked seizures result from treatable conditions, such as sleep deprivation, toxic exposure to stimulants, withdrawal from narcotics, barbiturates, or alcohol, fever, infection, metabolic disturbances, or SLE.

The approach to the evaluation of patients with a new-onset spell that may be a seizure, and the classification of seizures regardless of whether they are isolated seizures or part of a seizure disorder (e.g., epilepsy), are the same. The approach to treatment, however, is usually different. Although anticonvulsants are effective in controlling seizures acutely whether provoked or not, continuous prophylaxis is principally reserved for patients with epilepsy.

Seizures may occur with or without the loss of consciousness. Seizures are divided into *partial* and *generalized*. Partial seizures have clinical or electroencephalographic evidence of a focal onset; the abnormal discharge usually arises in a portion of one hemisphere and may spread to the rest of the brain during a seizure. Primary generalized seizures have no interictal evidence of focal onset on electroencephalogram (EEG). A generalized seizure can be primary or secondary.

a. Primary generalized seizures (bilaterally symmetric and without local onset).
   i. Tonic clonic (grand mal) or tonic or clonic.
   ii. Atonic or astatic seizures.
   iii. Absence seizures (petit mal).

Typical absences consist of abrupt onset and cessation of impairment of consciousness, with or without automatism, myoclonic jerks, tonic or autonomic components. A 3-Hz spike and wave discharge is usual EEG abnormality. Atypical absences have less abrupt onset and/or cessation of impaired consciousness and are more prolonged in tone with EEG abnormalities other than 3-Hz spike and wave discharge.

   iv. Myoclonic seizures.

(*Continued*)

Table 11 (*Continued*)

b. Partial or focal seizures (seizures beginning locally) (also referred to as Jacksonian, temporal lobe, or psychomotor seizure, according to type).

    i. Simple, without impairment of consciousness. Depending on anatomic site of origin of seizure discharge, initial symptom may be motor, sensory, aphasic, cognitive, affective, dysmnesic, illusional, olfactory, or psychological..

    ii. Complex, with partial impairment of consciousness, which may be simple at onset, followed by alteration or impairment of consciousness. Symptoms same as in i.

    iii. Simple or complex may evolve to secondary generalized tonic/clonic seizures. Sometimes secondary generalization is so rapid that there is no clinical evidence of partial onset, only electroencephalographic.

Diagnostic criteria:

a. Independent description by a reliable witness.

b. EEG abnormalities.[f]

Exclusions:

Seizure-like signs or symptoms or seizure from

- Vasovagal syncope.
- Cardiac syncope.
- Hysteria.
- Hyperventilation.
- Tics.
- Narcolepsy and cataplexy.
- Labyrinthitis.
- Alcohol and drug withdrawal.
- Medications: quinolones, imipenem.
- Subarachnoid hemorrhage.
- Trauma.
- Hypoglycemia.
- Panic attacks, conversion disorders, and malingering.

[a]*Acute confusional state* is equivalent to *delirium* as defined in the *Diagnostic and Statistical Manual of Mental Disorders, 4th edition* (DSM-IV) and the *International Statistical Classification of Diseases and Related Health Problems, 9th edition* (ICD-9), codes as an observable state of impaired consciousness, cognition (including perception), mood, affect, and behavior. The definitions of delirium in DSM-III, DSM-III-R, and DSM-IV have been tested for reliability, and the committee wanted a definition that would conform to ICD-9, World Health Organization, and DSM-IV.

Neurologists often use "encephalopathy," whereas psychiatrists use "delirium" to describe the same clinical state. Encephalopathy is defined in neurological texts as a diffuse cerebral dysfunction associated with a disturbance in consciousness, cognition, and mood, affect, and behavior. It implies a physiological etiology, and is usually used with descriptors of various metabolic disorders.

"Organic brain syndrome" is not recommended for usage because there is better studied terminology.

Acute confusional states are generally accompanied by cognitive deficits. If cognitive deficits are the only central nervous system manifestations, the illness should be recorded as "cognitive dysfunction."

[b]Preexisting cognitive deficits are not an exclusion. If acute confusional state is superimposed on preexisting cognitive deficits, diagnose both.

[c]Nerve conduction abnormalities may be subtle in early stages and may need to be repeated.

[d]In most patients with SLE, anxiety is a secondary stress reaction and not a direct manifestation of neuropsychiatric lupus syndromes.

[e]If mood disturbance occurs exclusively during an acute confusional state, classify as acute confusional state. If mood disturbance occurs exclusively during a psychotic disorder, classify as psychosis.

[f]EEG is a sensitive tool for diagnosis of epilepsy, but must be used with clinical data. Many epileptic patients have normal interictal EEG. Occasionally, using standard scalp leads, EEG may be normal during a partial simple seizure whereas during complex partial seizures subtle changes are almost always present. Approximately 2 to 3% of healthy individuals show paroxysmal EEG abnormalities.

(Adapted with permission from ACR Ad Hoc committee on neuropsychiatric lupus nomenclature: The American College of Rheumatology nomenclature and case definitions for neuropsychiatric lupus syndromes. Arthritis Rheum 1999;42:599–608, and from John Wiley and Sons.)

Table 12
1990 Criteria for the Classification of Takayasu's Arteritis from the American College of Rheumatology

1.	**Age at disease onset less than 40 years:** Development of symptoms or finding related to Takayasu's arteritis at age less than 40 years.
2.	**Claudication of extremities:** Development and worsening of fatigue and discomfort in muscles of 1 or more extremityy while in use, especially the upper extremities.
3.	**Decreased brachial artery pulse:** Decreased pulsation of 1 or both brachial arteries.
4.	**BP difference >10 mmHg:** Difference of >10 mmHg insystolic blood presure between arms.
5.	**Bruit over subclavian or aorta:** Bruit audible on auscultation over one or both subclavian arteries or abdominal aorta.
6.	**Arteriogram abnormality:** Arteriographic narrowing or occlusion of the entire aorta, its primary branches, or large arteries in the proximal upper or lower extremities; not resulting from arterioscerosis, fibromusular dysplasia, or similar causes; changes usually focal or segmental.

For purposes of classification, a patient shall be said to have Takayasu's arteritis if at least three of these six criteria are present. The presence of any three or more criteria yields a sensitivity of 90.5% and a specificity of 97.8%, BP = blood presure (systolic; difference between arms).

Adapted from Arend WP, Michel BA, Bloch DA, et al. The American College of Rheumatology 1990 criteria for the classification of Takayasu arteritis. Arthritis Rheum 1990 Aug; 33(8):1129–1134.

clinical judgment, but the criteria are useful in allowing physicians to clearly define the heretofore often-elusive concept of NPSLE.

TAKAYASU'S ARTERITIS

Takayasu's arteritis is a rare (one to two cases per million per year) inflammatory of medium- and large-sized arteries, with a strong predilection for the aortic for the aortic arch and its branches. It is also known as "aortic arch syndrome." It most often affects young women, and is found worldwide.

Pathologically there is a panarteritis with mononuclear infiltrates and sometimes giant cells. There may be stenosis and vessel occlusion with or without thrombosis. It may present as a nonspecific systemic illness, or with symptoms related to stenosis or occlusion of the aorta, its branches, or pulmonary arteries. Pulses are commonly absent in the involved vessels, particularly the subclavian artery. The diagnosis of Takayasu's arteritis should be suspected strongly in a young woman who develops a decrease or absence of peripheral pulses, discrepancies in blood presure, and arterial bruits. Table 12 lists diagnostic criteria from the American Rheumatological Association. Treatments include glucorticoids, angioplasty of affected arteries, and control of hypertension leading to organ injury.

TEMPORAL ARTERITIS (*SEE "POLYMYALGIA RHEUMATICA"*)

The primary manifestation of temporal arteritis is headache, although the major complication is acute, often irreversible visual loss. Polymyalgia rheumatica is the systemic form of temporal arteritis and has evolved separate diagnostic criteria, which are presented separately. Pathologically, biopsy of extracranial arteries (e.g., temporal artery) shows three major findings: granulomas with giant cells, often near remnants of the internal elastic membrane; nonspecific neutrophilic, eosinophilic, and lymphocytic infiltration of blood vessel wall; intimal fibrosis.

Temporal arteritis is among the most common of the vasculitides, with a strong age-related incidence. Several epidemiological studies have found that it may be becoming more common, although there is likely a strong secular trend because of better diagnostic awareness. There are differences in incidence between ethnic groups. It appears to be very rare in Asians, and relatively rare in Hispanic and African-American populations. In a retrospective study from the Mayo Clinic, the age- and gender-adjusted incidence was 18 per 100,000 per year over age 50. Incidence in women was 24 per 100,000 per year, and was 12 per 100,000 per year in men. Diagnostic criteria appearing Table 13.

Table 13

1990 Criteria for the Classification of Giant Cell (Temporal) Arteritis from the American College of Rheumatology

1. Age at disease onset at least 50 years
   Development of symptoms or findings beginning at age 50 or older.
2. New headache
   New onset of or new type of localized pain in the head.
3. Temporal artery abnormality
   Temporal artery tenderness to palpation or decreased pulsation, unrelated to arteriosclerosis of cervical arteries.
4. Elevated erythrocyte sedimentation rate
   Erythrocyte sedimentation rate ≥ 50 mm/hour by the Westergren method.
5. Abnormal artery biopsy
   Biopsy specimen with artery showing vasculitis characterized by a predominance of mononuclear cell infiltration or granulomatous inflammation, usually with multinucleated giant cells.

For purposes of classification, a patient shall be said to have giant cell (temporal) arteritis if at least three of these five criteria are present. The presence of any three or more criteria yields a sensitivity of 93.5% and a specificity of 91.2%.

(Adapted with permission from Hunder GG, Bloch DA, Michel BA, et al. The American College of Rheumatology 1990 criteria for the classification of giant cell arteritis. Arthritis Rheum 1990;33:1122–1128, and from John Wiley and Sons.)

Table 14

Diagnostic Criteria for Vogt-Koyanagi-Harada Disease

Complete Vogt-Koyanagi-Harada disease (criteria 1 to 5 must be present)
1. No history of penetrating ocular trauma or surgery preceding the initial onset of uveitis.
2. No clinical or laboratory evidence suggestive of other ocular disease entities.
3. Bilateral ocular involvement (a or b must be met, depending on the stage of disease when the patient is examined).
   a. Early manifestations of disease:
      i. There must be evidence of a diffuse choroiditis (with or without anterior uveitis, vitreous inflammatory reaction, or optic disk hyperemia), which may manifest as one of the following:
         (1) Focal areas of subretinal fluid, or
         (2) Bullous serous retinal detachments.
      ii. With equivocal fundus findings, both of the following must be present as well:
         (1) Focal areas of delay in choroidal perfusion, multifocal areas of pinpoint leakage, large placoid areas of hyperfluorescence, pooling within subretinal fluid, and optic nerve staining (listed in order of sequential appearance) by fluorescein angiography, and
         (2) Diffuse choroidal thickening, without evidence of posterior scleritis by ultrasonography.
   b. Late manifestations of disease:
      i. History suggestive of prior presence of findings from c.i, and either both ii and iii below, or multiple signs from c:
      ii. Ocular depigmentation (either of the following manifestations is sufficient):
         (1) Sunset glow fundus, or
         (2) Sugiura sign.
   c. Other ocular signs:
      i. Nummular chorioretinal depigmented scars, or
      ii. Retinal pigment epithelium clumping and/or migration, or
      iii. Recurrent or chronic anterior uveitis.
   d. Neurological/auditory findings (may have resolved by time of examination):
      i. Meningismus (malaise, fever, headache, nausea, abdominal pain, stiffness of the neck and back, or a combination of these factors; headache alone is not sufficient to meet definition of meningismus, however), or
      ii. Tinnitus, or
      iii. Cerebrospinal fluid pleocytosis.

(Continued)

Table 14 *(Continued)*

    e. Integumentary finding (not preceding onset of central nervous system or ocular disease):
        i. Alopecia, or
       ii. Poliosis, or
      iii. Vitiligo.

Incomplete Vogt-Koyanagi-Harada disease (criteria 1 to 3 and either 4 or 5 must be present)
1. No history of penetrating ocular trauma or surgery preceding the initial onset of uveitis, and
2. No clinical or laboratory evidence suggestive of other ocular disease entities, and
3. Bilateral ocular involvement.
4. Neurological/auditory findings; as defined for complete Vogt-Koyanagi-Harada disease above, or
5. Integumentary findings; as defined for complete Vogt-Koyanagi-Harada disease above

Probable Vogt-Koyanagi-Harada disease (isolated ocular disease; criteria 1 to 3 must be present)
1. No history of penetrating ocular trauma or surgery preceding the initial onset of uveitis.
2. No clinical or laboratory evidence suggestive of other ocular disease entities.
3. Bilateral ocular involvement as defined for complete Vogt-Koyanagi-Harada disease above.

Reprinted with permission from Read RW, Holland GN, Rao NA, et al. Revised diagnostic criteria for Vogt-Koyanagi-Harada disease: Report of an international committee on nomenclature. Am J Ophthalmol 2001;131:647–652, and from Elsevier.

VOGT-KOYANAGI-HARADA DISEASE

Vogt-Koyanagi-Harada disease is a chronic, bilateral, ocular and multisystem granulomatous disease of unknown origin. It is one of many known causes of uveitis with neurological findings, the differential of which includes infections (fungal, mycobacterial, syphilis, etc.), neoplasm (e.g., lymphoma), or other granulomatous disorders, such as sarcoidosis.

The criteria allow for diagnosis in both early and late stages. There is choroiditis with or without uveitis and ocular findings as detailed in Table 14. Neurological signs and symptoms include meningismus, a chronic meningeal reaction with cerebrospinal fluid pleocytosis, and tinnitus.

SOURCES

Acute Rheumatic Fever

American Heart Association. Jones criteria, updated. JAMA 1992;268:2069.

Neuro-Sweet Disease

Hisanaga K, Iwasaki Y, Itoyama Y, Neuro-Sweet Disease Study Group. Neuro-Sweet disease: clinical manifestations and criteria for diagnosis. Neurology. 2005; 64:1756–1761.

Paraneoplastic Syndromes

Graus F, Delattre JY, Antoine JC, et al. Recommended diagnostic criteria for paraneoplastic neurological syndromes. J Neurol Neurosurg Psychiatry 2004;5:1135–1140.

Polyarteritis Nodosa

Lightfoot RW Jr, Michel BA, Bloch DA, et al. The American College of Rheumatology 1990 criteria for the classification of polyarteritis nodosa. Arthritis Rheum 1990;33:1088–1093.

Polymyalgia Rheumatica

Bird HA, Esselinckx W, Dixon AS, Mowat AG, Wood PH. An evaluation of criteria for polymyalgia rheumatica. Ann Rheum Dis 1979;38:434–439.

Bird HA, Leeb BF, Montecucco CM, et al. A comparison of the sensitivity of diagnostic criteria for polymyalgia rheumatica. Ann Rheum Dis 2005;64:626–629.

Brooks RC, McGee SR. Diagnostic dilemmas in polymyalgia rheumatica. Arch Intern Med 1997;157:162–168.

Chuang TY, Hunder GG, Ilstrup DM, Kurland LT. Polymyalgia rheumatica: a 10-year epidemiologic and clinical study. Ann Intern Med. 1982;97:672–680.

Epperly TD, Moore KE, Harrover JD. Polymyalgia and temporal arteritis. Am Fam Physician 2000;62:789–796.

Jones JG, Hazleman BL. Prognosis and management of polymyalgia rheumatica. Ann Rheum Dis 1981;40:1–5.

Nobunaga M, Yoshioka K, Yasuda M, Shingu M. Clinical studies of polymyalgia rheumatica. A proposal of diagnostic criteria. Jpn J Med 1989;28:452–456.

Rheumatoid Arthritis

Arnett FC, Edworthy SM, Bloch DA, et al. The American Rheumatism Association 1987 revised criteria for the classification of rheumatoid arthritis. Arthritis Rheum 1988;31:315–324.

Sjögren's Syndrome

Vitali C, Moutsopoulos HM, Bombardieri S. The European Community Study Group on diagnostic criteria for Sjögren's syndrome. Sensitivity and specificity of tests for ocular and oral involvement in Sjögren's syndrome. Ann Rheum Dis 1994;53:637–647.

Vitali C, Bombardieri S, Moutsopoulos HM, et al. Assessment of the European classification criteria for Sjögren's syndrome in a series of clinically defined cases: results of a prospective multicentre study. The European Study Group on Diagnostic Criteria for Sjögren's Syndrome. Ann Rheum Dis 1996;55:116–121.

Vitali C, Bombardieri S, Jonsson R, et al. Classification criteria for Sjögren's syndrome: a revised version of the European criteria proposed by the American–European Consensus Group Ann Rheum Dis 2002;61:554–558.

Systemic Lupus Erythematosus

ACR Ad Hoc committee on Neuropsychiatric lupus nomenclature: The American College of Rheumatology nomenclature and case definitions for neuropsychiatric lupus syndromes. Arthritis Rheum 1999;42:599–608.

American College of Rheumatology. Arthritis and Rheumatism. Available at http://www.rheumatology.org/publications/ar/1999/aprilappendix.asp?aud=mem.

Tan EM, Cohen AS, Fries JF, et al. The 1982 revised criteria for the classification of systemic lupus erythematosus. Arthritis Rheum 1982;25:1271–1277.

Takayasu's Arteritis

Arend WP, Michel BA, Bloch DA, et al. The American College of Rheumatology 1990 criteria for the classification of Takayasu arteritis. Arthritis Rheum 1990;33:1129–1134.

Ishikawa K. Diagnostic approach and proposed criteria for the clinical diagnosis of Takayasu's arteriopathy. J Am Coll Cardiol 1988;12:964–972.

Temporal Arteritis

Friedman G, Friedman B, Benbassat J. Epidemiology of temporal arteritis in Israel. Isr J Med Sci 1982;18:241–244.

Hunder GG, Bloch DA, Michel BA, et al. The American College of Rheumatology 1990 criteria for the classification of giant cell arteritis. Arthritis Rheum 1990;33:1122–1128.

Johnson LN, Arnold AC. Incidence of nonarteritic and arteritic anterior ischemic optic neuropathy. Population-based study in the state of Missouri and Los Angeles County, California. J Neuroophthalmol 1994;14:38–44.

Liu NH, LaBree LD, Feldon SE, Rao NA. The epidemiology of giant cell arteritis: a 12-year retrospective study. Ophthalmology 2001;108:1145–1149.

Vogt-Koyanagi-Hamada Disease

Read RW, Holland GN, Rao NA, et al. Revised diagnostic criteria for Vogt-Koyanagi-Harada disease: Report of an international committee on nomenclature. Am J Ophthalmol 2001;131:647–652.

10
Infectious Diseases

AIDS

Although not a neurological disease *per se*, AIDS is included here because of its wide-ranging relevance to neurological practice and the multiple infections that can be associated with nervous system manifestations (Tables 1–3).

Table 1
Case Definition of AIDS-Defining Illnesses

The AIDS case definition includes a confirmed diagnosis of HIV-1 infection and one or more of the following AIDS-defining illnesses, diagnosed presumptively or definitively according to the criteria listed below:

Candidiasis of the bronchi, trachea, or lungs
Gross inspection by endoscopy or at autopsy or by microscopy (histology or cytology) on a specimen obtained directly from the tissues affected (including scrapings from the mucosal surface) not from a culture.

Candidiasis, esophageal
Definitive diagnosis:
Same as is for candidiasis of the bronchi, trachea, or lungs.
Presumptive diagnosis:
Recent onset of retrosternal pain on swallowing and oral candidiasis diagnosed by the gross appearance of white patches or plaques on an erythematous base or by the microscopic appearance of fungal mycelial filaments in an uncultured specimen scraped from the oral mucosa.

Cervical cancer, invasive
Histological evidence of cancer.

Coccidiomycosis, disseminated or extrapulmonary
Microscopy (histology or cytology), culture, or detection of antigen in a specimen obtained directly from the affected tissues or a fluid from those tissues.

Cryptococcosis, extrapulmonary
Microscopy (histology or cytology), culture, or detection of antigen in a specimen obtained directly from the affected tissues or a fluid from those tissues.

Cryptosporidiosis, more than 1 month's duration
Microscopy (histology or cytology), culture, or detection of antigen in a specimen obtained directly from the affected tissues or a fluid from those tissues.

Cytomegalovirus disease, other than liver, spleen, or nodes
Microscopy (histology or cytology), culture, or detection of antigen in a specimen obtained directly from the affected tissues or a fluid from those tissues.

Cytomegalovirus retinitis with loss of vision
Definitive diagnosis:
As for cytomegalovirus disease, other than liver, spleen, or lymph nodes.

(Continued)

From: *Current Clinical Neurology: Diagnostic Criteria in Neurology*
Edited by: A. J. Lerner © Humana Press Inc., Totowa, NJ

Table 1 *(Continued)*

Presumptive diagnosis:

A characteristic appearance on serial ophthalmoscopic examinations, for example discrete patches of retinal whitening with distinct borders, spreading in a centrifugal manner along the paths of blood vessels, progressing over several months, and frequently associated with retinal vasculitis, hemorrhage, and necrosis. Resolution of active disease leaves retinal scarring and atrophy with retinal pigment epithelial mottling.

Encephalopathy, HIV-related

Clinical findings of disabling cognitive or motor dysfunction interfering with occupation or activities of daily living, progressing over weeks to months, in the absence of a concurrent illness or condition other than HIV infection that could explain the findings. Methods to rule out such concurrent illness and conditions must include cerebrospinal fluid examination and either brain imaging (computed tomography or magnetic resonance) or autopsy.

Herpes simplex: chronic ulcer(s) of more than 1 month's duration, bronchitis, pneumonitis, or esophagitis

Microscopy (histology or cytology), culture, or detection of antigen in a specimen obtained directly from the affected tissues or a fluid from those tissues.

Histoplasmosis, disseminated or extrapulmonary

Microscopy (histology or cytology), culture, or detection of antigen in a specimen obtained directly from the affected tissues or a fluid from those tissues.

Isosporiasis, chronic intestinal, of more than 1 month's duration

Microscopy (histology or cytology), culture, or detection of antigen in a specimen obtained directly from the affected tissues or a fluid from those tissues.

Kaposi's sarcoma

Definitive diagnosis:

Microscopy (histology or cytology).

Presumptive diagnosis:

A characteristic gross appearance of an erythematous or violaceous plaque-like lesion on skin or mucous membrane.[a]

Lymphoma, Burkitt's

Microscopy (histology or cytology).

Lymphoma, immunoblastic

Microscopy (histology or cytology).

Lymphoma, primary, of brain

Microscopy (histology or cytology).

***Mycobacterium tuberculosis*, any site, pulmonary or extrapulmonary**

Definitive diagnosis:

Isolation of *M. tuberculosis*, *Mycobacterium bovis*, or *Mycobacterium africanum* from a clinical specimen

Presumptive diagnosis:

Demonstration of acid-fast bacilli in a clinical specimen or, when a culture is not available, in a histopathological lesion in a person with signs or symptoms compatible with tuberculosis, or evidence of resolution of disease where treatment with two or more antituberculosis medications have been prescribed and follow-up has been instigated.

Mycobacterial disease (other or unidentified species), disseminated or extrapulmonary

Definitive diagnosis:

Culture.

Presumptive diagnosis:

Microscopy of a specimen from stool or normally sterile body fluids, or tissue from a site other than lungs, skin, or cervical or hilar lymph nodes that shows acid-fast bacilli of a species not identified by culture.

***Pneumocystis carinii* pneumonia**

Definitive diagnosis:

Microscopy (histology or culture).

Presumptive diagnosis:

- A history of dyspnea on exertion or nonproductive cough of recent onset (within the past 3 months); and
- Chest X-ray evidence of diffuse bilateral interstitial infiltrates or evidence by gallium scan of diffuse bilateral pulmonary disease; and
- Arterial blood gas analysis showing arterial pO_2 less than 70 mmHg, or low respiratory diffusing capacity (less than 80% of predicted values), or an increase in the alveolar–arterial oxygen tension gradient; and
- No evidence of bacterial pneumonia.

(Continued)

Table 1 *(Continued)*

Pneumonia, recurrent bacterial
Definitive diagnosis:
Two or more episodes of acute pneumonia occurring within 12 months. Both episodes must have infection with a pathogen that typically causes pneumonia (other than *P. carinii* or *M. tuberculosis*) proven by culture or some other organism-specific diagnostic method and new (not present earlier) radiological evidence of pneumonia.
Presumptive diagnosis:
Two or more episodes occurring within 12 months of acute pneumonia (new symptoms, signs or X-ray evidence not present earlier), based on clinical or radiologic evidence.

Progressive multifocal leukoencephalopathy (*see* Table 4)
Microscopy (histology or cytology).

***Salmonella* septicemia, recurrent**
Culture-proven infection with *Salmonella* species.

Toxoplasmosis
Definitive diagnosis:
Microscopy (histology or cytology).
Presumptive diagnosis:
Toxoplasmosis of the brain, based on observation of:
- Recent onset of a focal neurological abnormality consistent with intracranial disease or a reduced level of consciousness; and
- Evidence by brain imaging (computed tomography or magnetic resonance imaging) of a lesion having a mass effect or the radiographic appearance of which is enhanced by injection of contrast medium; and
- Serum antibody to *Toxoplasma* or successful response to therapy for toxoplasmosis.

Wasting syndrome because of HIV infection
- Profound involuntary weight loss of more than 10% of baseline body weight; and
- Chronic diarrhea (at least two loose stools per day for 30 days) or chronic weakness and documented fever (for at least 30 days, intermittent or constant) in the absence of a concurrent illness or condition other than HIV infection, such as tuberculosis, cancer, cryptosporidiosis, or other specific enteritis, that could explain the findings.

Bacterial infection affecting a child less than 13 years of age
Laboratory diagnosis of multiple or recurrent bacterial infections (any combination of at least two within 2 years) of the following types: septicemia, pneumonia, meningitis, bone or joint infection, abscess of an internal organ or body cavity (excluding otitis media or superficial skin or mucosal abscesses) caused by *Haemophilus* spp., *Streptococcus pneumoniae* or other pyogenic bacteria.

Lymphoid interstitial pneumonia and/or pulmonary lymphoid hyperplasia affecting a child younger than 13 years of age
Definitive diagnosis:
Microscopy (histology or cytology).
Presumptive diagnosis:
Lymphoid interstitial pneumonia—bilateral, reticulonodular, interstitial pulmonary infiltrates present on chest X-ray for 2 months or more, with no pathogen identified and no response to antibiotic treatment. Other causes of interstitial infiltrates should be excluded, such as tuberculosis, *P. carinii* pneumonia, cytomegalovirus infection, and other viral or parasitic infections.

---

[a]A presumptive diagnosis of Kaposi's sarcoma should not be made by clinicians who have only seen few cases. (Adapted from AIDS and HIV surveillance case definition. MMWR 1999;48[RR13]:29–31.)

HIV-1-Associated Progressive Multifocal Leukoencephalopathy

Progressive multifocal leukoencephalopathy is caused by the JC virus, which is found widely. It occurs as a clinical infection in immunosuppressed individuals, for whom it is a recrudescent infection. The majority of cases of progressive multifocal leukoencephalopathy are now seen in patients with AIDS, where it may be the presenting opportunistic infection; it affects up to 5% of patients with AIDS. Giesen et al. proposed the criteria found in Table 4, but these diagnostic criteria have not been widely tested, and are based on an empirical series.

Table 2
US Centers for Disease Control 1993 Classification System
for HIV Infection and Expanded AIDS Surveillance Cases Definition
for Adolescents and Adults

	CD4+ T-cell count		
Clinical category	*>500 µL*	*200–499 µL*	*<200 µL*
(A) Asymptomatic, primary HIV, PGL	A1	A2	A3
(B) Symptomatic, not (A) or (C)	B1	B2	B3
(C) AIDS-defining conditions	C1	C2	C3

PGL, persistent generalized lymphadenopathy.
(Adapted from AIDS and HIV surveillance case definition. MMWR 1999;48[RR13]:29–31.)

Table 3
Revised Surveillance Case Definition for HIV Infection

This revised definition of HIV infection, which applies to any HIV (e.g., HIV-1 or HIV-2), is intended for public health surveillance only. It incorporates the reporting criteria for HIV infection and AIDS into a single case definition. The revised criteria for HIV infection update the definition of HIV infection implemented in 1993; the revised HIV criteria apply to AIDS-defining conditions for adults and children, which require laboratory evidence of HIV. This definition is not presented as a guide to clinical diagnosis or for other uses.

I.   In adults, adolescents, or children aged greater than or equal to 18 months,[a] a reportable case of HIV infection must meet at least one of the following criteria:
Laboratory criteria:
- Positive result on a screening test for HIV antibody (e.g., repeatedly reactive enzyme immunoassay), followed by a positive result on a confirmatory (sensitive and more specific) test for HIV antibody (e.g., Western blot or immunofluorescence antibody test); *or*
- Positive result or report of a detectable quantity on any of the following HIV virological (nonantibody) tests:
  o   HIV nucleic acid (DNA or RNA) detection (e.g., DNA polymerase chain reaction [PCR] or plasma HIV-1 RNA).[b]
  o   HIV p24 antigen test, including neutralization assay.
  o   HIV isolation (viral culture).
or
Clinical or other criteria (if the above laboratory criteria are not met):
- Diagnosis of HIV infection, based on the laboratory criteria above, that is documented in a medical record by a physician; or
- Conditions that meet criteria included in the case definition for AIDS.

II. In a child aged less than 18 months, a reportable case of HIV infection must meet at least one of the following criteria:
Laboratory criteria:
Definitive:
- Positive results on two separate specimens (excluding cord blood) using one or more of the following HIV virological (nonantibody) tests:
  o   HIV nucleic acid (DNA or RNA) detection.
  o   HIV p24 antigen test, including neutralization assay, in a child greater than or equal to 1 month of age.
  o   HIV isolation (viral culture).
or
Presumptive:
A child who does not meet the criteria for definitive HIV infection but who has:
- Positive results on only one specimen (excluding cord blood) using the above HIV virological tests and no subsequent negative HIV virological or negative HIV antibody tests
or
Clinical or other criteria (if the above definitive or presumptive laboratory criteria are not met):
- Diagnosis of HIV infection, based on the laboratory criteria above, that is documented in a medical record by a physician; or
- Conditions that meet criteria included in the 1987 pediatric surveillance case definition for AIDS.

(Continued)

Table 3 *(Continued)*

III. A child aged less than 18 months born to an HIV-infected mother will be categorized for surveillance purposes as "not infected with HIV" if the child does not meet the criteria for HIV infection but meets the following criteria:

Laboratory criteria:

Definitive:
- At least two negative HIV antibody tests from separate specimens obtained at age 6 months or older; or
- At least two negative HIV antibody tests from separate specimens obtained at age 6 months or older; or
- At least two negative HIV virological tests[a] from separate specimens, both of which were performed at greater than or equal to 1 month of age and one of which was performed at age 4 months or older

and
- No other laboratory or clinical evidence of HIV infection (i.e., has not had any positive virological tests, if performed, and has not had an AIDS-defining condition).

or

Presumptive:

A child who does not meet the above criteria for definitive "not infected" status but who has:
- One negative enzyme immunoassay HIV antibody test performed at age 6 months or older and NO positive HIV virological tests, if performed; or
- One negative HIV virological test[a] performed at age 4 months or older and NO positive HIV virological tests, if performed; or
- One positive HIV virological test with at least two subsequent negative virological tests,[c] at least one of which is at age 4 months or older; or negative HIV antibody test results, at least one of which is at age 6 months or older

and
- No other laboratory or clinical evidence of HIV infection (i.e., has not had any positive virological tests, if performed, and has not had an AIDS-defining condition)

or

Clinical or other criteria (if the above definitive or presumptive laboratory criteria are not met):
- Determined by a physician to be "not infected," and a physician has noted the results of the preceding HIV diagnostic tests in the medical record

and
- NO other laboratory or clinical evidence of HIV infection (i.e., has not had any positive virological tests, if performed, and has not had an AIDS-defining condition).

IV. A child aged less than 18 months born to an HIV-infected mother will be categorized as having perinatal exposure to HIV infection if the child does not meet the criteria for HIV infection (II) or the criteria for "not infected with HIV" (III).

Draft revised surveillance criteria for HIV infection were approved and recommended by the membership of the Council of State and Territorial Epidemiologists (CSTE) at the 1998 annual meeting. Draft versions of these criteria were previously reviewed by state HIV/AIDS surveillance staffs, Centers for Desease Control, CSTE, and laboratory experts. In addition, the pediatric criteria were reviewed by an expert panel of consultants.

[a]Children aged 18 months or older but younger than 13 years are categorized as "not infected with HIV" if they meet the criteria in III.

[b]In adults, adolescents, and children infected by other than perinatal exposure, plasma viral RNA nucleic acid tests should NOT be used in lieu of licensed HIV screening tests (e.g., repeatedly reactive enzyme immunoassay). In addition, a negative (i.e., undetectable) plasma HIV-1 RNA test result does not rule out the diagnosis of HIV infection.

[c]HIV nucleic acid (DNA or RNA) detection tests are the virological methods of choice to exclude infection in children aged younger than 18 months. Although HIV culture can be used for this purpose, it is more complex and expensive to perform and is less well standardized than nucleic acid detection tests. The use of p24 antigen testing to exclude infection in children aged less than 18 months is not recommended because of its lack of sensitivity.

(Adapted from AIDS and HIV surveillance case definition. MMWR 1999;48[RR13]:29–31. Available from the website of the Centers for Disease Control: http://www.cdc.gov/mmwr/preview/mmwrhtml/rr4813a2.htm.)

Table 4

Features Suggestive of Diagnosis of HIV-1-Associated Progressive Multifocal Leukoencephalopathy

A. Rapid onset of neurological symptoms in HIV-1 infection.
B. Male gender.
C. Multifocal clinical deficits.
D. Magnetic resonance imaging findings of white matter.
    1. Multifocal, asymmetric.
    2. No mass effect.
    3. No contrast enhancement.
    4. No concomitant brain atrophy.
    5. Location near white/grey junction.
E. Cerebrospinal fluid JC virus-positive by polymerase chain reaction.
F. Normal cerebrospinal fluid.

Cases fitting this clinical profile would meet diagnostic criteria for progressive multifocal leukoencephalopathy. If more than one of five criteria are missing, a stereotactic brain biopsy is suggested.

(Adapted with permission from Giesen HJ, Neuen-Jacob E, Dorries K, Jablonowski H, Roick H, Arendt G. Diagnsotic criteria and clinical procedures in HIV-1-associated progressive multifocal leukoencephalopathy. J Neurol Sci 1997;147:63–72, and from Elsevier.)

ARBOVIRAL ENCEPHALITIS OR MENINGITIS

Table 5

2001 Case Definition of Arboviral Infection From the Center for Disease Control (Includes California Serogroup, Eastern Equine, St. Louis, Western Equine, West Nile, Powassan Encephalitides/Meningitides)

Clinical description

Arboviral infections may be asymptomatic or may result in illnesses of variable severity sometimes associated with central nervous system (CNS) involvement. When the CNS is affected, clinical syndromes ranging from febrile headache to aseptic meningitis to encephalitis may occur, and these are usually indistinguishable from similar syndromes caused by other viruses. Arboviral meningitis is characterized by fever, headache, stiff neck, and pleocytosis. Arboviral encephalitis is characterized by fever, headache, and altered mental status ranging from confusion to coma with or without additional signs of brain dysfunction (e.g., paresis or paralysis, cranial nerve palsies, sensory deficits, abnormal reflexes, generalized convulsions, and abnormal movements).

Laboratory criteria for diagnosis

*   Fourfold or greater change in virus-specific serum antibody titer, or
*   Isolation of virus from or demonstration of specific viral antigen or genomic sequences in tissue, blood, cerebrospinal fluid (CSF), or other body fluid, or
*   Virus-specific immunoglobulin (Ig)M antibodies demonstrated in CSF by antibody-capture enzyme immunoassay (EIA), or
*   Virus-specific IgM antibodies demonstrated in serum by antibody-capture EIA and confirmed by demonstration of virus-specific serum IgG antibodies in the same or a later specimen by another serological assay (e.g., neutralization or hemagglutination inhibition).

Case classification

Probable: an encephalitis or meningitis case occurring during a period when arboviral transmission is likely, and with the following supportive serology: a single or stable (less than or equal to twofold change) but elevated titer of virus-specific serum antibodies, or serum IgM antibodies detected by antibody-capture EIA but with no available results of a confirmatory test for virus-specific serum IgG antibodies in the same or a later specimen.

Confirmed: an encephalitis or meningitis case that is laboratory confirmed.

Comment: Because closely related arboviruses exhibit serological crossreactivity, positive results of serological tests using antigens from a single arbovirus can be misleading. In some circumstances (e.g., in areas where two or more closely related arboviruses occur, or in imported arboviral disease cases), it may be epidemiologically important to attempt to pinpoint the infecting virus by conducting cross-neutralization tests using an appropriate battery of closely related viruses. This is essential, for example, in determining that

Table 5 *(Continued)*

antibodies detected against St. Louis encephalitis virus are not the result of an infection with West Nile (or dengue) virus, or vice versa, in areas where both of these viruses occur.

The seasonality of arboviral transmission is variable and depends on the geographic location of exposure, the specific cycles of viral transmission, and local climatic conditions. Reporting should be etiology-specific (*see* below; the six encephalitides/meningitides printed in boldface are nationally reportable to CDC):

St. Louis encephalitis/meningitis
West Nile encephalitis/meningitis
Powassan encephalitis/meningitis
Eastern equine encephalitis/meningitis
Western equine encephalitis/meningitis
California serogroup viral encephalitis/meningitis (includes infections with the following viruses: La Crosse, Jamestown Canyon, snowshoe hare, trivittatus, Keystone, and California encephalitis viruses).
Other viral CNS infections transmitted by mosquitoes, ticks, or midges (e.g., Venezuelan equine encephalitis/meningitis and Cache Valley encephalitis/meningitis).

Adapted from the website of the Centers for Disease Control. Available at http://www.cdc.gov/epo/dphsi/casedef/encephalitiscurrent.htm.

INFECTIVE ENDOCARDITIS

Infective endocarditis has numerous neurological manifestations including stroke, mycotic aneurysms, meningoencephalitis, and septic encephalopathy.

The diagnosis of infective endocarditis has changed since the original van Reyn diagnostic criteria were published in 1981. The major clinical criteria are the so-called Duke criteria shown in the Table 6. Modifications to these criteria have been proposed, which include use of molecular markers, positive blood cultures for suspect organisms, and identification of the organism in a metastatic lesion(s).

Table 6
Duke Criteria for Infective Endocarditis

Pathological criteria
Microorganisms demonstrated by culture or histological examination
Active endocarditis demonstrated by histological examination
Major criteria
Positive blood cultures
• Typical micro-organisms consistent with endocarditis from two separate blood cultures.
• Micro-organisms consistent with endocarditis from persistently positive blood cultures.
Evidence of endocardial involvement
• Echocardiography: oscillating structures, abscess formation, new partial dehiscence of prosthetic valve.
• New valvular regurgitation.
Minor criteria
• Predisposing heart disease.
• Fever higher than 38°C.
• Vascular phenomena.
• Immunological phenomena.
• Microbiological evidence (no major criterion).
• Suspect echocardiography (no major criterion).

Reprinted with permission from Prendergast BD. Diagnostic criteria and problems in infective endocarditis. Heart 2004;90:611–613.

Table 7
Categories of Infective Endocarditis by Duke Criteria

Definite:	Pathological criteria positive
	or two major criteria positive
	or one major and two minor criteria positive
	or five minor criteria positive
Possible:	All cases that cannot be classified as definite or rejected
Rejected:	Alternative diagnosis
	Resolution of the infection with antibiotic treatment in less than 4 days
	No histological evidence

Reprinted with permission from Prendergast BD. Diagnostic criteria and problems in infective endocarditis. Heart 2004;90:611–613, and from BMJ Publishing Group.

LYME DISEASE (INFECTION BECAUSE OF *BORRELIA BURGDORFERI*)

Table 8
1996 Case Definition for Lyme Disease From the Centers for Disease Control

Clinical description

A systemic, tick-borne disease with protean manifestations, including dermatological, rheumatological, neurological, and cardiac abnormalities. The best clinical marker for the disease is the initial skin lesion (i.e., erythema migrans [EM]) that occurs in 60–80% of patients.

Laboratory criteria for diagnosis

- Isolation of *Borrelia burgdorferi* from a clinical specimen, or
- Demonstration of diagnostic immunoglobulin M or immunoglobulin G antibodies to *B. burgdorferi* in serum or cerebrospinal fluid (CSF). A two-test approach using a sensitive enzyme immunoassay or immunofluorescence antibody followed by Western blot is recommended.

Case classification

Confirmed: a case with EM or a case with at least one late manifestation (as defined below) that is laboratory-confirmed.

Comment: This surveillance case definition was developed for national reporting of Lyme disease; it is not intended to be used in clinical diagnosis.

Definition of terms used in the clinical description and case definition:

- *EM*. For purposes of surveillance, EM is defined as a skin lesion that typically begins as a red macule or papule and expands over a period of days to weeks to form a large round lesion, often with partial central clearing. A single primary lesion must reach greater than or equal to 5 cm in size. Secondary lesions also may occur. Annular erythematous lesions occurring within several hours of a tick bite represent hypersensitivity reactions and do not qualify as EM. For most patients, the expanding EM lesion is accompanied by other acute symptoms, particularly fatigue, fever, headache, mildly stiff neck, arthralgia, or myalgia. These symptoms are typically intermittent. The diagnosis of EM must be made by a physician. Laboratory confirmation is recommended for persons with no known exposure.
- *Late manifestations*. Late manifestations include any of the following when an alternate explanation is not found:
  1. *Musculoskeletal system*. Recurrent, brief attacks (weeks or months) of objective joint swelling in one or a few joints, sometimes followed by chronic arthritis in one or a few joints. Manifestations not considered as criteria for diagnosis include chronic progressive arthritis not preceded by brief attacks and chronic symmetric polyarthritis. Additionally, arthralgia, myalgia, or fibromyalgia syndromes alone are not criteria for musculoskeletal involvement.
  2. *Nervous system*. Any of the following, alone or in combination: lymphocytic meningitis; cranial neuritis, particularly facial palsy (may be bilateral); radiculoneuropathy; or, rarely, encephalomyelitis. Encephalomyelitis must be confirmed by demonstration of antibody production against *B. burgdorferi* in the CSF, evidenced by a higher titer of antibody in CSF than in serum. Headache, fatigue, paresthesia, and mildly stiff neck alone are not criteria for neurological involvement.

(Continued)

Table 8 (*Continued*)

    3. *Cardiovascular system.* Acute onset of high-grade (second- or third-degree) atrioventricular conduction defects that resolve in days to weeks and are sometimes associated with myocarditis. Palpitations, bradycardia, bundle branch block, or myocarditis alone are not criteria for cardiovascular involvement.

- *Exposure.* Exposure is defined as having been (less than or equal to 30 days before onset of EM) in wooded, brushy, or grassy areas (i.e., potential tick habitats) in a county in which Lyme disease is endemic. A history of tick bite is not required.
- *Disease endemic to county.* A county in which Lyme disease is endemic is one in which at least two confirmed cases have been previously acquired or in which established populations of a known tick vector are infected with *B. burgdorferi.*

Adapted from the website of the Centers for Disease Control. Available at http://www.cdc.gov/epo/dphsi/print/lyme_disease_current.htm.

NEUROCYSTICERCOSIS

Table 9
Diagnostic Criteria for Neurocysticercosis

Categories of criteria	Criteria
Absolute	1. Histological demonstration of the parasite from biopsy of a brain or spinal cord lesion. 2. Cystic lesions showing the scolex on CT or MRI. 3. Direct visualization of subretinal parasites by funduscopic examination.
Major	1. Lesions highly suggestive of neurocysticercosis on neuroimaging studies.[a] 2. Positive serum EITB[b] for the detection of anticysticercal antibodies. 3. Resolution of intracranial cystic lesions after therapy with albendazole or praziquantel. 4. Spontaneous resolution of small single enhancing lesions.[c]
Minor	1. Lesions compatible with neurocysticercosis on neuroimaging studies.[d] 2. Clinical manifestations suggestive of neurocysticercosis.[e] 3. Positive CSF ELISA for detection of anticysticercal antibodies or cysticercal antigens. 4. Cysticercosis outside the CNS.[f]
Epidemiologic	1. Evidence of a household contact with *Taenia solium* infection. 2. Individuals coming from or living in an area where cysticercosis is endemic. 3. History of frequent travel to disease endemic areas.

   [a]CT or MRI showing cystic lesions without scolex, enhancing lesions, or typical parenchymal brain calcifications.

   [b]EITB assay using purified extracts of *Taenia solium* antigens, as developed by the Centers for Disease Control and Prevention (Atlanta, GA).

   [c]Solitary ring-enhancing lesions measuring less than 20 mm in diameter in patients presenting with seizures, a normal neurological examination, and no evidence of an active systemic disease.

   [d]CT or MRI showing hydrocephalus or abnormal enhancement of the leptomeninges, and myelograms showing multiple filling defects in the column of contrast medium.

   [e]Seizures, focal neurological signs, intracranial hypertension, and dementia.

   [f]Histologically confirmed subcutaneous or muscular cysticercosis, plain X-ray films showing "cigar-shaped" soft-tissue calcifications, or direct visualization of cysticerci in the anterior chamber of the eye.

   CT, computed tomography; MRI, magnetic resonance imaging; EITB, enzyme-linked immunotransfer blot; CSF, cerebrospinal fluid; ELISA, enzyme-linked immunosorbent assay; CNS, central nervous system.

   (Adapted with permission from Del Brutto OH, Rajshekhar V, White AC Jr, et al. Proposed diagnostic criteria for neurocysticercosis. Neurology 2001;57:177–183.)

Table 10
Degrees of Certainty for the Diagnosis of Neurocysticercosis

Diagnostic certainty	Criteria
Definitive	1. Presence of one absolute criterion.
	2. Presence of two major plus one minor and one epidemiological criterion.
Probable	1. Presence of one major plus two minor criteria.
	2. Presence of one major plus one minor and one epidemiological criterion.
	3. Presence of three minor plus one epidemiological criterion.

The presence of two different lesions is highly suggestive of neurocysticercosis on neuroimaging studies should be considered as two major diagnostic criteria. However, positive results in two separate types of antibody detection tests should be interpreted only based on the test failing in the highest category of diagnostic criteria.

(Adapted with permission from Del Brutto OH, Rajshekhar V, White AC Jr, et al. Proposed diagnostic criteria for neurocysticercosis Neurology 2001;57:177–183.)

NEUROSYPHILIS

Table 11
Diagnostic Criteria for Neurosyphilis

1. **Clinical description**
   - Evidence of central nervous system infection with *Treponema pallidum*.
2. **Laboratory criteria for diagnosis**
   - A reactive serological test for syphilis and reactive venereal disease research laboratory test in cerebrospinal fluid (CSF).
3. **Case classification**
   Probable: syphilis of any stage, a negative venereal disease research laboratory test in CSF, and both the following:
   - Elevated CSF protein or leukocyte count in the absence of other known causes of these abnormalities.
   - Clinical symptoms or signs consistent with neurosyphilis without other known causes for these clinical abnormalities.
   Confirmed: syphilis of any stage that meets the laboratory criteria for neurosyphilis.

Adapted from the website of the Centers for Disease Control. Available at http://www.cdc.gov/epo/dphsi/casedef/syphiliscurrent.htm#neuro.

HUMAN RABIES

Table 12
1997 Case Definition of Human Rabies From the Centers for Disease Control and Prevention

1. **Clinical description**
   Rabies is an acute encephalomyelitis that usually progresses to coma or death within 10 days after the first symptom.
2. **Laboratory criteria for diagnosis**
   - Detection by direct fluorescent antibody of viral antigens in a clinical specimen (preferably the brain or the nerves surrounding hair follicles in the nape of the neck), or
   - Isolation (in cell culture or in a laboratory animal) of rabies virus from saliva, cerebrospinal fluid, or central nervous system tissue, or
   - Identification of a rabies-neutralizing antibody titer greater than or equal to 5 (complete neutralization) in the serum or cerebrospinal fluid of an unvaccinated person
3. **Case classification**
   Confirmed: a clinically compatible case that is laboratory confirmed.

Laboratory confirmation by all of the above methods is strongly recommended.
(Adapted from the website of the Centers for Disease Control. Available at http://www.cdc.gov/epo/dphsi/print/rabies_human_current.htm.)

Table 13
Diagnostic Criteria for Subacute Sclerosing Panencephalitis

Major
  1 Elevated cerebrospinal fluid measles antibody titers.
  2 Typical or atypical clinical history.
  3 Typical: acute (rapidly) progressive, subacute progressive, chronic progressive, chronic remitting/relapsing.
  4 Atypical: seizures, prolonged stage I, unusual age (infancy, adulthood).
Minor
  5 Typical electroencephalography(periodic slow wave complexes).
  6 Cerebrospinal fluid immunoglobulin G increased.
  7 Brain biopsy: typical inflammatory pathology, extra-/intranuclear inclusions, neurofibrillary tangles.
Special
  8 Molecular diagnostic techniques to identify mutations of wild-type measles virus genome.
  9 The more atypical the case, the more criteria 5 and/or 6 are required.

Reprinted with permission from Gascon GG. Randomized treatment study of inosiplex versus combined inosiplex and intraventricular interferon-α in subacute sclerosing panencephalitis (SSPE): international multicenter study. J Child Neurol 2004;18:819–827, and from BC Decker.

SUBACUTE SCLEROSING PANENCEPHALITIS

This rare condition is caused by aberrant measles virus with nonproductive persistent infection of neural cells. It most often occurs in childhood or adolescence, although rare adult cases have been described. Males are more frequently affected than females, and the greatest risk occurs in children infected with measles in the first year of life.

The clinical course begins (stage I) with a slowly progressive dementia, often affecting behavior and associated with school performance decline. Stage II features include spasticity, weakness, and myoclonic jerks, and seizures occur. Optic manifestations are common and include a macular choreoretinitis and optic atrophy. There may be cerebellar ataxia and dystonia. Stage III is marked by stupor and coma, often with autonomic instability leading to marked fluctuations in body temperature and abnormal sweating.

Diagnosis may be made with the presence of one major and one minor criterion.

WHIPPLE'S DISEASE

Whipple's disease is caused by the bacterium *Tropheryma whipplei*. It most commonly affects the small intestine, where it produces a syndrome of chronic diarrhea and malabsorption. The central nervous system is sometimes also involved, and rarely is the only apparent site of disease. Within the nervous system, it may produce dementia and behavioral, visual changes, supranuclear gaze palsy, seizures, autonomic/hypothalamic disturbances, oculomasticatory myorhythmia, and oculofacial-skeletal myorhythmia. Other systemic symptoms of Whipple's disease include polyarthralgias and relapsing fever.

The diagnosis may be suspected on clinical grounds. Polymerase chain reaction on cerebrospinal fluid samples for *T. whipplei*, or histopathological identification on biopsy specimens is possible. Galldicks et al. described a novel combination of magnetic resonance imaging findings and positron-emission tomography scan results, but only in a single case. There was a nonenhancing, nonedematous lesion with an incomplete shell of fluid surrounding the lesion. Positron-emission tomography scanning showed very low tracer uptake. Treatment is with long-term antibiotics for up to 1 year in length.

Table 14
Diagnostic Criteria for Central Nervous System Whipple's Disease

  1. **Definite central nervous system (CNS) Whipple's disease**
      Must have one of the following three criteria:
      a. Oculomasticatory myorhythmia or oculofacial-skeletal myorhythmia.
      b. Positive tissue biopsy.
      c. Positive polymerase chain reaction (PCR) analysis.

(Continued)

Table 14 *(Continued)*

If the histological or PCR analysis was not performed on CNS tissue, then the patient must also demonstrate neurological signs. If the histological or PCR analysis is performed on CNS tissue, then the patient need not show neurological signs (i.e., asymptomatic CNS infection).

2. **Possible CNS Whipple's disease**

Must have one of four systemic symptoms, not because of another known etiology:
   a. Fever of unknown etiology.
   b. Gastrointestinal symptoms (steatorrhea, chronic diarrhea, abdominal distension, or pain).
   c. Chronic migratory arthralgias or polyarthralgias.
   d. Unexplained lymphadenopathy, night sweats, or malaise.

Also must have any one of four neurological signs, not because of another known etiology:
   a. Supranuclear vertical gaze palsy.
   b. Rhythmic myoclonus.
   c. Dementia with psychiatric symptoms.
   d. Hypothalamic manifestations.

Adapted with permission from Louis ED, Lynch T, Kaufmann P, Fahn S, Odel J. Diagnostic guidelines in central nervous system Whipple's disease. Ann Neurol 1996;40:561–568, and from John Wiley and Sons.

SOURCES

AIDS

AIDS and HIV surveillance case definition. MMWR 1999;48(RR13):29–31.

HIV-1-Associated Progressive Multifocal Leukoencephalopathy

Giesen HJ, Neuen-Jacob E, Dorries K, Jablonowski H, Roick H, Arendt G. Diagnsotic criteria and clinical procedures in HIV-1 associated progressive multifocal leukoencephalopathy. J Neurol Sci 1997;147:63–72.

Arboviral Encephalitis and Meningitis

Centers for Disease Control and Prevention, Division of Public Health Surveillance and Informatics. Encephalitis or Meningitis, Arboviral (includes California serogroup, Eastern equine, St. Louis, Western equine, West Nile, Powassan). Available at http://www.cdc.gov/epo/dphsi/casedef/encephalitiscurrent.htm.

Infective Endocarditis

Durack DT, Lukes AS, Bright DK, et al. New criteria for diagnosis of infective endocarditis: utilization of specific echo-cardiographic findings. Am J Med 1994;96:200–209.

Prendergast BD. Diagnostic criteria and problems in infective endocarditis. Heart 2004; 90:611–613.

van Reyn CF, Levy BS, Arbeit RD, et al. Infective endocarditis: an analysis based on strict case definitions. Ann Intern Med 1981;94:505–517.

Lyme Disease

Centers for Disease Control and Prevention, Division of Public Health Surveillance and Informatics. Lyme Disease (*Borrelia burgdorferi*). Available at http://www.cdc.gov/epo/dphsi/print/lyme_disease_current.htm.

Neurocysticercosis

Del Brutto OH, Rajshekhar V, White AC Jr, et al. Proposed diagnostic criteria for neurocysticercosis Neurology 2001;57:177–183.

Neurosyphilis

Centers for Disease Control and Prevention, Division of Public Health Surveillance and Informatics. Syphilis. Available at http://www.cdc.gov/epo/dphsi/casedef/syphiliscurrent.htm#neuro.

Human Rabies

Centers for Disease Control and Prevention, Division of Public Health Surveillance and Informatics. Rabies, Human. Available at http://www.cdc.gov/epo/dphsi/print/rabies_human_current.htm.

Subacute Sclerosing Panencephalitis

Gascon GG. Randomized treatment study of inosiplex versus combined inosiplex and intraventricular interferon-α in subacute sclerosing panencephalitis (SSPE): international multicenter study. J Child Neurol 2004;18:819–827.

Whipple's Disease

Galldiks N, Burghaus L, Vollmar S, et al. Novel neuroimaging findings in a patient with cerebral Whipple's disease: a magnetic resonance imaging and positron emission tomography study. J Neuroimaging 2004;14:372–376.

Halperin JJ, Landis DM, Kleinman GM. Whipple disease of the nervous system. Neurology 1982;32:612–617.

Louis ED. Whipple disease. Curr Neurol Neurosci Rep 2003;3:470–475.

Louis ED, Lynch T, Kaufmann P, Fahn S, Odel J. Diagnostic guidelines in central nervous system Whipple's disease. Ann Neurol 1996;40:561–568.

11

Movement Disorders

CORTICOBASAL DEGENERATION

First described in the 1960s, corticobasal degeneration is also known as cortical-basal ganglionic degeneration. It typically comes on as an asymmetric parkinsonian syndrome, most often in the sixth decade or later. Long considered a rare disorder, the description of additional cases and case series in recent years has widened the clinical spectrum.

Cortical manifestations of corticobasal degeneration include not only dementia and alien limb sign, but also apraxia and cortical sensory loss. The basal ganglionic component includes parkinsonism and limb dystonia. There may be postural tremor and a focal reflex myoclonus. Dementia may be the presenting sign. Not all patients exhibit the "alien limb" sign throughout the clinical course.

Two sets of diagnostic criteria derived from clinical case series are summarized in Table 1. Proposed research diagnostic criteria are listed in Table 2.

Table 1
Clinical Manifestations of Corticobasal Degeneration

Reference	Clinical manifestations
Riley et al., 1990	*Basal ganglia signs:* Akinesia, rigidity; limb dystonia; athetosis; postural instability, falls; orolingual dyskinesias. *Cerebral cortical signs:* Cortical sensory loss, alien limb phenomenon, dementia, apraxia, frontal release reflexes, dysphasia. *Other manifestations:* Postural-action tremor, hyperreflexia, impaired ocular motility, dysarthria, focal reflex myoclonus, impaired eyelid motion, dysphagia.
Watts et al., 1994, 1997	*Major:* Akinesia, rigidity, postural/gait disturbance; action/postural tremor; alien limb phenomenon; cortical signs; dystonia; myoclonus. *Minor:* Choreoathetosis, dementia, cerebellar signs, supranuclear gaze abnormalities, frontal release signs, blepharospasm.

Adapted with permission from Litvan I, Bhatia KP, Burn DJ, et al. SIC task force appraisal of clinical diagnostic criteria for Parkinsonian disorders. Mov Dis 2003;18:46–486, and from John Wiley and Sons.

Table 2
Proposed Research Criteria for Corticobasal Degeneration

Reference	Inclusion criteria	Exclusion criteria
Lang et al., 1994	Rigidity plus one cortical sign (apraxia, cortical sensory loss, or alien limb). *Or* Asymmetric rigidity, dystonia and focal reflex myoclonus.	Early dementia, early vertical gaze palsy, rest tremor, severe autonomic disturbances, sustained responsiveness to levodopa, lesions on imaging studies indicating another pathological condition.

(Continued)

From: *Current Clinical Neurology: Diagnostic Criteria in Neurology*
Edited by: A. J. Lerner © Humana Press Inc., Totowa, NJ

Table 2 *(Continued)*

Reference	Inclusion criteria	Exclusion criteria
Kumar et al., 1998	Chronic progressive course, asymmetric onset, presence of: "higher" cortical dysfunction (apraxia, cortical sensory loss, or alien limb). *And* Movement disorders: akinetic rigid syndrome-levodopa resistant, and limb dystonia and reflex; focal myoclonus.	

Qualification of clinical features: rigidity, easily detectable without reinforcement; apraxia, more than simple use of limb as an object, clear absence of cognitive or motor deficit; cortical sensory loss, asymmetric, with preserved primary sensation; alien limb phenomenon, more than simple levitation; dystonia, focal in limb, present at rest at onset; myoclonus, reflex myoclonus spreading beyond stimulated digits.

(Adapted with permission from Litvan I, Bhatia KP, Burn DJ, et al. SIC task force appraisal of clinical diagnostic criteria for Parkinsonian disorders. Mov Dis 2003;18:467–486, and from John Wiley and Sons.)

DYSTONIA OWING TO *DYT1* MUTATIONS

Table 3
Diagnostic Criteria for Dystonia Because of DYT1 Mutations

1.	Definite dystonia	Characteristic overt twisting or directional movements and postures that are consistently present.
2.	Probable dystonia	Postures or movements suggestive of dystonia that are insufficient in intensity or consistency to merit classification as definite (e.g., excessively tense and labored writing with minimal posturing, flurries of blinking, but no episodes of sustained closure, mild or intermittent head deviation).
3.	Possible dystonia	Muscle contractions not considered abnormal but remotely suggestive of dystonia (e.g., unusual hand grip with mild excess hand tension but normal flowing handwriting, increased blinking with no flurries or sustained contractions, clumsy rapid feet movements with intermittent overflow toe posturing).
4.	Additional features	Scoliosis and regular tremor (i.e., without sustained directionality) were not considered signs of dystonia for any category.
5.	"Unratable" characteristics	Individuals with neurological abnormalities, such as hemiparesis because of stroke, that could mask dystonia or etiological factors, such as neuroleptic exposure or birth injury, that obfuscate a diagnosis of primary torsion dystonia.

Adapted from Bressman, S. B., Raymond D, Wendt K, et al. Diagnostic criteria for dystonia in *DYT1* families. Neurology 2002;59:1780–1782.

ESSENTIAL TREMOR

Frequently familial in nature, essential tremor is one of the more common neurological disorders. There have been multiple diagnostic criteria used in studies reported in the medical literature, resulting in heterogeneity of definition. Because the majority of individuals have a small physiological tremor, inclusion of these individuals in studies affects reported prevalence estimates and may affect population studies of genetic markers in essential tremor.

A proposed set of diagnostic criteria was published by Louis et al., based on a comparison of 10 different criteria in their Washington Heights–Inwood Genetic Study of Essential Tremor. They emphasize the need not only to consider the form of the tremor, but also its severity in making the diagnosis of essential tremor.

Table 4
Tremor Rating Scale

0	No visible tremor.
1	Low amplitude, barely perceivable tremor, or present intermittently.
2	Moderate amplitude (1–2 cm), clearly oscillatory, and usually present.
3	Large amplitude (>2 cm), violent, jerky, affecting writing or spilling liquids.

Adapted with permission from Louis ED, Ford B, Lee H, Andrews H, Cameron B. Diagnostic criteria for essential tremor: a population perspective. Arch Neurol 1998;55:823–828.

Table 5
Diagnostic Criteria for Essential Tremor

Criteria for definite ET (all five must be true)

1. On examination, a + 2 postural tremor of at least one arm (a head tremor may also be present, but is not sufficient for the diagnosis).
2. On examination, there must be
   a. a + 2 kinetic tremor during at least four tasks, or
   b. a – 2 kinetic tremor on one task and a + 3 kinetic tremor on a second task; tasks include pouring water, using a spoon to drink water, drinking water, touching finger to nose, and drawing a spiral.
3. If on examination the tremor is present in the dominant hand, them by report it must interfere with at least one activity of daily living (eating, drinking, writing, or using the hands). If on examination the tremor is not present in the dominant hand, then this criterion is irrelevant.
4. Medications, alcohol, Parkinsonism, dystonia, other basal ganglionic discoders, and hyperthyroidism are not potential etiological factors.
5. Not psychogenic (bizarre features, inconsistent in character, changing, subject is distractable, or other psychiatric features on examination).

Criteria for probable ET (either 1a or 1b must be true; 2 and 3 must be true)

1. a. Same as 2 above (*see* definite ET).
   b. Head tremor is present on examination.
2. Use of medications, alcohol, Parkinsonism, dystonia, other basal ganglionic disorders, and hyperthyroidism are nor potential etiological factors.
3. Not psychogenic.

Criteria for possible ET

1. On examination, a + 2 kinetic tremor must be present on three tasks 0 to +3 Tremor ratings.
0. No visible tremor.
+1. Low amplitude, barely perceivable tremor, or intermittent tremor.
+2. Tremor is of moderate emplitude (1–2 cm) and usually present it is clearly oscillatory.
+3. Large amplitude (>2 cm), violent, jerky tremor resulting in difficulty completing the task owing to spilling or inability to hold a pen to paper.

ET, essential tremor.
(Reprinted with permission from Louis ED, Ford B, Lee H, Andrews H, Cameron B. Diagnostic criteria for essential tremor: a population persepective. Arch Neurol 1998;55:823–828 and from the American Medical Association.)

FAHR'S DISEASE

Fahr's disease is a condition associated with calcifications within the brain. An alternate name for this condition is idiopathic bilateral basal ganglia (or striatopallidodentate) calcinosis. Many of the described cases have been associated with disturbances of calcium and phosphorus homeostasis, such as hyperparathyroidism. Familial forms have also been described. The nosology of Fahr's disease is complicated by the lack of clinical–pathological correlations and speculation on the role of calcification in the etiology of the observed syndrome.

Diagnostic criteria have been proposed based on a series of 17 patients described by Shibayama et al., although their accuracy and reliability has not been examined. Additionally, the criteria do not mention the Parkinsonism that has been associated with Fahr's disease.

Table 6
Proposed Diagnostic Criteria for Fahr's Disease

1. Insidious onset.
2. Progressive impairment of memory.
3. Early personality change (loss of social and ethical awareness).
4. Disinhibition.
5. Early loss of insight.
6. Late in the course.
   a. Stereotyped and perseverative behavior and speech.
   b. Mutism.
7. Brain computer tomography shows bilateral frontal and temporal atrophy and calcification of the basal ganglia.

Adapted with permission from Shibayana H, Iwai K, Takeuchi T. Clinical diagnostic criteria for non-Alzheimer non-Pick dementia with Fahr's disease [NANPDF]. Neurobiol Aging 1996;17:S27, and Elsevier.

MULTIPLE-SYSTEM ATROPHY

Multiple-system atrophy is a progressive disorder with features of parkinsonism, cerebellar, autonomic, urinary, and corticospinal dysfunction. It is of unknown etiology. It most commonly affects middle-aged individuals, and both genders are affected equally. Disease course is variable and median survival from first symptoms is about 9 years.

The parkinsonian features are usually unresponsive to levodopa therapy. There may be gait and limb ataxia, orthostatic hypotension, erectile dysfunction, constipation, and decreased sweating. Whereas multiple-system atrophy is a distinct neuropathological entity, the consensus diagnostic criteria depend on specific clinical features. Pathologically, glial cytoplasmic inclusions and degeneration are found throughout the basal ganglia, substantia nigra, brainstem autonomic nuclei, and Purkinje cells of the cerebellum.

NEUROLEPTIC MALIGNANT SYNDROME

Neuroleptic malignant syndrome is usually thought of as a syndrome of fever and catatonic rigidity, with increased serum creatine phosphokinase levels in the setting of neuroleptic administration. The etiology of this disorder is obscure, and lack of consistent case definitions has hampered fuller study of this syndrome. The initial description of neuroleptic malignant syndrome referred to it as "pallor and hyperthermia" with isolated primary symptoms of fever, akinesia or stupor with hypertonicity, and pulmonary congestion. Since then, a number of diagnostic criteria have been proposed as summarized at length by Adityanjee, Mathews, and Aderibigbe in their 1999 review. In essence, the syndromic definitions stress the presence of rigidity, fever, and autonomic changes in the presence of neuroleptic exposure. Alteration in sensorium is also a common feature of several of these criteria.

Conditions with clinical similarity to neuroleptic malignant syndrome include malignant hyperthermia, drug toxicity (e.g., lithium), heat stroke, and related syndromes.

PANDAS SYNDROME

A heterogeneous clinical syndrome whose acronym stands for *p*ediatric *a*utoimmune *n*europsychiatric *d*isorders *a*ssociated with *s*treptococcal infections, the clinical recognition of PANDAS began with the observation of obsessive-compulsive disorder arising in individuals with Sydenham's chorea. In current usage, PANDAS primarily applies to children and adolescents with obsessive-compulsive or tic disorders occurring in association with streptococcal infections. The clinical spectrum of this "syndrome" may be widening, as recent case reports have included other movement disorders secondary to basal ganglia dysfunction with PANDAS, including dystonia, or chorea occurring after streptococcal infection. The common pathophysiology is felt to be antistreptococcal antibodies that crossreact with cellular structures in the basal ganglia, leading to neurological dysfunction.

Table 7
Clinical Domains, Features and Criteria Used in the Diagnosis of Multiple System Atrophy

I. Autonomic and urinary dysfunction
   A. Autonomic and urinary features
      1. Orthostatic hypotension (by 20 mmHg systolic or 10 mmHg diastolic).
      2. Urinary incontinence or incomplete bladder emptying.
   B. Criterion for autonomic failure or urinary dysfunction in MSA
      1. Orthostatic fall in blood pressure (by 30 mmHg systolic or 15 mmHg diastolic) or urinary incontinence (persistent, involuntary partial or total bladder emptying, accompanied by erectile dysfunction in men) or both.
II. Parkinsonism
   A. Parkinsonian features
      1. Bradykinesia (slowness of voluntary movement with progressive reduction in speed and amplitude during repetitive actions).
      2. Rigidity.
      3. Postural instability (not caused by primary visual, vestibular, cerebral, or proprioceptive dysfunction).
      4. Tremor (postural, resting, or both).
   B. Criterion for Parkinsonism in MSA
      1. Bradykinesia plus at least one of items 2 to 4.
III. Cerebellar dysfunction
   A. Cerebellar features
      1. Gait ataxia (wide-based stance with steps of irregular length and direction).
      2. Ataxic dysarthria.
      3. Limb ataxia.
      4. Sustained gaze-evoked nystagmus.
   B. Criterion for cerebellar dysfunction in MSA
      1. Gait ataxia plus at least one of items 2 to 4.
IV. Corticospinal tract dysfunction
   A. Corticospinal tract features
      1. Extensor plantar responses with hperreflexia.
   B. Corticospinal tract dysfunction in MSA: no corticospinal tract features are used in defining the diagnosis of MSA

A feature (A) is a characteristic of the disease and a criterion (B) is a defining feature or composite of features required for diagnosis.
MSA, multiple system atrophy.
(Reprinted from Gilman S, Low PA, Quinn N, et al. Consesus statement on the diagnosis of multiple system atrophy. J Neurol Sci 1999; 163:94–98 with permission from Elsevier).

Table 8
Diagnostic Categories of Multiple-System Atrophy

I. Possible MSA: one criterion plus two features from seperate domains. When the criterion is Parkinsonism, a poor levodopa response qualifies as one feature (hence only one additional future is required).
II. Probable MSA: criterion for autonomic failure/urinary dysfunction, plus poor levodopa-responsive Parkinsonism or cerebellar dysfunction.
III. Definite MSA: pathologically confirmed by the presence of a high density of glial cytoplasmic inclusions in association with a combination of degenerative changes in the nigrostriatal and olivopontocelebeller pathways.

The features and criteria for each clinical domain are shown in Table 7.
(Reprinted with permission from Gilman S, Low PA, Quinn N, et al. Consensus statement on the diagnosis of multiple system atrophy. J Neurol Sci 1999;163:94–98.)

PARKINSON'S DISEASE

Originally described by James Parkinson, Parkinson's disease (PD) is characterized by a combination of the cardinal symptoms of tremor, rigidity, bradykinesia, and postural instability. However, these

Table 9
Exclusion Criteria for the Diagnosis of MSA

I. History
    a. Symptomatic onset under 30 years of age.
    b. Family history of a similar disorder.
    c. Systemic diseases or other identifiable causes for features listed in Table 7.
    d. Hallucinations unrelated to medication.
II. Physical examination
    a. DSM criteria for dementia.
    b. Prominent slowing of vertical saccades or vertical supranuclear gaze plasy.[a]
    c. Evidence of focal cortical dysfunction such as aphasia, alien limb syndrome, and parietal dysfunction.
III. Laboratory investigation
    Metabolic, molecular, genetic, and imaging evidence of an alternative cause of feature listed in Table 7.

[a]In practice, multiple-system atrophy is most frequently confused with Parkinson's disease or progressive supranuclear palsy (PSP). Mild limitation of upward gaze alone is nonspecific, whereas a prominent (>50%) limitation of upward gaze of any limitation of downward gaze suggests PSP. Before the onset of vertical gaze limitation, a clinically obvious slowing of voluntary vertical saccades is usually easily detectable in PSP and assists in the early differentiation of these two disorders.
DSM, *Diagnostic and Statistical Manual of Psychiatric Disorders*.
(Reprinted with permission from Gilman S, Low PA, Quinn N, et al. Consesus statement on the diagnosis of multiple system atrophy. J Neurol Sci 1999;163:94–98, and Elsevier.)

Table 10
Neuroleptic Malignant Syndrome: Diagnostic Criteria (Levenson, 1985)

A. Major manifestations
    1. Fever.
    2. Rigidity.
    3. Elevated creatine phosphokinase levels.
    4. Altered consciousness.
    5. Diaphoresis.
    6. Leukocytosis.
B. Minor manifestations
    1. Tachycardia.
    2. Abnormal blood pressure.
    3. Tachypnea.

The presence of all three major or two major and four minor manifestations indicates a high probability of the presence of neuroleptic malignant syndrome, if supported by clinical history (e.g., not indicative of malignant hyperthermia).
(Adapted with permission from Adityanjee, Mathews T, Aderibighe YA. Proposed research diagnostic criteria for neuroleptic malignant syndrome. Int J Neuropsychopharmacol 1999;2:129–144.)

Table 11
Neuroleptic Malignant Syndrome: Diagnostic Criteria (Addonizio et al., 1986)

    1. Elevated temperature: at least 37.5°C in the absence of other systemic illness.
    2. Rigidity.
    3. Tremor.
    4. Tachycardia (at least 100 beats/min).
    5. Elevated blood pressure (at least 150/100 mmHg).
    6. Diaphoresis.
    7. Incontinence.
    8. Leukocytosis (>10,800 cells/mm^3).
    9. Confusion.
    10. Elevated creatine phosphokinase levels (>83 U/L).

The occurrence of 5 out of 10 symptoms in the same 48-hour period is used to identify an episode. The absence of fever and extra pyramidal symptoms preclude the diagnosis of neuroleptic malignant syndrome.
(Adapted with permission from Adityanjee, Mathews T, Aderibighe YA. Proposed research diagnostic criteria for neuroleptic malignant syndrome. Int J Neuropsychopharmacol 1999;2:129–144.)

Table 12
Neuroleptic Malignant Syndrome: Diagnostic Criteria

1. Hyperthermia:
   Oral temperature of at least 38°C[a] in the absence of other etiology.
2. Extrapyramidal symptoms (at least two of the following):
   a. Leadpipe rigidity.
   b. Trismus.
   c. Cogwheel rigidity.
   d. Dysphagia.
   e. Sialorrhea.
   f. Chorea.
   g. Oclogyric crisis.
   h. Dyskinetic movements.
   i. Retrocollis.
   j. Festinating gate.
   k. Opisthotonos.
   l. Flexor–extensor posturing.
3. Autonomic dysfunction (at least two of the following):
   a. Hypertension (at least 20 mmHg diastolic above the baseline).
   b. Tachycardia (at least 30 beats above baseline).
   c. Tachypnea (at least 25 breaths/min).
   d. Profuse sweating.
   e. Incontinence.
4. For retrospective diagnosis:
   If documentation of one of the above criteria is inadequate, diagnosis of probable neuroleptic malignant syndrome is permissible if the remaining two criteria are met, plus one of the following: clouded consciousness, delirium, mutism, stupor or coma, leukocytosis (white blood count > 15,000 cells/mm^3), serum creatine kinase level greater than 1000 U/L.

[a]The original criteria of Pope et al. permitted a diagnosis of neuroleptic malignant syndrome with oral hyperthermia of only 37.5°C.
(Pope et al. 1986; modified by Keck et al. 1989) (Adapted with permission from Adityanjee, Mathews T, Aderibighe YA. Proposed research diagnostic criteria for neuroleptic malignant syndrome. Int J Neuropsychopharmacol 1999;2:129–144.)

signs occur in a large number of other conditions, and occasionally all may occur in parkinsonian syndromes that are nonetheless distinct from PD.

Other symptoms that may occur in the course of PD, but are generally not included in its diagnosis include dementia, depression (with or without psychosis), and autonomic phenomena.

Response to medication (levodopa or dopamine agonists) has been increasingly recognized as part of the diagnosis. However useful, this limits prospective identification of individuals presenting to a physician for initial diagnosis.

Gelb, Oliver, and Gilman proposed clinical diagnostic criteria. They separated the cardinal symptoms—"group A" for the above-mentioned cardinal symptoms, and "group B" for symptoms suggestive of other possible diagnoses—and then added "possible," "probable," and "definite" classifications; they also proposed histopathological criteria for PD.

Other diagnostic criteria schema have been proposed. Albanese expands the list of exclusion criteria to include specific features, such as known cerebral vascular diseases with stepwise deterioration, head injuries, encephalitis, oculogyric crises, neuroleptic use at onset, Babinski signs, cerebellar signs, along with negative response to levodopa. The literature, however, has isolated cases with many of these symptoms, or cases that fulfill diagnostic criteria for PD while manifesting other conditions and confirmed by autopsy.

PAROXYSMAL KINESIEGENIC DYSKINESIA

A rare syndrome where there are involuntary movements associated with quick voluntary movements. Paroxysmal kinesiegenic dyskinesia (PKD) occurs either as an idiopathic or secondary disorder.

Table 13
Diagnostic Criteria of Neuroleptic Malignant Syndrome (Adityanjee et al., 1988)

Essential clinical criteria (all four of the following must be present):
1. Altered sensorium (any of the following):
   a. Confusion.
   b. Clouding of consciousness.
   c. Disorientation.
   d. Mutism.
   e. Stupor.
   f. Coma.

Should be documented by at least two independent observers on at least 2 consecutive days.
Nonspecific changes in mental state, e.g., restlessness or agitation, should not be equated with altered sensorium
2. Muscular rigidity.
3. Hyperpyrexia of unknown origin:
   a. Should be greater than 38°C orally.
   b. Should be more than 24 hours in duration.
   c. No concurrent physical cause for hyperpyrexia.
4. Autonomic dysfunction (at least two of the following):
   a. Rapid pulse (more than 90 beats/min).
   b. Rapid respiration (more than 25 breaths/min).
   c. Blood pressure fluctuations (at least a change of 30 mmHg in systolic pressure or 15 mmHg in diastolic pressure).
   d. Excessive sweating.
   e. Incontinence.
   f. Supportive features:
      i. Elevations in serum creatine phosphokinase levels.
      ii. Leukocytosis.

These should be considered as inessential features only as they are nonspecific and not of much diagnostic value.

(Adapted from Adityanjee, Mathews T, Aderibighe YA. Proposed research diagnostic criteria for neuroleptic malignant syndrome. Int J Neuropsychopharmacol 1999;2:129–144, with permission.)

Table 14
Neuroleptic Malignant Syndrome: Diagnostic Criteria (Caroff et al., 1991; Caroff and Mann, 1993; Lazarus et al., 1989)

All five items required concurrently:
1. Treatment with neuroleptics within 7 days of onset (2–4 weeks for depot neuroleptics).
2. Hyperthermia (38°C or more).
3. Muscle rigidity.
4. Five of the following:
   a. Change in mental status.
   b. Tremor.
   c. Tachycardia.
   d. Incontinence.
   e. Hypotension or hypertension creatine phosphokinase elevation or myoglobinuria.
   f. Tachypnea or hypoxia.
   g. Leukocytosis.
   h. Diaphoresis or sialorrhea metabolic acidosis.
   i. Dysarthria or dysphagia.
5. Exclusion of other drug-induced, systemic, or neuropsychiatric illness.

(Adapted from Adityanjee, Mathews T, Aderibighe YA. Proposed research diagnostic criteria for neuroleptic malignant syndrome. Int J Neuropsychopharmacol 1999;2:129–144, with permission.)

Table 15
Research Diagnostic Criteria for Neuroleptic Malignant Syndrome

1. Altered sensorium (any one of the following):
   a. Confusion.
   b. Clouding of consciousness.
   c. Mutism.
   d. Stupor.
   e. Coma.
   Rating of severity should be done by at least two independent observers on Glasgow Coma Scale on at least 2 consecutive days. Nonspecific changes in mental state, e.g., restlessness or agitation, should not be equated with altered sensorium.
2. Extrapyramidal motor symptoms (any one of the following):
   a. Muscular rigidity.
   b. Dysphagia.
   c. Dystonia.
   d. Motor symptoms should be rated on the Simpson-Angus (extrapyramidal symptoms) Rating Scale.
3. Hyperpyrexia of unknown origin:
   a. Should be greater than 38.5°C orally.
   b. Should be sustained for at least 48 hours in duration.
   c. No concurrent physical/medical cause for hyperpyrexia.
4. Autonomic dysfunction (at least two of the following):
   a. Tachycardia (pulse more than 100 beats/min).
   b. Tachypnea (respiration more than 25 breaths/min).
   c. Blood pressure fluctuations (at least a change of 30 mmHg in systolic pressure or 15 mmHg in diastolic pressure).
   d. Excessive sweating (diaphoresis).
   e. New-onset incontinence.
5. Relationship of onset of symptoms with exposure event defined by any one of the following:
   a. Oral ingestion or parenteral administration (dose increase, dose decrease, discontinuation) of an antipsychotic drug (typical or atypical), a dopamine depleter (e.g., tetrabenazine) dopamine blocker (e.g., metoclopramide) or a psychostimulant drug (e.g., cocaine) during the previous 2 weeks.
   b. Withdrawal of antiparkinsonian (e.g., amantidine) or anticholinergic drug during previous week.
   c. Intramuscular administration of a long-acting depot antipsychotic medication during the previous 8 weeks.
6. Exclusion criteria:
   Symptoms not caused by any other existing or new general medical (secondary to substance abuse, infectious illnesses, metabolic, delirium, etc.), neurological (encephalitis, epilepsy, brain tumors, etc.) or psychiatric disorder (e.g., catatonic schizophrenia, mood disorder with catatonic features).
7. Supportive features (any two of the following):
   a. Elevations in serum creatine phosphokinase levels.
   b. Leukocytosis.
   c. Low serum iron levels.
   d. Elevation of liver enzymes.
   e. Myoglobinuria.

Type I NMS
   Criteria 1–6 must be present for making a research diagnosis.

Type II NMS
   Criteria 1 and 3 and 4–6, and any one item from criterion 7 must be present for the diagnosis. Criterion 2 is not necessary for making diagnosis.

Standardized assessment
   All the patients with a suspected diagnosis should be rated on the following: Glasgow Coma Scale, Simpson-Angus (extrapyramidal symptoms) Rating Scale, and Bush-Francis Catatonia Rating Scale.

Adapted with permission from Adityanjee, Mathews T, Aderibighe YA. Proposed research diagnostic criteria for neuroleptic malignant syndrome. Int J Neuropsychopharmacol 1999;2:129–144.

Table 16
Diagnostic Criteria for Pediatric Autoimmune Neuropsychiatric Disorders Associated With Streptococcal Infections Syndrome

1.	Presence of obsessive-compulsive disorder and/or a tic disorder.
2.	Pediatric onset of symptoms (age 3 years to puberty).
3.	Episodic course of symptom severity.
4.	Association with group A β-hemolytic streptococcal infection (a positive throat culture for strep throat or history of scarlet fever).
5.	Association with neurological abnormalities (motoric hyperactivity or adventitious movements, such as choreiform movements).

Adapted from Frequently asked questions about PANDAS. Pediatric Autoimmune Neuropsychiatric Disorders Associated with Streptococcal Infections. Available via http://intramural.nimh.nih.gov/pdn/faqs.htm.

Secondary cases may be seen in association with multiple sclerosis, metabolic derangements (hypo- or hyperglycemia), cerebrovascular disease, or after trauma.

The exact gene has not been identified, but PKD may be seen in conjunction with the syndrome of infantile convulsions and choreoathetosis, which is linked to the pericentric region of chromosome 16. However, cases linked to loci elsewhere on chromosome 16 or other chromosomes have been reported. PKD has also been seen in episodic ataxia type 1, which suggests that it may be a channelopathy.

PROGRESSIVE SUPRANUCLEAR PALSY

First described by Steele, Richardson, and Olzweski in 1964, progressive supranuclear palsy (PSP) is also known by its acronym. The original descriptions focused on the parkinsonian movement disorder with progressive eye movement abnormality and frequent falls. Dementia also occurs as part of the clinical expression of PSP. PSP is almost never familial in nature. More recent investigations have tended to widen the scope of the clinical spectrum, and clinical overlaps occur, particularly with corticobasal degeneration. PSP may be misdiagnosed as PD or vascular dementia. False-negative diagnoses confirmed pathologically may include not only corticobasal degeneration but also multiple-system atrophy, central nervous system Whipple's disease, diffuse Lewy body disease, subcortical gliosis, and prion diseases.

Of some difficulty in diagnosis is that the characteristic eye movements may not be present initially, although there is good agreement that slowed vertical saccades are the most consistent early eye movement abnormality.

There have been a number of sets of diagnostic criteria proposed, mostly on clinical grounds. These are shown in Table 19. The validity and reliability of these criteria have been investigated in several studies, and the results are summarized in Table 20.

The latest set of diagnostic criteria is the National Institute of Neurological Disorders and Stroke-PSP clinical criteria and is included in Table 21.

STIFF-PERSON SYNDROME

Stiff-person syndrome is problematic in terms of its proper classification. It could be placed among movement disorders, neuromuscular disorders, or immune-based conditions. A paraneoplastic form of this disorder also exists. It is most commonly an autoimmune condition, with circulating antibodies to glutamic acid decarboxylase. Other conditions, such as Batten's disease, may also have autoantibodies to glutamic acid decarboxylase, although the specific antibody epitope on the protein molecule may be different.

Diagnostic criteria for the stiff-person syndrome are adapted from those of Lorish et al. (who also considered a positive response to intravenous or oral diazepam a prerequisite for the diagnosis of the stiff-person syndrome).

Table 17
Proposed Diagnostic Criteria for Parkinson's Disease

I. Clinical features according to diagnostic utility
    A. Group A: Characteristic of Parkinson's disease
        1. Resting tremor.
        2. Rigidity.
        3. Bradykinesia.
        4. Asymmetric onset.
    B. Group B: Suggestive of other diseases
        1. Features unusual early in the disease:
            a. Prominent postural instability within the first 3 years of the disease.
            b. Freezing phenomena in the first 3 years.
            c. Hallucinations unrelated to medications in the first 3 years.
            d. Dementia preceding motor symptoms or in the first year:
                i. Supranuclear gaze palsy (other than upgaze restriction) or slowing of saccades.
                ii. Severe, symptomatic dysautonomia unrelated to medications.
                iii. Documentation of a lesion or condition associated with parkinsonism and plausibly connected to the patient's symptom (e.g., focal brain lesion or recent neuroleptic exposure).
II. Possible Parkinson's disease
    A. At least two of four group A symptoms, at least one of which is tremor or bradykinesia
    And
    B. *Either* no group B symptoms
    Or
    Symptoms less than 3 years duration, and none of the group B symptoms are present to date
    And
    C. *Either* substantial and sustained response to levodopa or a dopamine agonist has been documented
    Or
    Patient has not had an adequate trial of levodopa or a dopamine agonist.
III. Probable Parkinson's disease
    A. At least three group A symptoms are present
    And
    B. No group B symptoms present for those with symptoms over 3 years
    And
    C. Substantial and sustained response to levodopa or a dopamine agonist has been documented.
IV. Definite Parkinson's disease
    A. All criteria for *possible* or *probable* Parkinson's disease are met
    And
    B. Histopathological confirmation of the diagnosis

Adapted with permission from Gelb DJ, Oliver E, Gilman S. Diagnostic criteria for Parkinson's disease. Arch Neurol 1999;56:33–39.

TOURETTE SYNDROME AND TIC DISORDERS

A *tic* is an involuntary, rapid, recurrent, nonrhythmic motor movement (usually involving circumscribed muscle groups), or vocal production that is of sudden onset and serves no apparent purpose. Tics are often described as "irresistible," but they can usually be suppressed for varying periods. Tics can be motor or vocal tics, and may be simple or complex, although the boundaries are not well defined. Examples of simple tics include eye blinking, neck jerking, shoulder shrugging, and facial grimacing. Common simple vocal tics include throat clearing, barking, sniffing, and hissing. Complex tics include hitting oneself, jumping, and hopping. Common complex vocal tics include the repetition of particular words, and sometimes coprolalia (cursing), and palilalia, which is the repetition of one's own sounds or words. Coprolalia is not an explicit or compulsory diagnostic criteria.

Table 18
Proposed Clinical Criteria for Paroxysmal Kinesiegenic Dyskinesia

1. Identified kinesigenic trigger for the attacks.
2. Short duration of attacks (<1 minute).
3. No loss of consciousness or pain during attacks.
4. Exclusion of other organic diseases and normal neurological examination.
5. Control of attacks with phenytoin or carbamazepine, if tried.
6. Age at onset between 1 and 20 years, if no family history of PKD.

Adapted from Bruno MK, Hallett M, Gwinn-Hardy K, et al. Clinical evaluation of idiopathic paroxysmal kinesigenic dyskinesia: new diagnostic criteria. Neurology. 2004;63:2280–2287.

Table 19
Published Diagnostic Criteria for Progressive Supranuclear Palsy

Reference	Derivation and use
Lees, 1987	Defined as progressive nonfamilial disorder beginning in middle- or old age with SNO and exhibits two of five "cardinal features."[a]
Blin et al., 1990	Defined as "probable" if all of nine criteria are met or "possible" if seven of nine are fulfilled.[a]
Duvoisin, 1992	Criteria divided into four sections—essential for diagnosis, confirmatory manifestations, manifestations consistent with but not diagnostic of PSP and features inconsistent with PSP.[a]
Golbe, 1993	Defined as onset after age 40, progressive course bradykinesia and SNO, plus three of six further features, plus absence of three "inconsistent" clinical features.[a]
Tolosa et al., 1994	Defined as a nonfamilial disorder of onset after age 40, progressive course and SNO, plus three of five further features for "probable" and two of five for "possible," plus absence of five "inconsistent" clinical features.[a]
Collins et al., 1995	Retrospectively from review of 12 pathologically confirmed cases; algorithm-based, including prerequisites and exclusionary criteria; SNO and/or prominent postural instability, plus a number of other specified signs.
Litvan et al., 1996	Systematic literature review, logistic regression and CART analysis; validated using data from postmortem confirmed cases; "definite," "probable," and "possible" categories described.

Features among different set of criteria overlap.

[a]Based on the experience of the investigator.

SNO, supranuclear ophthalmoparesis; PSP, progressive supranuclear palsy; CART, classification and regression tree analysis.

(Adapted with permission from Litvan I, Bhatia KP, Burn DJ, et al. SIC task force appraisal of clinical diagnostic criteria for Parkinsonian disorders. Mov Dis 2003;18:467–486.)

Tourette syndrome is often associated with attention deficit hyperactivity disorder and has genetic overlap in families with obsessive-compulsive disorder.

Diagnostic Guidelines

Tics need to be distinguished from other movement disorders, including chorea, tremor, dystonia, and myoclonus. Unlike these basic movement disorder types, tics are unique in that they may be suppressed by the patient. Tics also need to be distinguished from stereotypes seen in autism or mental retardation. The lack of rhythmicity of tics helps in this differentiation. Obsessive-compulsive activities may resemble complex tics but differ in that the former are purposeful (such as tapping or turning a number of times).

Table 20
National Institute of Neurological Disorders and Stroke and Society for Progressive Supranuclear Palsy, Clinical Criteria for the Diagnosis of Progressive Supranuclear Palsy

Diagnostic categories	Inclusion criteria	Exclusion criteria	Supportive criteria
	For possible and probable: Gradually progressive disorder with age at onset at 40 or later	*For possible and probable:* Recent history of encephalitis; alien limb syndrome; cortical sensory deficits; focal frontal or temporoparietal atrophy; hallucinations or delusions unrelated to dopaminergic therapy; cortical dementia of Alzheimer's type; prominent, early cerebellar symptoms or unexplained dysautonomia; or evidence of other diseases that could explain the clinical features	Symmetric akinesia or rigidity, proximal more than distal; abnormal neck posture, especially retrocollis; poor or absent response of parkinsonism to levodopa; early dysphagia and dysarthria; early onset of cognitive impairment including more than two of apathy, impairment in abstract thought, decreased verbal fluency, utilization or imitation behavior, or frontal release signs
Possible	Either vertical supranuclear palsy or both slowing of vertical saccades and postural instability with falls within 1 year of disease onset		
Probable	Vertical supranuclear palsy and prominent postural instability with falls within first year of disease onset[a]		
Definite	All criteria for possible or probable PSP are met and histopathological confirmation at autopsy		

[a]Later defined as falls or the tendency to fall (patients are able to stabilize themselves).
PSP, progressive supranuclear palsy.
(Adapted with permission from Litvan I, Bhatia KP, Burn DJ, et al. SIC task force appraisal of clinical diagnostic criteria for Parkinsonian disorders. Mov Dis 2003;18:467–486.)

Gilles de la Tourette Syndrome

Two sets of diagnostic criteria are currently used. (*Note* in Table 23 that the *Diagnostic and Statistical Manual of Mental Disorders, 4th edition*, has dropped the criteria that tic severity be such that social or occupational functioning is impaired because of the tics.)

ICD-10

The ICD-10 refers to the disorder as "combined vocal and multiple motor tic disorder (de la Tourette syndrome)" (*Note* in Table 24 the difference in age of onset criteria.)

This is a form of tic disorder in which there are, or have been, multiple motor tics and one or more vocal tics, although these need not have occurred concurrently. Onset is usually in childhood or adolescence. A history of motor tics before development of vocal tics is common; the symptoms frequently worsen during adolescence, and it is common for the disorder to persist into adult life.

Table 21
Validity and Reliability of Diagnostic Criteria for Progressive Supranuclear Palsy

Reference	PSP cases/all cases	Diagnostic criteria	Sens. (%)	Spec. (%)	PPV (%)	NPV (%)	κ	Comments and recommendations
Litvan et al., 1996	24/105	Lees	53	95	77	88	0.81	Diagnosis of six neurologists using these criteria when evaluating clinical vignettes (values reported are from the first clinical evaluation)
		Blin et al. Probable	13	100	100	80	0.71	
		Blin et al. Possible	55	94	73	87	0.78	
		Golbe	49	97	85	87	0.74	
Litvan et al., 1997	24/83	Lees	58	95	82			Features extracted from 83 cases with detailed clinical information
		Blin et al. Probable	21	100	100			
		Blin et al. Possible	63	85	63			
		Golbe	50	98	92			
		Tolosa et al. Possible	54	98	93			
		Tolosa et al.	54	98	93			
		Collins Verified	25	100	100			
		Collins et al. Possible	42	92	67			
		NINDS-SPSP Probable	50	100	100			
		NINDS-SPSP Possible	83	93	83			
Lopez et al., 1999	8/40	NINDS-SPSP Probable	62	100	100	92	0.72 through 0.91	Diagnosis of four physicians reviewing the first clinical evaluation of patients with dementia and/or Parkinsonism
		NINDS-SPSP Possible	75	99	96	95		

Sens., sensitivity; Spec., specificity; PPV, positive predictive value; NPV, negative predictive value; κ, kappa statistic (interrater reliability); NINDS-SPSP, National Institute of Neurological Disorders and Stroke and Society for Progressive Supranuclear Palsy, Inc.; PSP, progressive supranuclear palsy.

Three published studies have reported the diagnostic accuracy of the PSP. Two of the studies used overlapping cases but different methodology (Litvan et al., 1996; Litvan et al., 1997). Validity values are given in percentages.

(Adapted with permission from Litvan I, Bhatia KP, Burn DJ, et al. SIC task force appraisal of clinical diagnostic criteria for Parkinsonian disorders. Mov Dis 2003;18:467–486.)

Table 22
Diagnostic Criteria for Stiff-Person Syndrome

1. Stiffness and rigidity in axial muscles (proximal limb muscles may also be sometimes involved).
2. Abnormal axial posture (usually an exaggeration of the normal lumbar lordosis).
3. Superimposed spasms precipitated by voluntary movement, emotional upsets and unexpected auditory and somaesthetic stimuli.
4. Absence of brainstem, pyramidal, extrapyramidal, and lower motor neuron signs, sphincter and sensory disturbance, and cognitive involvement (epilepsy may occur).
5. Continuous motor unit activity in at least one axial muscle.

Adapted with permission from Lorish TR, Thorsteinsson G, Howard FM. Stiff-man syndrome updated. Mayo Clin Proc 1989;64:629–636.

Table 23
Diagnostic and Statistical Manual of Mental Disorders, 4th edition, **Diagnostic Criteria for Tourette Syndrome**

1. Both multiple motor tics and one or more vocal tics must be present at the same time, although not necessarily concurrently.
2. The tics must occur many times a day (usually in bouts) nearly every day or intermittently over more than 1 year, during which time there must not have been a tic-free period of more than 3 consecutive months.
3. The age at onset must be less than 18 years.
4. The disturbance must not be caused by the direct physiological effects of a substance (e.g., stimulants) or a general medical condition (e.g., Huntington's disease or postviral encephalitis).

Adapted from American Psychiatric Association. Diagnostic and Statistical Manual of Mental Disorders, 4th rev. ed. Washington, DC: American Psychiatric Association, 1994.

Table 24
Diagnostic and Statistical Manual of Mental Disorders, 4th edition, **Diagnostic Criteria for Transient Tic Disorder**

1. Single or multiple motor and/or vocal tics occurring daily for at least 2 weeks but for no longer than 1 year.
2. Tics occur many times a day, nearly every day for at least 4 weeks, but no longer than 12 consecutive months.
3. Onset before age 18.
4. The disturbance must not be the result of the direct physiological effects of a substance (e.g., stimulants) or a general medical condition (e.g., Huntington's disease or postviral encephalitis).

Adapted from American Psychiatric Association. Diagnostic and Statistical Manual of Mental Disorders, 4th rev. ed. Washington, DC: American Psychiatric Association, 1994.

Table 25
Diagnostic and Statistical Manual of Mental Disorders, 4th edition, **Diagnostic Criteria for Chronic Motor/Vocal Tic Disorder**

1. Single or multiple motor or vocal tics, but not both, have been present during the disorder.
2. Tics occur many times a day, nearly every day for more than 1 year, without an intervening tic-free period of more than 3 months.
3. Onset before age 18.
4. The disturbance must not be because of the direct physiological effects of a substance (e.g., stimulants) or a general medical condition (e.g., Huntington's disease or postviral encephalitis).

Adapted from American Psychiatric Association. Diagnostic and Statistical Manual of Mental Disorders, 4th rev. ed. Washington, DC: American Psychiatric Association, 1994.

The vocal tics are often multiple with explosive repetitive vocalizations, throat clearing, and grunting, and there may be the use of obscene words or phrases. Sometimes there is associated gestural echopraxia, which also may be of an obscene nature (copropraxia). As with motor tics, the vocal tics may be voluntarily suppressed for short periods, be exacerbated by stress, and disappear during sleep.

The *Diagnostic and Statistical Manual of Mental Disorders, 4th edition*, recognizes two more circumscribed tic disorders, of which transient tic disorder is relatively common in childhood, affecting from 5 to 24% of school children.

SOURCES

Corticobasal Degeneration

Boeve BF, Maraganore DM, Parisi JE, et al. Pathologic heterogeneity in clinically diagnosed corticobasal degeneration. Neurology 1999;53:795–800.

Grimes DA, Lang AE, Bergeron CB. Dementia as the most common presentation of cortical-basal ganglionic degeneration. Neurology 1999;53:1969–1974.

Kompoliti K, Goetz CG, Boeve BF, et al. Clinical presentation and pharmacological therapy in corticobasal degeneration. Arch Neurol 1998;55:957–961.

Kumar R, Bergeron C, Pollanen MS, Lang AE. Cortical basal ganglionic degeneration. In: Jankovic J, Tolosa E, eds. Parkinson's Disease and Movement Disorders. Baltimore: Williams and Wilkins, 1998;297–316.

Lang AE, Riley DE, Bergeron C. Cortico-basal ganglionic degeneration. In: Calne DB, ed. Neurodegenerative Diseases. Philadelphia: WB Saunders, 1994;877–894.

Litvan I, Bhatia KP, Burn DJ, et al. SIC task force appraisal of clinical diagnostic criteria for Parkinsonian disorders. Mov Dis 2003;18:467–486.

Riley DE, Lang AE, Lewis A, et al. Cortical-basal ganglionic degeneration. Neurology 1990;40:1203–1212.

Riley DE, Lang AE. Clinical diagnostic criteria. Adv Neurol 2000;82:29–34.

Riley DE, Lang AE. Cortico-basal ganglionic degeneration. In: Stern MB, Koller WC, eds. Parkinsonian Syndromes. New York: Dekker, 1993;379–392.

Rinne JO, Lee MS, Thompson PD, Marsden CD. Corticobasal degeneration. A clinical study of 36 cases. Brain 1994;117:1183–1196.

Watts RL, Brewer RP, Schneider JA, Mirra S. Corticobasal degeneration. In: Watts RL, Koller WC, eds. Movement Disorders: Neurologic Principles and Practice. New York: McGraw Hill, 1997;611–621.

Watts RL, Mirra S. Corticobasal ganglionic degeneration. In: Marsden CD, Fahn S, eds. Movement Disorders 3. London: Butterworths, 1994;282–299.

Dystonia Because of DYT1 Mutations

Bressman SB, Raymond D, Wendt K, et al. Diagnostic criteria for dystonia in *DYT1* families. Neurology 2002;59:1780–1782.

Essential Tremor

Fahn S, Tolosa E, Martin C. Clinical rating scale for tremor. In: Jankovic J, Tolosa E, eds. Parkinson's Disease and Movement Disorders. Baltimore: Williams and Wilkins, 1993;271–280.

Louis ED, Ford B, Lee H, Andrews H, Cameron B. Diagnostic criteria for essential tremor: a population perspective. Arch Neurol 1998;55:823–828.

Fahr's Disease

Benke T, Karner E, Seppi K, et al. Subacute dementia and imaging correlates in a case of Fahr's disease. J Neurol Neurosurg Psychiatry 2004;75:1163–1165.

Lang AE. Corticobasal degeneration syndrome with basal ganglia calcification: Fahr's disease as a corticobasal look-alike? Mov Dis 2002;17:563–567.

Lauterbach EC, Cummings JL, Duffy J, et al. Neuropsychiatric correlates and treatment of lenticulostriatal diseases: a review of the literature and overview of research opportunities in Huntington's, Wilson's, and Fahr's diseases. A report of the ANPA committee on research, American Neuropsychiatric Association. J Neuropsychiatry Clin Neurosci 1999;11:4.

Shibayana H, Iwai K, Takeuchi T. Clinical diagnostic criteria for non-Alzheimer non-Pick dementia with Fahr's disease (NAN-PDF). Neurobiol Aging 1996;17:S27.

Multiple System Atrophy

Gilman S, Low PA, Quinn N, et al. Consensus statement on the diagnosis of multiple system atrophy. J Neurol Sci 1999;163:94–98.

Neuroleptic Malignant Syndrome

Addonizio G, Susman VL, Roth SD. Symptoms of neuroleptic malignant syndrome in 82 consecutive inpatients. Am J Psychiatry 1986;143:1587–1590.

Adityanjee. The spectrum concept and prevalence of neuroleptic malignant syndrome (letter). Am J Psychiatry 1988;145:1041.

Adityanjee, Aderibigbe YA, Mathews T. Epidemiology of neuroleptic malignant syndrome. Clin Neuropharmacol 1999;22:151–158.

Adityanjee, Mathews T, Aderibighe YA. Proposed research diagnostic criteria for neuroleptic malignant syndrome. Int J Neuropsychopharmacol 1999;2:129–144.

Caroff SN, Mann SC. Neuroleptic malignant syndrome. Med Clin North Am 1993;77:185–202.

Caroff SN, Mann SC, Lazarus A, Sullivan K, MacFadden W. Neuroleptic malignant syndrome: diagnostic issues. Psychiatric Ann 1991;21:130–147.

Delay J, Deniker P, Drug-induced extrapyramidal syndromes. In: Pinken D, Gruyn S, eds. Handbook of Clinical Neurology. New York: Elsevier, 1968.

Keck PE Jr, Sebastianelli J, Pope HG Jr, McElroy SL. Frequency and presentation of neuroleptic malignant syndrome in a large psychiatric hospital. J Clin Psychiatry 1989;50:352–355.

Lazarus A, Mann SC, Caroff SN. The Neuroleptic Malignant Syndrome and Related Conditions. Washington, DC: American Psychiatric Press, 1989.

Levinson DF, Simpson GM. Neuroleptic-induced extrapyramidal symptoms with fever heterogeneity of neuroleptic malignant syndrome. Arch Gen Psychiatry 1986;43:839–848.

Pope HG, Check PE, Miserly SL. Frequency and presentation of neuroleptic malignant syndrome in a large psychiatric hospital. Am J Psychiatry 1986;143:1227–1233.

PANDAS Syndrome

Murphy TK, Petitto JM, Voeller KK. Goodman WK. Obsessive compulsive disorder: is there an association with childhood streptococcal infections and altered immune function? Semin Clin Neuropsychiatry 2001;6:266–276.

Snider LA, Swedo SE. Post-streptococcal autoimmune disorders of the central nervous system. Curr Opin Neurol 2003;16:359–365.

Parkinson's Disease

Albanese A, Diagnostic criteria for Parkinson's disease. Neurol Sci, 2003;24:S23–S26.

Gelb DJ, Oliver E, Gilman S. Diagnostic criteria for Parkinson's disease. Arch Neurol 1999;56:33–39.

Hedera P, Lerner AJ, Castellani R, Friedland RP. Concurrence of Alzheimer's disease, Parkinson's disease, diffuse Lewy body disease, and amyotrophic lateral sclerosis. J Neurol Sci 1995;128:219–224.

Kompoliti K, Goetz CG, Boeve BF, et al. Clinical presentation and pharmacological therapy in corticobasal degeneration. Arch Neurol 1998;55:957–961.

Riley DE, Chelimsky TC. Autonomic nervous system testing may not distinguish multiple system atrophy from Parkinson's disease. J Neurol Neurosurg Psychiatry 2003;74:56–60.

Paroxysmal Kinesiegenic Dyskinesia

Bruno MK, Hallett M, Gwinn-Hardy K, et al. Clinical evaluation of idiopathic paroxysmal kinesigenic dyskinesia: new diagnostic criteria. Neurology. 2004;63:2280–2287.

Progressive Supranuclear Palsy

Bhidayasiri R, Riley DE, Somers JT, Lerner AJ, Buttner-Ennever JA, Leigh RJ. Pathophysiology of slow vertical saccades in progressive supranuclear palsy. Neurology 2001;57:2070–2077.

Blin J, Baron JC, Dubois B, et al. Positron-emission tomography study in progressive supranuclear palsy. Brain hypometabolic pattern and clinicometabolic correlations. Arch Neurol 1990;47:747–752.

Collins SJ, Ahlskog JE, Parisi JE, Maraganore DM. Progressive supranuclear palsy: neuropathologically based diagnostic clinical criteria. J Neurol Neurosurg Psychiatry 1995;58:167–173.

Duvoisin RC. Clinical diagnosis. In: Litvan I, Agid Y, eds. Progressive Supranuclear Palsy: Clinical and Research Approaches. New York: Oxford University Press, 1992;15–33.

Golbe LI. Progressive supranuclear palsy. In: Jankovic J, Tolosa E, eds. Parkinson's Disease and Movement Disorders. Baltimore: Williams and Wilkins, 1993;145–161.

Kuniyoshi S, Riley DE, Zee DS, Reich SG, Whitney C, Leigh RJ. Distinguishing progressive supranuclear palsy from other forms of Parkinson's disease: evaluation of new signs. Ann NY Acad Sci 2002;956:484–486.

Lees A. The Steele-Richardson-Olszewski syndrome (progressive supranuclear palsy). In: Marsden CD, Fahn S, eds. Movement Disorders 2. London: Butterworths, 1987;272–287.

Leigh RJ, Riley DE. Eye movements in Parkinsonism: It's saccadic speed that counts. Neurology 2000;54:1018, 1019.

Litvan I, Agid Y, Calne D, et al. Clinical research criteria for the diagnosis of progressive supranuclear palsy (Steele-Richardson-Olszewski syndrome): report of the NINDS-SPSP international workshop. Neurology 1996;47:1–9.

Litvan I, Agid Y, Jankovic J, et al. Accuracy of clinical criteria for the diagnosis of progressive supranuclear palsy (Steele-Richardson-Olszewski syndrome). Neurology 1996;46:922–930.

Litvan I, Campbell G, Mangone CA, et al. Which clinical features differentiate progressive supranuclear palsy (Steele-Richardson-Olszewski syndrome) from related disorders? A clinicopathological study. Brain 1997;120:65–74.

Litvan I, Bhatia KP, Burn DJ, et al. SIC task force appraisal of clinical diagnostic criteria for Parkinsonian disorders. Mov Dis 2003;18:467–486.

Tolosa E, Valldeoriola F, Marti MJ. Clinical diagnosis and diagnostic criteria of progressive supranuclear palsy (Steele-Richardson-Olszewski syndrome). J Neural Transm Suppl 1994;42:15–31.

Stiff-Person Syndrome

Brown P, Marsden CD. The stiff man and stiff man plus syndromes. J Neurol 1999;246:648–652.

Lorish TR, Thorsteinsson G, Howard FM. Stiff-man syndrome updated. Mayo Clin Proc 1989;64:629–636.

Tourette Syndrome and Tic Disorders

American Psychiatric Association. Task Force on DSM-IV. Diagnostic and statistical manual of mental disorders, 4th ed. Washington, DC: American Psychiatric Association, 1994.

Tourette disorder information and support site. Available via http://www.tourettes-disorder.com/.

12
Neuromuscular Disorders

CEREBRAL PALSY

The diagnosis of cerebral palsy is a clinical one, consisting of the clinical history of the mother and infant and the pediatric and neurological examination of the infant. The diagnosis is dependent on two key findings: evidence of nonprogressive damage to the developing brain and the presence of a resulting impairment of the motor (neuromuscular) control system of the body, the latter usually accompanied by a physiological impairment and functional disability.

These clinical findings can be enriched by a number of laboratory investigations. These include structural and functional neuroimaging, electroencephalogram, and gait-analysis tools. The findings on these tests may suggest a different diagnosis, and their correlation with motor findings and disability from such are variable.

CHRONIC INFLAMMATORY DEMYELINATING POLYNEUROPATHY

Chronic inflammatory demyelinating polyneuropathy (CIDP) is an immune-based neuropathy of unknown cause. Both cellular and humoral components of the immune response appear to be important in pathogenesis, although the precipitating antigen (or antigens) is unknown. There is breakdown of the blood–nerve barrier, and recruitment of macrophages. Secretion of toxic factors then damage myelin sheaths and may produce axonal injury.

CIDP may occur at any age, and separate criteria for adults and children have been proposed. In HIV-positive patients, there may be as many as 50 white blood cells/mm^3. CIDP may also occur in connection with other autoimmune disorders, and in cases of monoclonal gammopathy of unknown significance. Successful treatment of CIDP with corticosteroids, immunoglobulin infusions, plasmapheresis, and immunosuppressants has been reported.

The American Academy of Neurology (AAN) has published both clinical and electrophysiological criteria for the diagnosis of CIDP (Table 1). The basic AAN criteria here have begun to be studied in terms of their sensitivity and specificity, and various authors have proposed modification to enhance the sensitivity of the electrophysiological criteria. The AAN criteria strongly depend on the presence of severe demyelinating features; they are insensitive to mild cases of CIDP, or those with extensive axonal loss. The presence of clinical variants has led some authors to find that more than half of CIDP cases do not fulfill criteria completely.

Because of these restrictions in the AAN criteria and their lack of sensitivity, Hughes et al. proposed similar criteria that they felt to be more sensitive (Table 2). For CIDP in the setting of monoclonal gammopathy of unknown significance, related criteria have been proposed (Table 3). Similar criteria have also been developed for childhood CIDP (Table 4).

From: *Current Clinical Neurology: Diagnostic Criteria in Neurology*
Edited by: A. J. Lerner © Humana Press Inc., Totowa, NJ

Table 1

American Academy of Neurology Diagnostic Criteria for Chronic Inflammatory Demyelinating Polyneuropathy

Chronic inflammatory demyelinating polyneuropathy (CIDP) is a diagnosis of pattern recognition based on clinical signs and symptoms, electrodiagnostic studies, cerebrospinal fluid examination, laboratory tests appropriate to the specific clinical situation, and, on occasions, results from nerve biopsy.

Four features are used as the basis of diagnosis: clinical, electrodiagnostic, pathological, and cerebrospinal fluid (CSF) studies. These are further divided into mandatory, supportive, and exclusion. Mandatory features are those required for diagnosis and should be present for all definite cases. Supportive features are helpful in clinical diagnosis, but by themselves, do not make a diagnosis and are not part of the diagnostic categories. Exclusion features strongly suggest alternative diagnoses.

I. **Clinical**
  A. Mandatory
    1. Progressive or relapsing motor and sensory, rarely, only motor or sensory, dysfunction of more than one limb of a peripheral nerve nature, developing over at least 2 months.
    2. Hypo- or areflexia. This usually involves all four limbs.
  B. Supportive
    1. Large-fiber sensory loss predominates over small-fiber sensory loss.
  C. Exclusion
    1. Mutilation of hands or feet, retinitis pigmentosa, ichthyosis, appropriate history of drug or toxic exposure known to cause a similar peripheral neuropathy, or family history of an inherited peripheral neuropathy.
    2. Sensory level.
    3. Unequivocal sphincter disturbance.

II. **Electrodiagnostic studies**
  A. Mandatory
    1. Nerve conduction studies, including studies of proximal nerve segments in which the predominant process is demyelination.
    2. *Must have three of four*
      a. Reduction of conduction velocity (CV) in two or more motor nerves.
        i. <80% of lower limit of normal (LLN) if amplitude is >80% of LLN.
        ii. <70% of LLN if amplitude is <80% of LLN.
      b. Partial conduction block or abnormal temporal dispersion in one or more motor nerves: either peroneal nerve between ankle and fibular head, median nerve between wrist and elbow, or ulnar nerve between wrist and below elbow.
      c. Prolonged distal latencies in two or more nerves.
        i. >125% of upper limit of normal (ULN) if amplitude >80% of LLN.
        ii. >150% of ULN if amplitude <80% of LLN.
      d. Absent F waves or prolonged minimum F-wave latencies (10–15 trials) in two or more motor nerves.
        i. >120% of ULN if amplitude >80% of LLN.
        ii. >150% of ULN if amplitude <80% of LLN.
    3. Supportive
      a. Reduction in sensory CV <80% of LLN.
      b. Absent H reflexes.

III. **CSF studies**
  A. Mandatory
    1. Cell count <10/mm^3 if HIV-seronegative or <50/mm^3 if HIV-seropositive.
    2. Negative syphilis serology.
  B. Supportive
    1. Elevated protein.

IV. **Pathological features**
  A. Mandatory
    1. Nerve biopsy showing unequivocal evidence of demyelination and remyelination.
  B. Supportive
    1. Subperineurial and endoneurial edema.
    2. Mononuclear cell infiltration.

(Continued)

Table 1 *(Continued)*

      3. Onion bulb formation.

      4. Prominent variation in the degree of demyelination between fascicles.

  C. Exclusion

      1. Vasculitis, neurofilamentous swollen axons, amyloid deposits, or intracytoplasmic inclusions in Schwann cells or macrophages including adrenoleukodystrophy, metachromatic leukodystrophy, globoid cell leukodystrophy, or evidence of specific pathology.

Diagnostic categories for research purposes

Definite: Clinical A and C, electrodiagnosis A, CSF A, and pathology A and C.

Probable: Clinical A and C, electrodiagnosis A, and CSF A.

Possible: Clinical A and C and electrodiagnosis A.

Laboratory studies

Depending on the results of the laboratory tests, those patients meeting the criteria above are classified into groups listed below. The following studies are suggested: complete blood count, erythrocyte sedimentation rate, chemistry profile, creatine kinase, antinuclear antibody, thyroid functions, serum and urine immunoglobulin studies (to include either immunofixation electrophoresis or immunoelectrophoresis, and HIV and hepatitis serology. The list of laboratory studies is not comprehensive. For instance, in certain clinical circumstances, other studies may be indicated, such as phytanic acid, long-chain fatty acids, porphyrins, urine heavy metals, α-lipoprotein, β-lipoprotein, glucose tolerance test, imaging studies of the central nervous system, and lymph node or bone marrow biopsy.

Classification of CIDP

  A. Idiopathic CIDP; no concurrent disease.

  B. Concurrent disease with CIDP (depending on laboratory studies or other clinical features)

      1. Systemic lupus erythematosus.

      2. HIV infection.

      3. Monoclonal or biclonal gammopathy (macroglobulinemia, POEMS syndrome, osteosclerotic myeloma).

      4. Castleman's disease.

      5. Monoclonal gammopathies of undetermined significance.

      6. Diabetes.

      7. Central nervous system demyelinating disease.

POEMS, *p*olyneuropathy, *o*rganomegaly, *e*ndocrinopathy, *m*onoclonal gammopathy, and *s*kin changes.

(Adapted from Research criteria for diagnosis of chronic inflammatory demyelinating polyneuropathy [CIDP]. Report from an Ad Hoc Subcommittee of the American Academy of Neurology AIDS Task Force. Neurology 1991;41:617–618.)

DYSTROPHINOPATHIES

This comprises both Duchenne's muscular dystrophy and the milder Becker's form of muscular dystrophy. Both of these are caused by mutations on chromosome Xp21.

FACIOSCAPULOHUMERAL MUSCULAR DYSTROPHY

Facioscapulohumeral muscular dystrophy (FSHD) is a dominantly inherited muscular dystrophy affecting about 1 in 20,000 individuals. The weakness is not restricted to areas named in the disease name; weakness may occur in hip girdle, ankle dorsiflexors, and occasionally oropharynx. Extramuscular manifestations of this slowly progressing myopathy may include hearing loss and retinal vasculopathy. All patients with a confirmed diagnosis of FSHD carry a chromosomal rearrangement within the subtelomeric region of chromosome 4q (4q35). This subtelomeric region is composed mainly of a polymorphic repeat structure consisting of 3.3-kb repeated elements (D4Z4). The number of repeat units varies from 10 to more than 100 in the population, and, in patients with FSHD, an allele of 1 to 10 residual units is observed because of the deletion of an integral number of these units.

GUILLAIN-BARRE SYNDROME

Guillain-Barre Syndrome (GBS) is also known as acute inflammatory demyelinating polyneuropathy. It is a distinct syndrome from CIDP. Many cases follow a nonspecific illness, such as an upper

Table 2

Inflammatory Neuropathy Cause and Treatment: Neurophysiological Criteria for Diagnosis of Chronic Inflammatory Demyelinating Polyneuropathy

Either:

1. Partial conduction block or abnormal temporal dispersion of conduction must be present in at least two nerves, and there must be significantly reduced conduction velocity, significantly prolonged distal motor latency, or absent or significantly prolonged minimum F-wave latency in at least one other nerve
    OR
2. In the absence of block or dispersion, significantly reduced conduction velocity, significantly prolonged distal motor latency, or absent or significantly prolonged minimum F-wave latency must be present in at least three nerves
    OR
3. In the presence of significant neurophysiological abnormalities in only two nerves, unequivocal histological evidence of demyelinating or demyelinated nerve fibers in a nerve biopsy must also be present.

Recording technique

The following nerves were tested on both sides (unless the criteria are fulfilled by studying a smaller number of nerves or points):

*   Median (wrist, elbow, axilla).
*   Ulnar (wrist, elbow, axilla, Erb's point).
*   Peroneal (ankle, below fibular head, above fibular head).
*   Tibial (ankle, popliteal fossa).
*   Ten consecutive F waves were recorded from each nerve, and the minimal latency was measured.

Definitions

Partial conduction block: A ≤15% change in duration between proximal and distal sites and >20% drop in negative peak area and peak to peak amplitude.

Abnormal temporal dispersion and possible conduction block: A ≥15% change in duration between proximal and distal sites and >20% drop in negative peak area or peak-to-peak amplitude between proximal and distal sites; additional studies, such as stimulation across short segments or recording of individual motor units, required for confirmation.

Significantly reduced conduction velocity: ≤80% of lower limit of normal or, if distal motor compound muscle action potential amplitude <80% of normal, <70% of lower limit of normal.

Significantly prolonged distal motor latency: ≥125% of upper limit of normal or, if amplitude <80% of normal, >150% of upper limit of normal.

Significantly delayed minimum F-wave latency: ≥120% of upper limit of normal or, if amplitude <80% of normal, >150% of upper limit of normal.

These criteria have been compared with those of the Ad Hoc Subcommittee and found to be more sensitive.

Adapted from Hughes R, Bensa S, Willison H, et al. Randomized controlled trial of intravenous immunoglobulin versus oral prednisolone in chronic inflammatory demyelinating polyradiculoneuropathy. Ann Neurol 2001;50:195–201, with permission of John Wiley and Sons, Inc.

respiratory infection. Cases of GBS, especially those associated with *Campylobacter jejuni* infection, may have axonal injury in addition to demyelinating features. The presence of axonal injury and loss also affects prognosis. The majority of individuals affected with GBS recover, and similar degrees of improvement rate are seen with both γ-globulin infusions as with plasmapheresis.

Table 8 presents the basic diagnostic criteria used for GBS. Subtypes of GBS are listed with clinical summaries in Table 9.

INCLUSION BODY MYOSITIS

Inclusion body myositis (IBM) is usually classified among the inflammatory myopathies because the clinical picture may resemble polymyositis (PM) or dermatomyositis (DM). The diagnosis is established based on the histopathological evaluation of muscle biopsy specimens.

Table 3
Proposal for Criteria for Demyelinating Polyneuropathy Associated With Monoclonal Gammopathy of Undetermined Significance

A causal relation between chronic inflammatory demyelinating polyneuropathy and monoclonal gammopathy of undetermined significance should be considered in patients with:
1. Demyelinating polyneuropathy according to the electrodiagnostic American Academy of Neurology criteria for idiopathic chronic inflammatory demyelinating polyneuropathy.
2. Presence of an M protein (immunoglobulin [Ig]M, IgG, or IgA), without evidence of malignant plasma cell dyscrasias, such as multiple myeloma, lymphoma, Waldenstrom's macroglobulinemia, or amyloidosis.
3. Family history negative for neuropathy.
4. Age over 30 years.

The relation is definite when the following is present:
1. IgM M protein with antimyelin-associated glycoprotein (MAG) antibodies.

The relation is probable when at least three of the following are present in a patient without anti-MAG antibodies:
1. Time to peak of the neuropathy greater than 2 years.
2. Chronic, slowly progressive course without relapsing or remitting periods.
3. Symmetric distal polyneuropathy.
4. Sensory symptoms and signs predominate over motor features.

A causal relation is unlikely when at least three of the following are present in a patient without anti-MAG antibodies:
1. Median time to peak of the neuropathy is within 1 year.
2. Clinical course is relapsing and remitting or monophasic.
3. Cranial nerves are involved.
4. Neuropathy is asymmetric.
5. Motor symptoms and signs predominate.
6. History of preceding infection.
7. Presence of abnormal median sensory nerve action potential in combination with normal sural sensory nerve action potential.

Adapted from Notermans NC, Franssen H, Eurelings M, Van der Graaf Y, Wokke JH. Diagnostic criteria for demyelinating polyneuropathy associated with monoclonal gammopathy. Muscle Nerve 2000;23:73–79, with permission of John Wiley and Sons, Inc.

IBM is a disease of adults, most commonly over age 50. It affects men more than it does women. In contrast to PM/DM, the weakness may be asymmetric. The pattern of weakness, with prominent early involvement of quadriceps, finger and wrist flexors, and ankle dorsiflexors (*see* Table 1), contrasts with proximal greater than distal weakness in PM/DM, and is useful in raising clinical suspicion. The weakness is usually slowly progressive, and many patients are not diagnosed for years after onset.

The nature of the inclusion bodies, and the finding of β-amyloid in muscle fibers has led to theories that IBM may be a degenerative disorder of muscle (with homologies to Alzheimer's disease) or possibly of viral origin.

MOTOR NEURON DISEASE

Amyotrophic Lateral Sclerosis

Amyotrophic lateral sclerosis (ALS) is also known as motor neuron disease, and popularly, as Lou Gehrig's disease. Motor neuron diseases occur throughout life, with different syndromes having different eponyms. One of the distinguishing features of motor neuron diseases is their varying combinations of both upper motor and lower neuron features. Other neurological features may occur, such as dementia or retinal degeneration ("ALS-Plus"). Motor neuron disease may also occur as part of other disorders, such as Creutzfeldt-Jakob disease, frontotemporal dementia, and spinocerebellar degeneration. ALS may be mimicked by delayed postpoliomyelitis, multifocal motor neuropathy with or without conduction block, endocrinopathies, lead intoxication, or infections. Motor neuron diseases may occur

Table 4
Revised Diagnostic Criteria for Childhood Chronic Inflammatory Demyelinating Polyneuropathy

Mandatory clinical criteria:
1. Progression of muscle weakness in proximal and distal muscles of upper and lower extremities over at least 4 weeks, or alternatively when rapid progression (Guillain-Barre syndrome-like presentation) is followed by relapsing or protracted course (more than 1 year).
2. Areflexia or hyporeflexia.

A.1. Major laboratory features
A.1.1. Electrophysiological criteria
Must demonstrate at least three of the following four major abnormalities in motor nerves (or two of the major plus two of the supportive criteria):

A.1.1.1. Major
1. Conduction block or abnormal temporal dispersion in one or more motor nerves at sites not prone to compression.
   a. Conduction block: at least 50% drop in negative peak area or peak-to-peak amplitude of proximal compound muscle action potential (CMAP) if duration of negative peak of proximal CMAP is <130% of distal CMAP duration.
   b. Temporal dispersion: abnormal if duration of negative peak of proximal CMAP is >130% of distal CMAP duration.
      Recommendations:
      • Conduction block and temporal dispersion can be assessed only in nerves where amplitude of distal CMAP is >1 mV.
      • Supramaximal stimulation should always be used.
2. Reduction in conduction velocity (CV) in two or more nerves is <75% of the mean –2 standard deviations (SD) CV value for age.
3. Prolonged distal latency in two or more nerves: >130% of the mean +2 SD distal latency value for age.
4. Absent F waves or prolonged F-wave minimal latency in two or more nerves: >130% of the mean +2 SD F-wave minimal latency for age.
5. Recommendation: F-wave study should include a minimum of 10 trials.

A.1.1.2. Supportive
1. When conduction block is absent, the following abnormal electrophysiological parameters are indicative of nonuniform slowing and thus of an acquired neuropathy:
   a. Abnormal median sensory nerve action potential, whereas the sural nerve sensory nerve action potential is normal.
   b. Abnormal minimal latency index.
   c. Difference of >10 m/second in motor CVs between nerves of upper or lower limbs (either different nerves from the same limb: for example, left median versus left ulnar; or the same nerve from different sides, for example, left versus right ulnar nerves).

A.1.2. Cerebrospinal fluid (CSF studies) CSF protein >35 mg/dL, Cell count <10 cells/mm³
A.1.3. Nerve biopsy features
Nerve biopsy with predominant features of demyelination.

A.1.3.1. Exclusion criteria
1. Clinical features or history of a hereditary neuropathy, other diseases, or exposure to drugs or toxins that are known to cause peripheral neuropathy.
2. Laboratory findings (including nerve biopsy or DNA studies) that show evidence for a different etiology other than CIDP.
3. Electrodiagnostic features of abnormal neuromuscular transmission, myopathy, or anterior horn cell disease.

A.1.3.2. Diagnostic criteria (must have no exclusion criteria):
1. Confirmed CIDP
   a. Mandatory clinical features.
   b. Electrodiagnostic and CSF features.
2. Possible CIDP
   a. Mandatory clinical features.
   b. One of the three laboratory findings.

Adapted from Nevo Y, Topaloglu H. 88th ENMC International Workshop: Childhood chronic inflammatory demyelinating polyneuropathy (including revised diagnostic criteria), Naarden, The Netherlands, 8–10 December 2000. Neuromuscu Dis 2002;12:195–200, with permission from Elsevier.

Table 5
Criteria for the Diagnosis of Duchenne's Muscular Dystrophy

Elements
1. Symptoms are present before the age of 5.
2. Clinical signs comprise progressive symmetric muscular weakness: proximal limb muscles more than distal muscles; initially only lower limb muscles. Calf hypertrophy is often present.
3. Exclusions: fasciculations, loss of sensory modalities.
4. Wheelchair dependency before the age of 13.
5. There is at least a 10-fold increase of serum creatine kinase activity (in relation to age and mobility).
6. Muscle biopsy: abnormal variation in diameter of the muscle fibers (atrophic and hypertrophic fibers), (foci of) necrotic and regenerative fibers, hyalin fibers, increase of endomysial connective and fat tissue.
7. Muscle biopsy: almost no dystrophin demonstrable, except for an occasional muscle fiber (less than 5% of fibers).
8. DNA: Duchenne type (frameshift) deletion within the *dystrophin* gene; identical deletion or identical haplotype, involving closely linked markers, as in previous cases in the family.
9. Positive family history, compatible with X-linked recessive inheritance.

Assessment of Duchenne's Muscular Dystrophy
The diagnosis is definite when:
1. First case in a family:
   a. Age <5 years: (2), 3, 5, 6, 7, (8) all present.
   b. Age 5–12 years: 1, 2, 3, 4, 5 (at least once), 6, 7, 8, or all present.
   c. Age >12 years: (1), 2, 3, 4, 5 (at least once), 8 (or 6 and 7), all present.
2. Another case in the family (according to element 9) complies with the criteria under 1:
   a. Age <5 years: 5 and 9 present.
   b. Age 5–12 years: 1, 2, 3, 5 (at least once) all present.
   c. Age >12 years: (1), 2, 3, 4, 5 (at least once), all present.

Reprinted from Jennekens FGI, ten Kate LP, de Visser M, Wintzen AR. Diagnostic criteria for Duchenne and Becker muscular dystrophy and myotonic dystrophy. Neuromuscul Dis 1991;1:389–391, with permission from Elsevier.

Table 6
Criteria for the Diagnosis of Becker's Muscular Dystrophy

Elements
1. Clinical signs comprise progressive symmetric muscular weakness and atrophy of proximal limb muscles more than distal muscles; initially only lower limb muscles. Calf hypertrophy is often present. Weakness of the quadriceps femoris may be the only manifestation for a long time. Some patients have cramps that are mostly induced by activity. Contractures of the elbow flexors occur late in the course of the disease.
2. Exclusions: fasciculations, loss of sensory modalities.
3. No wheelchair dependency before 16th birthday.
4. There is a more than a fivefold increase of serum creatine kinase activity (in relation to age and mobility).
5. Electromyography: short duration, low amplitude, polyphasic action potentials, fibrillations, and positive waves. Normal motor and sensory nerve conduction velocities.
6. Muscle biopsy: abnormal variation in diameter of the muscle fibers (disseminated or small groups of atrophic and hypertrophic fibers), (foci of) regenerative fibers, mostly disseminated necrotic fibers. Dependent on stage and course of the disease, there may be a minor degree of grouping of histochemical fiber types and increase of connective and fat tissue.
7. Muscle biopsy: dystrophin present.
8. DNA: Becket type (in frame) deletion within the *dystrophin* gene, identical deletion or identical haplotype, involving closely linked markers, as in previous case in the family.
9. Positive family history, compatible with X-linked recessive inheritance.

Assessment of Becker's Muscular Dystrophy
The diagnosis is definite when:
1. First case in a family: (1), 2, 3, 4, 5, and either 8 or 6 and 7 all present.
2. Another case in the family (according to element 9) complies with the criteria under 1:
   a. The case is a first-degree relative: 4 (at least twice) present.
   b. In other situations: (1), 2, 3, 4, 5 and either 8 or 6 and 7 all present.

Reprinted from Jennekens FGI, ten Kate LP, de Visser M, Wintzen AR. Diagnostic criteria for Duchenne and Becker muscular dystrophy and myotonic dystrophy. Neuromuscul Dis 1991;1:389–391, with permission from Elsevier.

Table 7
Diagnostic Criteria for Facioscapulohumeral Muscular Dystrophy

I. **Inclusion:**
   Weakness of facial muscles.
   Weakness of scapular stabilizing muscles and ankle dorsiflexors.

II. **Exclusion:**
   Autosomal recessive or X-linked inheritance.
   Diffuse severe contractures.
   Cardiomyopathy.
   Extraocular and bubar weakness.
   Sensory loss.
   Neurogenic electromyography.
   Biopsy suggestive of another disorder.
   Skin rash suggestive of dermatomyositis.

III. **Supportive features:**
   Prominent asymmetry.
   Descending sequence of involvement.
   Sparing of deltoids.
   Early involvement of abdominal muscles (Beevor's sign).
   Selective involvement of lower trapezius.
   Typical shoulder appearance, with straight clavicles and forward-sloping shoulders.
   Relative sparing of neck flexors.
   High-frequency hearing loss or retinal vasculopathy.

Adapted from Tawil R, Figlewicz DA, Griggs RC, Weiffenbach B. FSH Consortium Facioscapulohumeral dystrophy: a distinct regional myopathy with a novel molecular pathogenesis. Ann Neurol 1988;43:279–282, with permission from John Wiley and Sons, Inc.

Table 8
Diagnostic Criteria for Guillain-Barre Syndrome

Features required for diagnosis
1. Progressive weakness in both arms and legs.
2. Areflexia.
3. Features strongly supporting diagnosis.
4. Progression of symptoms over days, up to 4 weeks.
5. Relative symmetry of symptoms.
6. Mild sensory symptoms or signs.
7. Cranial nerve involvement, especially bilateral diplegia.
8. Recovery beginning two to four weeks after progression ceases.
9. Autonomic dysfunction.
10. Absence of fever at onset.

Features excluding diagnosis
1. Diagnosis of botulism, myasthenia, poliomyelitis, or toxic neuropathy.
2. Abnormal porphyrin metabolism.
3. Recent diphtheria.
4. Laboratory criteria.
5. High concentration of protein in cerebrospinal fluid with fewer than 10 cells/mm^3.

Electrodiagnostic features (three of four)
1. Reduction in conduction velocity of two or more motor nerves with <80% of lower limit of normal (LLN) if amplitude is >80% of LLN; <70% of LLN if amplitude is <80% of LLN.
2. Prolonged distal latencies in two or more motor nerves >125% of upper limit of normal (ULN) if amplitude is >80% of LLN; >150% of ULN if amplitude is <80%.
3. Absent or prolonged F-waves in two or more motor nerves, >120% of ULN if amplitude is >LLN; >150% of ULN if amplitude is <80% of LLN.
4. Conduction block or abnormal temporal dispersion (>20% drop in amplitude or >15% change in duration between proximal and distal sites) in one or more motor nerves.

Adapted from Asbury AK, Cornblath DR. Assessment of current diagnostic criteria for Guillain-Barre syndrome. Ann Neurol 1990;27:S21–S24, with permission from John Wiley and Sons, Inc.

Table 9
Subtypes of Guillain-Barre Syndrome

1. **Acute inflammatory demyelinating polyradiculoneuropathy**
   a. Autoimmune disorder, antibody-mediated.
   b. Triggered by antecedent viral or bacterial infection.
   c. Electrophysiological findings demonstrate demyelination.
   d. Inflammatory demyelination may be accompanied by axonal nerve loss.
   e. Remyelination occurs after the immune reaction stops.
2. **Acute motor axonal neuropathy**
   a. Pure motor axonal form of neuropathy.
   b. Sixty-seven percent of patients are seropositive for campylobacteriosis.
   c. Electrophysiological studies are normal in sensory nerves; reduced or absent in motor nerves.
   d. Recovery is typically more rapid.
   e. High proportion of pediatric patients.
3. **Acute motor sensory axonal neuropathy**
   a. Wallerian-like degeneration of myelinated motor and sensory fibers.
   b. Minimal inflammation and demyelination.
   c. Similar to acute motor axonal neuropathy, except acute motor sensory axonal neuropathy affects sensory nerves and roots.
   d. Typically affects adults.
4. **Miller Fisher syndrome**
   a. Rare disorder.
   b. Rapidly evolving ataxia, areflexia, mild limb weakness, and ophthalmoplegia.
   c. Sensory loss unusual, but proprioception may be impaired.
   d. Demyelination and inflammation of cranial nerve III and VI, spinal ganglia, and peripheral nerves.
   e. Reduced or absent sensory nerve action potentials; tibial H reflex is usually absent.
   f. Resolution occurs in 1–3 months.
5. **Acute panautonomic neuropathy**
   a. Rarest of all the variants.
   b. Sympathetic, parasympathetic nervous systems are involved.
   c. Cardiovascular involvement is common (postural hypotension, tachycardia, hypertension, dysrhythmias).
   d. Blurry vision, dry eyes, and anhydrosis.
   e. Recovery is gradual and often incomplete.
   f. Often combined with sensory features.

Adapted from Newswanger DL, Warren CR. Guillain-Barre Syndrome. Am Fam Physician 2004;15:2405–2410. Available online at http://www.aafp.org/afp/20040515/2405.html.

as a familial condition in up to 20% of cases. The prototypical disorder is adult onset ALS, for which the El Escorial criteria are the most widely used at present (Table 12).

Primary Lateral Sclerosis

Primary lateral sclerosis is a pure upper motor neuron variant of motor neuron disease. Patients presenting with primary lateral sclerosis may evolve into a more typical picture of ALS over the course of several years. Differential diagnosis would include other pure upper motor neuron disorders, such as hereditary spastic paraparesis, or myelopathies because of intrinsic or extrinsic lesions of the cord. It is most common in the fifth decade of life, and usually involves spasticity more in the legs than arms. Pseudobulbar signs or frontal lobe signs may be present. Bladder involvement occurs late, and sensory systems should be spared.

MULTIFOCAL MOTOR NEUROPATHY

Multifocal motor neuropathy is an acquired demyelinating neuropathy that may resemble both chronic inflammatory demyelinating polyneuropathy or motor neuron disease. Recognition of multifocal

Table 10
Diagnostic Criteria and Classification for Inclusion Body Myositis

I. **Characteristic features—inclusion criteria**
  A. **Clinical features**
    1. Duration of illness >6 months.
    2. Age of onset >30 years old.
    3. Muscle weakness.
    4. Must affect proximal and distal muscles of arms and legs and patient must exhibit at least one of the following features:
       a. Finger flexor weakness.
       b. Wrist flexor weakness greater than wrist extensor weakness.
       c. Quadriceps muscle weakness (equal to or less than Medical Research Council grade 4).
  B. **Laboratory features**
    1. Serum creatine kinase <12 times normal value.
    2. Muscle biopsy.
       a. Inflammatory myopathy characterized by mononuclear cell invasion of nonnecrotic muscle fibers.
       b. Vacuolated muscle fibers.
       c. Either:
          i. Intracellular amyloid deposits (must use fluorescent method of identification before excluding the presence of amyloid), or
          ii. 15- to 18-nm tubulofilaments by electron microscopy.
    3. Electromyography must be consistent with features of an inflammatory myopathy (however, long-duration potentials are commonly observed and do not exclude diagnosis of sporadic inclusion body myositis).
  C. **Family history**
    Rarely, inclusion body myositis may be observed in families. This condition is different from hereditary inclusion body myopathy without inflammation. The diagnosis of familial inclusion body myositis requires specific documentation of the inflammatory component by muscle biopsy in addition to vacuolated muscle fibers, intracellular (within muscle fibers) amyloid, and 15- to 18-nm tubulofilaments.
II. **Associated disorders**
    Inclusion body myositis occurs with a variety of other, especially immune-mediated, conditions. An associated condition does not preclude a diagnosis of inclusion body myositis if diagnostic criteria (below) are fulfilled.
III. **Diagnostic criteria for inclusion body myositis**
  A. **Definite inclusion body myositis**
    Patient must exhibit all muscle biopsy features, including invasion of nonnecrotic fibers by mononuclear cells, vacuolated muscle fibers, and intracellular (within muscle fibers) amyloid deposits or 15- to 18-nm tubulofilaments. None of the other clinical or laboratory features is mandatory if muscle biopsy features are diagnostic.
  B. **Possible inclusion body myositis**
    If the muscle biopsy shows only inflammation (invasion of nonnecrotic muscle fibers by mononuclear cells) without other pathological features of inclusion body myositis, then a diagnosis of possible inclusion body myositis can be given if the patient exhibits the characteristic clinical (A1–A3) and laboratory (B1, B3) features.

Adapted from Mendell J, Barohn R, Askanas V, et al. Inclusion body myositis and myopathies. Ann Neurol 1995;38:705–713, with permission from John Wiley and Sons, Inc.

motor neuropathy is important because of its treatment implications, including response to intravenous immunoglobulin infusions or other immunosuppressive treatment regimes.

MYASTHENIA GRAVIS

For myasthenia gravis, there are not so much diagnostic criteria as a set of diagnostic tests with varying sensitivity and specificity. These tests include characteristic clinical course, response to

Table 11
Clinical Classification of Motor Neuron Disorders (Adult Onset, 15–50 Years; Elderly Onset, Over 50 Years)

Disorder	Age at onset	Inheritance
Combined upper and lower motor neuron involvement		
Amyotrophic lateral sclerosis		
Sporadic	Adult, elderly	
Familial adult onset	Adult	Autosomal-dominant
Familial juvenile onset	Childhood	Autosomal-recessive
Pure lower motor neuron involvement		
Proximal hereditary motor neuronopathy		
Acute infantile form (Werdnig-Hoffmann)	Infantile	Autosomal-recessive
Chronic childhood form (Kugelberg-Welander)	Infantile, childhood	Autosomal-recessive
Adult onset forms	Adult	Autosomal-recessive, Autosomal-dominant
Hereditary bulbar palsy		
X-linked bulbospinal neuronopathy (Kennedy)	Adult, elderly	Sex-linked-recessive
With deafness (Brown-Violetta-Van Laere)	Childhood, adult	?
Without deafness (Fazio-Londe)	Childhood	Autosomal-recessive
Hexosaminidase deficiency	Childhood, adult	Autosomal-recessive
Multifocal motor neuropathies	Adult, elderly	
Postpolio syndrome	Elderly	
Postirradiation syndrome	Adult, elderly	
Monomelic, focal, or segmental spinal muscular atrophy	Adult	
Pure upper motor neuron involvement		
Primary lateral sclerosis	Adult, elderly	
Hereditary spastic paraplegia	Adult, elderly	Autosomal-recessive
Neurolathyrism	Adult	
Konzo	Adult	

Adapted from Donaghy M. Classification and clinical features of motor neurone diseases and motor neuropathies in adults. J Neurology 1999;246:331–333, with permission from Springer Verlag.

anticholinesterase medications, antibody testing (acetylcholine receptor antibody is the most specific, but only 50% of ocular myasthenics are positive), electromyography (repetitive stimulation and single-fiber electromyogram as appropriate). The differential diagnosis includes other conditions that can produce generalized weakness and/or weakness of ocular muscles. These include Lambert-Eaton myasthenic syndrome, congenital myasthenia, drug-induced myasthenia, hyperthyroidism, Graves' disease, mitochondrial myopathies, motor neuron disease, and central nervous system lesions. There are specific tests for each of these, but it is important to recall that diagnostic testing, such as injection of an anticholinesterase (e.g., Tensilon [edrophonium] testing), may yield false-positives.

In the diagnostic criteria for neuropsychiatric systemic lupus erythematosus (one of many disorders associated with myasthenia gravis), there are diagnostic criteria for myasthenia gravis, but the extent to which the wider medical community or specialists in neuromuscular diseases adhere to this case definition is unclear.

MYOTONIC DYSTROPHY

The most frequent adult dystrophy, myotonic dystrophy is often recognized easily in adults by the characteristic face, muscle myotonia with hand grip for example, or percussion myotonia, and distal weakness. Endocrinopathies and cardiomyopathies are associated with myotonic dystrophy but do not form part of the core diagnostic criteria.

Table 12
The El Escorial Diagnostic Criteria for Amyotrophic Lateral Sclerosis

I. Requirements for the diagnosis of amyotrophic lateral sclerosis (ALS)
    The diagnosis of ALS requires:
    A. The *presence* of:
        1. Evidence of *lower motor neuron (LMN) degeneration* by clinical, electrophysiological or neuropathological examination,
        2. Evidence of *upper motor neuron (UMN) degeneration* by clinical examination, and
        3. *Progressive spread of symptoms or signs* within a region or to other regions, as determined by history or examination, together with.
    B. The *absence* of:
        1. *Electrophysiological and pathological evidence of other disease processes* that might explain the signs of LMN and/or UMN degeneration, and
        2. *Neuroimaging evidence of other disease processes* that might explain the observed clinical and electrophysiological signs.
II. Clinical studies in the diagnosis of ALS
    A careful history, physical and neurological examination must search for clinical evidence of UMN and LMN signs in four regions (brainstem, cervical, thoracic, or lumbosacral spinal cord of the central nervous system). Ancillary tests should be reasonably applied, as clinically indicated, to exclude other disease processes. These should include electrodiagnostic, neurophysiological, neuroimaging, and clinical laboratory studies.
    Clinical evidence of LMN and UMN degeneration is required for the diagnosis of ALS.
    The clinical diagnosis of ALS, without pathological confirmation, may be categorized into various levels of certainty by clinical assessment alone depending on the presence of UMN and LMN signs together in the same topographical anatomic region in either the brainstem (bulbar cranial motor neurons), cervical, thoracic, or lumbosacral spinal cord (anterior horn motor neurons). The terms *clinical definite ALS* and *clinically probable ALS* are used to describe these categories of clinical diagnostic certainty on clinical criteria alone (Table 13).

Reprinted with permission from Subcommittee on Motor Neuron Diseases of World Federation of Neurology Research Group on Neuromuscular Diseases, El Escorial "Clinical Limits of ALS" Workshop Contributors. El Escorial World Federation of Neurology criteria for the diagnosis of amyotrophic lateral sclerosis, J Neurol Sci 124:96–107.

POLYMYOSITIS AND DERMATOMYOSITIS

Inflammatory myopathies of unknown etiology, PM and DM are generally still diagnosed according to the criteria of Peter and Bohan, first proposed in 1975 (Table 19). (Note that the criteria include a histopathological component, thus hopefully increasing the specificity of the criteria. This will also help in differentiating these conditions from the other inflammatory myopathy, IBM [*see* "Inclusion Body Myositis"].)

DM is a disorder allied to PM. It is characterized by the presence of skin changes that may occur on the face and trunk. There may also be subcutaneous calcific nodules, although these are more common in childhood DM. Systemic involvement in PM and DM may include lung disorders, such as interstitial thickening, and cardiac involvement with electrocardiogram changes, pericarditis, and congestive heart failure. There may also be a gastrointestinal bleeding and a malabsorption syndrome secondary to microvasculitis in the gut. Other connective tissue diseases occur in about 20% of cases of inflammatory myopathies. The exact relationship of DM to malignancy is also unclear, although it may be the presenting feature of a neoplasm, thus making it also classifiable as a paraneoplastic disorder.

Diagnostic criteria from the rheumatological literature, with sensitivity and specificity higher than 90% are shown in Table 20. There has been recent controversy in the neurological literature as to whether PM is overdiagnosed. Van der Meulen and colleagues, reviewing a large case series found that many cases of inflammatory myositis, could not be diagnosed even with muscle biopsy, and that only a few were "definite " PM cases. Surprisingly, five out of nine of these PM cases were later found to have IBM. This may say something about secular changes in diagnostic patterns, as well as the relatively

Table 13
Subtypes of Amyotrophic Lateral Sclerosis

Clinically definite amyotrophic lateral sclerosis (ALS)
Clinical evidence alone of the presence of upper motor neuron (UMN), as well as lower motor neuron (LMN) signs, in three regions.

Clinically probable ALS
Clinical evidence alone by UMN and LMN signs in at least two regions with some UMN signs necessarily rostral to (above) the LMN signs.

Clinically probable, laboratory-supported ALS
Clinical signs of UMN and LMN dysfunction are in only one region, or when UMN signs alone are present in one region, and LMN signs defined by electromyogram criteria are present in at least two limbs, with proper application of neuroimaging and clinical laboratory protocols to exclude other causes.

Clinically possible ALS
Defined when clinical signs of UMN and LMN dysfunction are found together in only one region or UMN signs are found alone in two or more regions; or LMN signs are found rostral to UMN signs and the diagnosis of clinically probable, laboratory-supported ALS cannot be proven by evidence on clinical grounds in conjunction with electrodiagnostic, neurophysiological, neuroimaging or clinical laboratory studies. Other diagnoses must have been excluded to accept a diagnosis of clinically possible ALS.

Clinically suspected ALS
A pure LMN syndrome, wherein the diagnosis of ALS could not be regarded as sufficiently certain to include the patient in a research study. Hence, this category is deleted from the revised El Escorial Criteria for the Diagnosis of ALS.

Reprinted from Subcommittee on Motor Neuron Diseases of World Federation of Neurology Research Group on Neuromuscular Diseases, El Escorial "Clinical Limits of ALS" Workshop Contributors. El Escorial World Federation of Neurology criteria for the diagnosis of amyotrophic lateral sclerosis. J Neurol Sci 124:96–107, with permission from Elsevier.

Table 14
Proposed Diagnostic Criteria for Primary Lateral Sclerosis

I. **Clinical**
   A. Insidious onset of spastic paresis, usually beginning in the lower extremities but occasionally arms or bulbar.
   B. Adult onset, usually fifth decade or later.
   C. Absence of family history.
   E. Gradually progressive course (not step-like).
   F. Duration at least 3 years.
   G. Clinical findings usually limited to those associated with corticospinal dysfunction.
   H. Symmetric distribution, ultimately developing severe spastic spinobulbar paresis.

II. **Laboratory** (help in excluding other diagnoses)
   A. Normal serum chemistries including normal vitamin B_{12} level.
   B. Negative serological test for syphilis.
   C. In endemic areas, negative Lyme and human T-cell lymphotropic virus-1 serologies.
   D. Normal cerebrospinal fluid parameters, including absence of oligoclonal bands.
   E. Absent denervation potentials on electromyogram, or at most occasional fibrillation and increased activity in a few muscles (late and minor).
   F. Absence of compressive lesions of cervical spine or foramen magnum (spinal magnetic resonance imaging [MRI] scanning recommended).
   G. Absence of high-signal lesions on MRI similar to those seen in multiple sclerosis.

III. **Additionally suggestive of primary lateral sclerosis**
   A. Preserved bladder function.
   B. Absent or very prolonged latency on corticomotor-evoked responses in the presence of normal peripheral stimulus-evoked maximum compound muscle potentials.
   C. Focal atrophy of precentral gyrus on MRI.
   D. Decreased glucose consumption in paricentral region on positron-emission tomography scan.

Adapted from Pringle CE, Hudson AJ, Munoz DG, et al. Primary lateral sclerosis. Clinical features, neuropathology and diagnostic criteria. Brain 1992;115:495–520, with permission of Oxford University Press.

Table 15
Diagnostic Criteria for Multifocal Motor Neuropathy

Definite multifocal motor neuropathy
1. Weakness without objective sensory loss in the distribution of two or more named nerves. During the early stages of symptomatic weakness, the historical or physical finding of diffuse, symmetric weakness excludes multifocal motor neuropathy.
2. Definite conduction block is present in two or more nerves outside of common entrapment sites.[a]
3. Normal sensory nerve conduction velocity across the same segments with demonstrated motor conduction block.
4. Normal results for sensory nerve conduction studies on all tested nerves, with a minimum of three nerves tested. The absence of each of the following upper motor neuron signs: spastic tone, clonus, extensor plantar response, and pseudobulbar palsy.

Probable multifocal motor neuropathy
1. Weakness without objective sensory loss in the distribution of two or more named nerves. During the initial weeks of symptomatic weakness, the presence of diffuse, symmetric weakness excludes multifocal motor neuropathy.
2. The presence of either:
   a. Probable conduction block in two or more motor nerve segments that are not common entrapment sites, or
   b. Definite conduction block in one motor nerve segment and probable conduction block in a different motor nerve segment, neither of which segments are common entrapment sites.
3. Normal sensory nerve conduction velocity across the same segments with demonstrated motor conduction block when this segment is technically feasible for study (i.e., this is not required for segments proximal to axilla or popliteal fossa).
4. Normal results for sensory nerve conduction studies on all tested nerves, with a minimum of three nerves tested.
5. The absence of each of the following upper motor neuron signs: spastic tone, clonus, extensor plantar response, and pseudobulbar palsy.

[a]Median nerve at wrist, ulnar nerve at elbow or wrist, peroneal nerve at fibular head.
(Adapted from Olney RK, Lewis RA, Putnam TD, Campellone JV. Consensus criteria for the diagnosis of multifocal motor neuropathy. Muscle Nerve 2003;27:117–121, with permission from John Wiley and Sons, Inc.)

Table 16
Diagnostic Criteria for Myasthenia Gravis From the Case Definitions for Neuropsychiatric Syndromes in Systemic Lupus Erythematosus

A. Characteristic signs and symptoms
   One or more of the following:
   1. Diplopia, ptosis, dysarthria, weakness in chewing, difficulty in swallowing, muscle weakness with preserved deep tendon reflexes, and, less commonly, weakness of neck extension and flexion, and weakness of trunk muscles.
   2. Increased weakness during exercise and repetitive use with at least partially restored strength after periods of rest.
   3. Dramatic improvement in strength following administration of anticholinesterase drug (edrophonium and neostigmine).
   And one or more of the following:
B. Electromyogram and repetitive stimulation of a peripheral nerve: In myasthenia gravis repetitive stimulation at a rate of two per second shows characteristic decremental response that is reversed by edrophonium or neostigmine. Single-fiber studies show increased jitter.
C. Antibodies to acetylcholine receptors.

Adapted from American College of Rheumatology. Arthritis and rheumatism: Appendix A: Case definitions for neuropsychiatric syndromes in systemic lupus erythematosus. Available via http://www.rheumatology.org/publications/ar/1999/499ap9.asp?aud=mem.

Table 17
Diagnostic Criteria for Myotonic Dystrophy

The clinical picture depends on the age of onset:
1. Congenital and infantile myotonic dystrophy, age <10 years.
2. Juvenile/adult myotonic dystrophy, age 10–50 years.
3. Late-adult/senile myotonic dystrophy, age >50 years.

Elements
1.
    a. Congenital myotonic dystrophy
        i. Stillbirth or generalized severe muscular weakness (including the face) and hypotonia with sucking, swallowing, and sometimes, respiratory insufficiency. Absence of tendon reflexes. Club feet.
        ii. Symptoms of myotonic dystrophy (*see* 2) in the mother.
        iii. If mother asymptomatic: immature fibers in the muscle biopsy.
    b. Infantile myotonic dystrophy
        i. Mental retardation.
        ii. Generalized weakness, especially of the face and distal limbs; myotonia starts usually between age 5 and 10 years.
        iii. Electromyography[a]: myotonic volleys in several muscles.
        iv. Symptoms of myotonic dystrophy in one of the parents.
        v. Same haplotype, involving closely linked markers, as affected first-degree relative.
2. Juvenile/adult myotonic dystrophy
    a. Myotonia of grip and/or percussion myotonia of thenar muscles.
    b. Weakness of one or more of the following:
        i. Orbicularis oculi.
        ii. Pharyngeal muscles.
        iii. Distal limb muscles.
    Atrophy of masticatory muscles and/or distal limb muscles may be obvious.
    c. Cortical cataract (slit-lamp examination mandatory).[b]
    d. Electromyography:[a] myotonic volleys in several muscles.
    e. Positive family history compatible with autosomal-dominant inheritance.
    f. Same haplotype, involving closely linked markers, as affected first-degree relative.
3. Late adult/senile myotonic dystrophy
    a. Cortical cataract.[b]
    b. Rarely neuromuscular symptoms (*see* 2).
    c. Electromyography:[a] myotonic volleys in several muscles.
    d. Positive family history compatible with autosomal-dominant inheritance.
    e. Same haplotype, involving closely linked markers, as affected first-degree relative.
    f. Asymptomatic heterozygotes occur, even in old age.

---

[a]Electromyography: myotonic volleys ("dive bomber") resemble repetitive denervation potentials, with inconstant frequency 20–120 Hz, duration at least 0.5 seconds.

[b]Cataract should be cortical, assessed by experienced ophthalmologist with slit-lamp and should not be used as criterion if no first-degree family member is affected.

(Adapted from Jennekens FGI, ten Kate LP, de Visser M, Wintzen AR. Diagnostic criteria for Duchenne and Becker muscular dystrophy and myotonic dystrophy. Neuromuscul Dis 1991;1:389–391, with permission from Elsevier.)

low specificity built into the Peter and Bohan criteria. Additionally, muscle pathology standards have changed over the decades of observation in this report, and it is now appreciated that many congenital myopathies may have inflammatory infiltrates and be mistaken for PM.

Table 18
Degrees of Ascertainment of the Diagnosis of Myotonic Dystrophy (Based on Criteria in Table 17)

	A. First case in the family	B. There is a first-degree relative who complies with the criteria under A[a]
la	i, ii, (iii) all present	i, ii, (iii) all present
2a	(i), ii, (iii), iv, (i), ii, (iii), iv (v) all present	(v) all present
2	i, iii,(v) i, 22 or ii, iii, iv, (v) 22 or i, ii, (v) iii or vi present	iv or vi present
3	More than one element or iv present	i or ii or iv present

[a]When family history is positive and B is not valid, one should rule as under A.

(Adapted from Jennekens FGI, ten Kate LP, de Visser M, Wintzen AR. Diagnostic criteria for Duchenne and Becker muscular dystrophy and myotonic dystrophy. Neuromuscul Dis 1991;1:389–391, with permission from Elsevier.)

Table 19
Peter and Bohan Diagnostic Criteria for Polymyositis and Dermatomyositis

Symmetric proximal muscle weakness.
Typical rash of dermatomyositis.
Elevated serum muscle enzymes.
Myopathic changes on electromyography.
Characteristic muscle biopsy abnormalities and the absence of histopathological signs of other myopathies.

Adapted from Bohan A, Peter JB. Polymyositis and dermatomyositis (first of two parts). N Engl J Med 1975; 292:344–347.

POST-POLIO SYNDROME

Now also known as post-polio muscle dysfunction, the etiology of this disorder is unclear. A consensus workshop in 1996 proposed the diagnostic criteria in Table 21.

SPINAL MUSCULAR ATROPHY

Spinal muscular atrophy (SMA) refers to a group of disorders with lower motor neuron dysfunction because of loss of anterior horn cells. The syndromes may present in infancy (Werdnig-Hoffman syndrome: SMA I), childhood (chronic infantile: SMA II), adolescence (Kugelberg-Welander disease: SMA III), or adulthood (SMA IV). Developmental arrest and limited survival are features of SMA types I and II. Spinal muscular atrophy is one of the commonest autosomal-recessive disorders, with an incidence of about 1 per 10,000 live births, so that carrier frequency is 1 in 50.

The differentiation of these complex disorders is increasingly being done by genetic analysis. The autosomal-recessive proximal spinal muscular atrophies have been linked to mutations or deletions in the survival motor neuron gene on chromosome 5q11.12-13.3. Variants of SMA also linked to chromosome 5q include SMA with arthrogryposis, and a very severe form with survival measured in weeks after birth.

There are also SMA syndromes, often with other neurological features, that are not linked to 5q mutations. These include Kennedy's disease (X-linked bulbospinal muscular atrophy with androgen resistance), Fazio-Londe (a progressive bulbar atrophy of childhood), late-onset Tay-Sachs disease, focal atrophy syndromes, and distal spinal muscular atrophies ("spinal" Charcot-Marie-Tooth disease), and autosomal-dominant adult-onset SMA.

For clinical recognition purposes, the clinical criteria have been revised by an international workshop published in 1999.

Table 20
Diagnostic Criteria for Polymyositis and Dermatomyositis

Patients presenting at least one item from the first criterion and four items from the second through ninth criteria are said to have dermatomyositis. Patients presenting no items from the first criterion and at least four items from the second through ninth criteria are said to have polymyositis.

1. Skin lesions
   - Heliotrope rash (red-purple edematous erythema on the upper palpebra).
   - Gottron's sign (red-purple keratotic, atrophic erythema, or macules on the extensor surface of finger joints).
   - Erythema on the extensor surface of extremity joints: slightly raised red-purple erythema over elbows or knees.
2. Proximal muscle weakness (upper or lower extremity and trunk).
3. Elevated serum creatine kinase or aldolase level.
4. Muscle pain on grasping or spontaneous pain.
5. Myogenic changes on electromyogram (short-duration, polyphasic motor unit potentials with spontaneous fibrillation potentials).
6. Positive anti-Jo-1 (histadyl tRNA synthetase) antibody.
7. Nondestructive arthritis or arthralgias.
8. Systemic inflammatory signs (fever: more than 37°C at axilla, elevated serum C-reactive protein level or accelerated erythrocyte sedimentation rate of more than 20 mm/hour by the Westergren method).
9. Pathological findings compatible with inflammatory myositis (inflammatory infiltration of skeletal evidence of active regeneration may be seen).

At least one item from 1 and at least four items from criteria 2 to 9 are required for diagnosis of dermatomyositis. Sensitivity is 94.1% (127/135), and specificity of skin lesions against systemic lupus erythematosus and systemic sclerosis is 90.3% (214/237). At least four items from criteria 2 to 9 are required for diagnosis of polymyositis. Sensitivity is 98.9% (180/182), and specificity of polymyositis and dermatomyositis against all control diseases combined is 95.2% (373/392).

Adapted with permission from: Tanimoto K, Nakano K, Kano S, et al. Classification criteria for polymyositis and dermatomyositis. J Rheumatol 1995;22:668–674.

Table 21
Consensus Workshop Diagnostic Criteria for Post-Polio Syndrome

1. History of paralytic polio: confirmed or not confirmed, partial or fairly complete functional recovery.
2. After a period of functional stability of at least 15 years, development of new muscle dysfunction:
   - Muscle weakness.
   - Muscle atrophy.
   - Muscle pain.
   - Fatigue.
3. Neurological examination compatible with prior poliomyelitis:
   - Lower motor neuron lesion.
   - Decreased or absent tendon reflexes.
   - No sensory loss.
   - Compatible findings on electromyogram and/or magnetic resonance imaging.

Adapted from Borg K. Post-polio muscle dysfunction 29th ENMC workshop: 14–16 October 1994, Naarden, The Netherlands. Neuromuscul Dis 1996;6:75–80, with permission from Elsevier.

Table 22
Diagnostic Criteria of Proximal Spinal Muscular Atrophy

Clinical criteria

1. **Age at onset**
   In spinal muscular atrophy (SMA) type I (severe form), onset age ranges from prenatal period to 6 months.
   In SMA type II (intermediate form), onset before the age of 18 months.
   In SMA type III (mild form), onset is usually after the age of 18 months.
2. **Muscle weakness**
   Inclusion Muscle weakness of the trunk and limbs (proximal more than distal; lower limbs weaker than upper); symmetric.

(Continued)

Table 22 *(Continued)*

Exclusion: Weakness of extraocular muscles, diaphragm and the myocardium, or marked facial weakness.
Comments:
   a. There are rare congenital-onset cases of SMA whose clinical picture also includes external ophthalmoplegia, facial diplegia, and early respiratory insufficiency.
   b. Wasting, if often not conspicuous, in SMA type I.

3. **Other associated features**
   Inclusion: Fasciculations of tongue and tremor of hands.
   Comment: Tremor of the hands is frequently observed in SMA types II and III.
   Exclusion: Sensory disturbances. Central nervous system dysfunction.
   Comment: Arthrogryposis of the major joints is a rare finding in a severe form of SMA type I. In SMA type I, some mild limitation of abduction of the hips or extension of the knees or elbows is common.
   Exclusion: Involvement of other neurological systems or organs, i.e., hearing or vision.

4. **Course/life expectancy**
   Inclusion: In SMA type I and II, there is an arrest of development of motor milestones. Children with SMA type I are never able to sit without support. Children with SMA type II are unable to stand or walk without aid. In SMA type III, the ability to walk will be achieved.
   Inclusion: In SMA type I, the majority of patients have a life expectancy less than 2 years.
   In SMA type II, survival into adolescence or adulthood is common.
   In SMA type III, life expectancy is most likely normal.
   Comment: There will be certain patients who do not clearly fit any one category.

5. **Laboratory criteria: molecular genetics**
   Inclusion: The homozygous absence/mutation of the telomeric SMN gene (*SMNT*) in the presence of clinical symptoms is diagnostic.
   Comment: In cases with absence/mutation of the *SMNT*, further diagnostic procedures, such as electromyogram (EMG) and muscle biopsy, are no longer needed.
   Comment: The presence of both copies of *SMNT* argues strongly against the diagnosis.

6. **Biochemistry**
   Comment: Creatine kinase usually more than five times the upper limit of normal.

7. **Electrophysiology**
   Inclusion: Abnormal spontaneous activity, e.g., fibrillations, positive sharp waves, and fasciculations by EMG. Increased mean duration and amplitude of motor unit action potentials by EMG.
   Exclusion: In SMA types II and III, reduction of motor nerve conduction velocities (MNCVs) less than 70% of lower limit.
   Comment: MNCVs may be markedly reduced in SMA type I.
   Exclusion: Abnormal sensory nerve action potentials in SMA types II and III.
   Comment: There is a rare congenital-onset SMA with death within the first weeks of life in which MNCVs are very long and sensory nerve action potentials are absent.

8. **Histopathology of muscle**
   Characteristic features are the following:
   Inclusion: Groups of atrophic fibers of both types. Hypertrophic fibers of type I. Type grouping (chronic cases).
   Comment: In early-onset cases of SMA type I, these characteristic features may not be present; instead, there are small fibers of both types. In SMA III, there may be a concomitant myopathic pattern.

Adapted from Zerres K, Davies KE. 59th ENMC International Workshop: Spinal Muscular Atrophies: recent progress and revised diagnostic criteria 17–19 April 1998, Soestduinen, The Netherlands. Neuromuscul Dis 1999;9:272–278, with permission from Elsevier.

SOURCES

Amyotrophic Lateral Sclerosis

Donaghy M. Classification and clinical features of motor neurone diseases and motor neuropathies in adults. J Neurol 1999;246:331–333.

Subcommittee on Motor Neuron Diseases of World Federation of Neurology Research Group on Neuromuscular Diseases, El Escorial "Clinical Limits of ALS" Workshop Contributors. El Escorial World Federation of Neurology criteria for the diagnosis of amyotrophic lateral sclerosis. J Neurol Sci 1994;124:96–107.

Talbot K. Motor neurone disease. Postgrad Med J 2002;78:513–519.

Cerebral Palsy

Cornblath DR, Feasby TE, Hahn AF, et al. Research criteria for diagnosis of chronic inflammatory demyelinating polyneuropathy (CIDP). Neurology 1991;41:617–618.

Chronic Inflammatory Demyelinating Polyneuropathy

Hughes R, Bensa S, Willison H, et al. Randomized controlled trial of intravenous immunoglobulin versus oral prednisolone in chronic inflammatory demyelinating polyradiculoneuropathy. Ann Neurol 2001;50:195–201.

Molenaar DS, Vermeulen M, de Haan R. Diagnostic value of sural nerve biopsy in chronic inflammatory demyelinating polyneuropathy. J Neurol Neurosurg Psychiatry 1998;64:84–89.

Nevo Y, Topaloglu H. 88th ENMC International Workshop: childhood chronic inflammatory demyelinating polyneuropathy (including revised diagnostic criteria), Naarden, The Netherlands, 8–10 December 2000. Neuromuscul Dis 2002;12: 195–200.

Nicolas G, Maisonobe T, Le Forestier N, Leger JM, Bouche P. Proposed revised electrophysiological criteria for chronic inflammatory demyelinating polyradiculoneuropathy. Muscle Nerve 2002;25:26–30.

Notermans NC, Franssen H, Eurelings M, Van der Graaf Y, Wokke JH. Diagnostic criteria for demyelinating polyneuropathy associated with monoclonal gammopathy. Muscle Nerve 2000;23:73–79.

Research criteria for diagnosis of chronic inflammatory demyelinating polyneuropathy (CIDP). Report from an Ad Hoc Subcommittee of the American Academy of Neurology AIDS Task Force. Neurology 1991;41:617–618.

Sander HW, Latov N. Research criteria for defining patients with CIDP. Neurology 2003;60:S8–S15.

Saperstein DS, Katz JS, Amato AA, Barohn RJ. Clinical spectrum of chronic acquired demyelinating polyneuropathies. Muscle Nerve 2001;24:311–324.

Thaisetthawatkul P, Logigian EL, Herrmann DN. Dispersion of the distal compound muscle action potential as a diagnostic criterion for chronic inflammatory demyelinating polyneuropathy. Neurology 2002;59:1526–1532.

United Cerebral Palsy Research and Educational Foundation, 2002. Avaialbe via www.ucp.org.

Van den Bergh PY, Pieret F. Electrodiagnostic criteria for acute and chronic inflammatory demyelinating polyradiculoneuropathy. Muscle Nerve 2004;29:565–574.

Dystrophinopathies

Jennekens FGI, ten Kate LP, de Visser M, Wintzen AR. Diagnostic criteria for Duchenne and Becker muscular dystrophy and myotonic dystrophy. Neuromuscul Dis 1991;1:389–391.

Facioscapulohumeral Dystrophy

Awerbuch GI, Nigro MA, Wishnow R. Beevor's sign and facioscapulohumeral dystrophy. Arch Neurol 1990;47:1208–1209.

Brouwer OF, Padberg GW, Ruys CJM, Brand R, de Laat JAPM, Grote JJ. Hearing loss in facioscapulohumeral muscular dystrophy. Neurology 1991;41:1878–1881.

Fitzsimons RB, Gurwin EB, Bird AC. Retinal vascular abnormalities in facioscapulohumeral muscular dystrophy: a general association with genetic and therapeutic implications. Brain 1987;110:631–648.

Tawil R, McDermott MP, Mendell JR, et al. Facioscapulohumeral muscular dystrophy (FSHD); design of natural history and results of baseline testing. Neurology 1994;44:442–446.

Tawil R, Figlewicz DA, Griggs RC, Weiffenbach B. FSH Consortium Facioscapulohumeral dystrophy: a distinct regional myopathy with a novel molecular pathogenesis. Ann Neurol 1988;43:279–282.

van der Kooi AJ, Visser MC, Rosenberg N, et al. Extension of the clinical range of facioscapulohumeral dystrophy: report of six cases. J Neurol Neurosurg Psychiatry 2000;69:114–116.

Wijmenga C, Hewitt JE, Sandkuijl LA, et al. Chromosome 4q DNA rearrangements associated with facioscapulohumeral muscular dystrophy. Nature Genet 1992;2:26–30.

Guillain-Barre Syndrome

Annals of Neurology. Criteria for diagnosis of Guillain-Barre syndrome. Ann Neurol 1978;3:565–566.

Asbury AK, Cornblath DR. Assessment of current diagnostic criteria for Guillain-Barre syndrome. Ann Neurol 1990;27: S21–S24.

Newswanger DL, Warren CR. Guillain-Barre Syndrome. Am Fam Physician 2004;15:2405–2410. Available online at http://www.aafp.org/afp/20040515/2405.html.

Inclusion Body Myositis

Amato AA, Barohn RJ. Idiopathic inflammatory myopathies. In: Pourmand R, ed. Acquired Neuromuscular Diseases, Neurologic Clinics, vol. 15(3). Philadelphia: WB Saunders, 1977.

Mendell J, Barohn R, Askanas V, et al. Inclusion body myositis and myopathies. Ann Neurol 1995;38:705–713.

Multifocal Motor Neuropathy

Olney RK, Lewis RA, Putnam TD, Campellone JV. Consensus criteria for the diagnosis of multifocal motor neuropathy; Muscle Nerve 2003;27:117–121.

Myasthenia Gravis

ACR Ad Hoc Committee on Neuropsychiatric Lupus Nomenclature. The American College of Rheumatology nomenclature and case definitions for neuropsychiatric lupus syndromes. Arthritis Rheum 1999;42:599–608.

Kaminski HJ. Myasthenia Gravis and Related Disorders. Totowa: Humana Press, 2003.

Vincent A, Palace J, Hilton-Jones D. Myasthenia gravis. Lancet 2001;357:2122–2128.

Myotonic Dystrophy

Jennekens FGI, ten Kate LP, de Visser M, Wintzen AR. Diagnostic criteria for Duchenne and Becker muscular dystrophy and myotonic dystrophy. Neuromuscul Dis 1991;1:389–391.

Polymyositis and Dermatomyositis

Amato AA, Barohn RJ. Idiopathic inflammatory myopathies. Neur Clin 1997;15:615–648.

Bohan A, Peter JB. Polymyositis and dermatomyositis (first of two parts). N Engl J Med 1975;292:344–347.

Bohan A, Peter JB. Polymyositis and dermatomyositis (second of two parts). N Engl J Med 1975;292:403–407.

Chad DA. Inflammatory myopathies. In: Katirji B, Kaminski HJ, Preston DC, Ruff RL, Shapiro BE, eds. Neuromuscular Disorders in Clinical Practice. Boston: Butterworth Heinemann, 2002.

Tanimoto K, Nakano K, Kano S, et al. Classification criteria for polymyositis and dermatomyositis. J Rheumatol 1995;22:668–674.

van der Meulen MF, Bronner IM, Hoogendijk JE, et al. Polymyositis: an overdiagnosed entity. Neurology 2003;61:316–321.

Post-Polio Syndrome

Borg K. Post-polio muscle dysfunction, 29th ENMC workshop: 14–16 October 1994, Naarden, The Netherlands. Neuromuscul Dis 1996;6:75–80.

Primary Lateral Sclerosis

Pringle CE, Hudson AJ, Munoz DG, Kiernan JA, Brown WF, Ebers GC. Primary lateral sclerosis. Clinical features, neuropathology and diagnostic criteria. Brain 1992;115:495–520.

Spinal Muscular Atrophy

Bingham PM, Shen N, Rennert H, et al. Arthrogryposis due to infantile neuronal degeneration associated with deletion of the *SMNT* gene. Neurology 1997;49:848–851.

Brahe C, Servidei S, Zappata S, et al. Genetic homogeneity between childhood-onset and adult-onset autosomal recessive spinal muscularatrophy. Lancet 1995;346:741–742.

Devriendt K, Lammens M, Schollen E, et al. Clinical and molecular genetic features of congenital spinal muscular atrophy. Ann Neurol 1996;40:731–738.

Korinthenberg R, Sauer M, Ketelsen UP, et al. Congenital axonal neuropathy caused by deletions in the spinal muscular atrophy region. Ann Neurol 1997;42:364–368.

Lefebvre S, Bürglen L, Frézal J, Munnich A, Melki J. The role of the *SMN* gene in proximal spinal muscular atrophy. Hum Mol Genet 1998;7:1531-1536.

Ogino S, Wilson RB. Spinal muscular atrophy: molecular genetics and diagnostics. Expert Rev Mol Diagn 2004;4:15–29.

Prasad AN, Prasad C. The floppy infant: contribution of genetic and metabolic disorders. Brain Dev 2003;7:457–476.

Rietschel M, Rudnik-Schöneborn S, Zerres K. Clinical variability of autosomal dominant spinal muscular atrophy. J Neurol Sci 1992;107:65–73.

Russman BS. Spinal muscular atrophies. In: Katirji B, Kaminski HJ, Preston DC, Ruff RL, Shapiro BE, eds. Neuromuscular Disorders in Clinical Practice. Boston: Butterworth Heinemann, 2002.

Zerres K, Davies KE. 59th ENMC International Workshop: Spinal Muscular Atrophies: recent progress and revised diagnostic criteria 17–19 April 1998, Soestduinen, The Netherlands. Neuromuscul Dis 1999;9:272–278.

Zerres K, Rudnik-Schöneborn S, Forkert R, Wirth B. Genetic basis of adult-onset autosomal recessive spinal muscular atrophy. Lancet 1995;346:741–742.

Zerres K, Wirth B, Rudnik-Schöneborn S. Spinal muscular atrophy—clinical and genetic correlations. Neuromusc Dis 1997;7:202–207.

CANCER-RELATED FATIGUE

Neurological function figures prominently in essentially all of the 11 symptoms related to cancer-related fatigue in the proposed diagnostic criteria. Some studies have suggested that quality-of-life measures may be as important as predictors of survival in cancer as is response to chemotherapy.

CHRONIC FATIGUE SYNDROME

The criteria for diagnosing chronic fatigue syndrome were officially defined by the Centers for Disease Control in 1988 and revised in 2001. The Oxford criteria differ slightly. The British criteria insist on the presence of mental fatigue, although the American criteria include a requirement for several physical symptoms, reflecting the belief that chronic fatigue syndrome has an underlying immune or infectious pathology.

There may be overlaps between individuals satisfying diagnostic criteria for chronic fatigue syndrome and those meeting criteria for possibly related syndromes, such as fibromyalgia.

COMPLEX REGIONAL PAIN SYNDROME

Complex regional pain syndrome (CRPS) was formerly known as reflex sympathetic dystrophy or causalgia. It is now split into CRPS types I and II. One reason for the change in the nomenclature is that it is not always clear that the pain is mediated by the sympathetic nervous system. However, the new diagnostic criteria for CRPS retain the presence of autonomic changes at some point during the illness evolution, usually early in the course. The major distinguishing feature between the types is whether there is a history of nerve injury. Thus, CRPS type I is synonymous with reflex sympathetic dystrophy (no discrete nerve injury), whereas CRPS type II is synonymous with causalgia (with nerve injury). The injured nerve is generally a large named nerve such as median, sciatic, femoral, and so on. Weakness may be present, in the form of paralysis or dystonia, but is not a diagnostic feature of CRPS.

Modifications and proposed research diagnostic criteria were published in 1999 and are summarized in Tables 7 and 8. The authors found that the above-listed criteria, when used in isolation, lacked specificity and led to overdiagnosis. Using these modifications, diagnostic accuracy rates of about 85% were achieved for both CRPS and non-CRPS pain syndromes.

FATIGUE IN MULTIPLE SCLEROSIS

Fatigue in multiple sclerosis has been defined by the 1998 Paralyzed Veterans of America Multiple Sclerosis Council for Clinical Practice Guidelines as "a subjective lack of physical and/or mental energy that is perceived by the individual or caregivers to interfere with usual or desired activities."

Acute fatigue is defined as new or significant increase in fatigue within the last 6 weeks and as a fatigue that limits functional activities or quality of life.

From: *Current Clinical Neurology: Diagnostic Criteria in Neurology*
Edited by: A. J. Lerner © Humana Press Inc., Totowa, NJ

Table 1
Proposed (1998 Draft) International Statistical Classification of Diseases and Related Health Problems, 10th Edition, Criteria for Cancer-Related Fatigue

Six (or more) of the following symptoms have been present every day or nearly every day during the same 2-week period in the past month, and at least one of the symptoms is (A1) significant fatigue.

A.
  1. Significant fatigue, diminished energy, or increased need to rest, disproportionate to any recent change in activity level.
  2. Complaints of generalized weakness or limb heaviness.
  3. Diminished concentration or attention.
  4. Decreased motivation or interest to engage in usual activities.
  5. Insomnia or hypersomnia.
  6. Experience of sleep as unrefreshing or nonrestorative.
  7. Perceived need to struggle to overcome inactivity.
  8. Marked emotional reactivity (e.g., sadness, frustration, or irritability) to feeling fatigued.
  9. Difficulty completing daily tasks attributed to feeling fatigued.
  10. Perceived problems with short-term memory.
  11. Postexertional malaise lasting several hours.
B. The symptoms cause clinically significant distress or impairment in social, occupational, or other important areas of functioning.
C. There is evidence from the history, physical examination, or laboratory findings that the symptoms are a consequence of cancer or cancer therapy.
D. The symptoms are not primarily a consequence of comorbid psychiatric disorders, such as major depression, somatization disorder, somatoform disorder, or delirium.

Adapted with permission from Cella D, Peterman A, Passik S, et al. Progress toward guidelines for the management of fatigue. Oncology 1998;12:S369–S377.

Table 2
Centers for Disease Control Criteria for Chronic Fatigue Syndrome

Clinically evaluated, unexplained, persistent, or relapsing fatigue that is:
- Of new or definite onset.
- Not a result of ongoing exertion.
- Not alleviated by rest.
- Results in a substantial reduction in previous levels of occupational, social, or personal activity.

Four or more of the following symptoms that persist or recur during six or more consecutive months of illness and that do not predate the fatigue:
- Self-reported impairment of short-term memory or concentration.
- Sore throat.
- Tender lymph nodes.
- Muscle pain.
- Multijoint pain without swelling or redness.
- Headaches of a new type, pattern, or severity.
- Unrefreshing and/or interrupted sleep.
- Postexertion malaise (a feeling of general discomfort or uneasiness) lasting more than 24 hours.

Exclusion criteria:
1. Any active medical condition that may explain the presence of chronic fatigue, such as untreated hypothyroidism, sleep apnea and narcolepsy, and iatrogenic conditions, such as side effects of medication.
2. Some diagnosable illnesses may relapse or may not have completely resolved during treatment. If the persistence of such a condition could explain the presence of chronic fatigue, and if it cannot be clearly established that the original condition has completely resolved with treatment, then such patients should not be classified as having chronic fatigue syndrome. Examples of illnesses that can present such a picture include some types of malignancies and chronic cases of hepatitis B or C virus infection.
3. Any past or current diagnosis of a major depressive disorder with psychotic or melancholic features such as:
   a. Bipolar affective disorders.
   b. Schizophrenia of any subtype.

(Continued)

Table 2 *(Continued)*

    c. Delusional disorders of any subtype.

    d. Dementias of any subtype.

    e. Anorexia nervosa.

    f. Bulimia nervosa.

4. Alcohol or other substance abuse, occurring within 2 years of the onset of chronic fatigue and any time afterwards.

5. Severe obesity as defined by a body mass index (body mass index = weight in kilograms/[height in meters] × 2) equal to or greater than 45. (*Note:* Body mass index values vary considerably among different age groups and populations. No "normal" or "average" range of values can be suggested in a meaningful fashion. The range of 45 or greater was selected because it falls clearly within the range of severe obesity.)

Adapted from the website of the Centers for Disease Control and Prevention. Available at http://www.cdc.gov/ncidod/diseases/cfs/index.htm.

Table 3
Oxford (British) Criteria for Chronic Fatigue Syndrome

Severe disabling fatigue of at least a 6-month duration that:
- Affects both physical and mental functioning.
- Is present for more than 50% of the time.

Other symptoms, particularly myalgia and sleep and mood disturbances, may be present.

Exclusion criteria:
- Active, unresolved, or suspected disease that is likely to cause fatigue.
- Psychotic, melancholic, or bipolar depression (but not uncomplicated major depression).
- Psychotic disorders.
- Dementia.
- Anorexia or bulimia nervosa.

Adapted from Archard L, Banatvala JE, et al. A report—chronic fatigue syndrome: guidelines for research. J R Soc Med 1991;84:118–121.

Table 4
Additional Symptoms Frequent Among Patients With Chronic Fatigue Syndrome

Although the symptoms heretofore listed are the official diagnostic criteria, many patients with chronic fatigue syndrome present a variety of other symptoms, including:
- Pain (almost universal in chronic fatigue).
- Allergies.
- Chemical sensitivities.
- Secondary infections, including *Candida* and viral infections
- Cognitive impairment, including short-term memory loss, difficulty concentrating and doing word searches and math problems.
- Digestive disturbances, such as chronic constipation or diarrhea.
- Night sweats or spontaneous daytime sweats, unaccompanied by fever.
- Headaches, migraines.
- Weakness (paresis), muscle fatigue, and pain (fibromyalgia).
- Premenstrual syndrome.
- Sleep disorders, including excessive sleep (hypersomnia), light sleep, or an inability to sleep for more than an hour (hyposomnia), disturbing nightmares.
- A period of 1–3 hours after awakening, during which patients are too exhausted to get out of bed.
- Cystitis (inflammation of the urinary bladder), particularly interstitial cystitis in which urine cultures are negative.
- Vision and eye problems, including sensitivity to light (photophobia), dry eyes, tunnel vision, night blindness, and difficulty focusing.

An initial office examination may also find the following signs:
- Low blood pressure, particularly on standing (orthostatic hypotension).

(Continued)

Table 4 *(Continued)*

- Low oral temperatures (less than 97°F).
- Slightly elevated oral temperatures (but less than 100°F), which are part of persistent flu-like symptoms.
- Increased heart rate (tachycardia).
- A positive Romberg test (unsteadiness when standing with eyes closed).

Adapted from the website of the Centers for Disease Control and Prevention. Available at http://www.cdc.gov/ncidod/diseases/cfs/index.htm.

Table 5
Tests for Screening of Chronic Fatigue Syndrome Laboratory Tests for Evaluation of Possible Chronic Fatigue Syndrome

- Complete blood count with differential.
- Complete metabolic panel.
- Erythrocyte sedimentation rate.
- Urinalysis.

Optional tests include:
- Antinuclear antibodies and rheumatoid factor.
- Thyroid tests (T3, T4, thyroid-stimulating hormone).
- Adrenal tests (AM and PM cortisol levels).
- Lyme titers and HIV serology.

Specific tests that support (but do not necessarily confirm) a diagnosis of chronic fatigue include:
- Tests for viral infections, such as cytomegalovirus, Epstein-Barr virus, human herpesvirus 6, and Coxsackie virus.
- Immune system tests, including low natural-killer cell counts, elevated interferon-α, tumor necrosis-α, interleukins 1 and 2, T-cell activation, altered T4/T8 cell ratios, low T-cell suppressor cell count, fluctuating B- and T-cell counts, antinuclear antibodies, immunoglobulin deficiency, and antithyroid antibodies.
- Exercise testing may show decreased cortisol levels after exercise, decreased cerebral blood flow after exercise, inefficient glucose utilization, and erratic breathing patterns.

Adapted from the website of the Centers for Disease Control and Prevention. Available at http://www.cdc.gov/ncidod/diseases/cfs/index.htm.

Table 6
Diagnostic Criteria for Complex Regional Pain Syndrome

I. *Type I (reflex sympathetic dystrophy)*
   A. The presence of an initiating noxious event, or a cause of immobilization.
   B. Ongoing spontaneous pain, allodynia, or hyperalgesia is disproportionate to any inciting event and is not limited to the distribution of a single peripheral nerve.
   C. Evidence at some time of autonomic dysfunction, such as edema, changes in skin blood flow, hyperhidrosis, or abnormal sudomotor activity in the region of the pain.
   D. The diagnosis is excluded by the existence of conditions that would otherwise account for the degree of pain and dysfunction.
II. *Complex regional pain syndrome type II (causalgia)*
   A. Type II is a syndrome that develops after a nerve injury. Spontaneous pain or allodynia/hyperalgesia occurs and is not necessarily limited to the territory of the injured nerve.
   B. There is or has been evidence of edema, skin blood-flow abnormality, or abnormal sudomotor activity in the region of the pain since the inciting event.
   C. This diagnosis is excluded by the existence of conditions that would otherwise account for the degree of pain and dysfunction.

Adapted from Stanton-Hicks M, Janig W, Hassenbusch S, Haddox JD, Boas R, Wilson P. Reflex sympathetic dystrophy: changing concepts and taxonomy. Pain 1995;63:127–133, with permission from Elsevier.

Table 7
Signs and/or Symptoms on Complex Regional Pain Syndrome Checklist

1. "Burning" pain.
2. Hyperesthesia.
3. Temperature asymmetry.
4. Color changes.
5. Sweating changes.
6. Edema.
7. Nail changes.
8. Hair changes.
9. Skin changes.
10. Weakness.
11. Tremor.
12. Dystonia.
13. Decreased range of motion.
14. Hyperalgesia.
15. Allodynia.

Adapted from Bruehl S, Harden RN, Galer BS, et al. External validation of IASP diagnostic criteria for complex regional pain syndrome and proposed research diagnostic criteria. Pain 1999;81:147–154.

Table 8
Proposed Modified Research Diagnostic Criteria for Complex Regional Pain Syndrome

1. Continuing pain that is disproportionate to any inciting event.
2. Must report at least one symptom in each of four following categories:
   a. Sensory
      i. Reported hyperesthesia.
   b. Vasomotor
      i. Temperature asymmetry.
      ii. Skin color changes.
      iii. Skin color asymmetry.
   c. Sudomotor/edema
      i. Edema.
      ii. Sweating changes.
      iii. Sweating asymmetry.
   d. Motor/trophic
      i. Decreased range of motion.
      ii. Motor dysfunction
         (1) Weakness.
         (2) Tremor.
         (3) Dystonia.
      i. Trophic changes
         (1) Skin.
         (2) Nails.
         (3) Hair.
3. Must display at least one sign in two or more of the following categories:
   a. Sensory
      i. Hyperalgesia to pinprick.
      ii. Allodynia to light touch.
      iii. Vasomotor
         (1) Evidence of temperature asymmetry.
         (2) Evidence of skin color changes or asymmetry.
   b. Sudomotor/edema
      i. Evidence of edema.
      ii. Evidence of sweating changes.
      iii. Evidence of sweating asymmetry.

(Continued)

Table 8 *(Continued)*

  c. Motor/trophic
      i. Evidence of decreased range of motion.
      ii. Evidence of motor dysfunction
          (1) Tremor.
          (2) Weakness.
          (3) Dystonia.
  d. Evidence of trophic changes
      i. Skin.
      ii. Nails.
      iii. Hair.

Adapted from Bruehl S, Harden RN, Galer BS, et al. External validation of IASP diagnostic criteria for complex regional pain syndrome and proposed research diagnostic criteria. Pain 1999;81:147–154, with permission from Elsevier.

Chronic persistent fatigue is defined as fatigue that is present for any amount of time on 50% of the days for 6 weeks and fatigue that limits functional activities or quality of life.

FIBROMYALGIA

Table 9
1990 Criteria for the Classification of Fibromyalgia

  1. History of widespread pain
Definition: Pain is considered widespread when all of the following are present: pain in the left side of the body, pain in the right side of the body, pain above the waist, and pain below the waist. In addition, axial skeletal pain (cervical spine or anterior chest or thoracic spine or low back) must be present. In this definition, shoulder and buttock pain is considered as pain for each involved side. "Low back pain" is considered lower-segment pain.
  2. Pain in 11 of 18 tender point sites on digital palpation
Definition: Pain, on digital palpation, must be present in at least 11 of the following 18 sites:
Occiput: bilateral, at the suboccipital muscle insertions.
Low cervical: bilateral, at the anterior aspects of the intertransverse spaces at C5–C7.
Trapezius: bilateral, at the midpoint of the upper border.
Supraspinatus: bilateral, at origins above the scapula spine near the medial border.
Second rib: bilateral, at the second costochondral junctions, just lateral to the junctions on upper surfaces.
Lateral epicondyle: bilateral, 2 cm distal to the epicondyles.
Gluteal: bilateral, in upper outer quadrants of buttocks in anterior fold of muscle.
Greater trochanter: bilateral, posterior to the trochanteric prominence.
Knee: bilateral, at the medial fat pad proximal to the joint line.
Digital palpation should be performed with an approximate force of 4 kg.
For a tender point to be considered "positive," the subject must state that the palpation was painful. "Tender" is not to be considered "painful."

For classification purposes, patients will be said to have fibromyalgia if both criteria are satisfied. Widespread pain must have been present for at least 3 months. The presence of a second clinical disorder does not exclude the diagnosis of fibromyalgia.

(Adapted from Wolfe F, Smythe HA, Yunus MB, et al. The American College of Rheumatology 1990 criteria for the classification of fibromyalgia: report of the multicenter criteria committee. Arthritis Rheum 1999;33:160–172, with permission from John Wiley and Sons, Inc.)

MINOR HEAD INJURY

Despite being one of the most common conditions involving trauma and the nervous system, there remains wide variability in diagnostic criteria for minor head trauma. One method of categorizing head trauma is by using the initial Glasgow Coma Scale. Minimal head injury corresponds to a score of 15, without loss of consciousness. A score of 14 to 15, with loss of consciousness lasting less than 5 minutes, constitutes mild head injury and no neurological deficit. Those with scores of 13 would be considered

Table 10
Diagnostic Criteria for Minor Head Injury

Criterion	n	Percentage
Loss of consciousness	58	82
Posttraumatic amnesia	30	42
Impaired level of consciousness	5	7
Absence of focal neurological deficit	6	8
Other signs and symptoms[a]	29	41
No definition	8	11

In all, 64 hospitals listed which diagnostic criteria they used to define minor head injury.
[a]Vertigo, nausea, vomiting, headache, confusion.
(Adapted with permission from Bellner J, Jensen S-M, Romner B. Diagnostic criteria and use of ICD-10 codes to define and classify minor head injury. J Neurol Neurosurg Psychiatry 2003;74:351–352.)

Table 11
Recommended Definitions for Mild Traumatic Brain Injury

Incident cases of mild traumatic brain injury (MTBI)
The conceptual definition of MTBI is an injury to the head as a result of blunt trauma or acceleration or deceleration forces that result in one or more of the following conditions:
- Any period of observed or self-reported:
  o Transient confusion, disorientation, or impaired consciousness.
  o Dysfunction of memory around the time of injury.
  o Loss of consciousness lasting less than 30 minutes.
- Observed signs of neurological or neuropsychological dysfunction, such as:
  o Seizures acutely following injury to the head.
  o Among infants and very young children: irritability, lethargy, or vomiting following head injury.
  o Symptoms among older children and adults such as headache, dizziness, irritability, fatigue, or poor concentration, when identified soon after injury, can be used to support the diagnosis of MTBI, but cannot be used to make the diagnosis in the absence of loss of consciousness or altered consciousness. Research may provide additional guidance in this area.
Based on this conceptual definition, separate operational definitions of MTBI are recommended for cases identified from interviews and surveys, administrative health care datasets, and patient medical records.

Adapted from Center for Disease Control and Prevention, National Center for Injury Prevention and Control. Report to Congress on mild traumatic brain injury in the United States: steps to prevent a serious public health problem. September 2003. Available at http://www.cdc.gov/Migrated_Content/Report/TBI_Report_to_Congress_on_MTBI_Sept_2003.pdf.

to have moderate head injury. However, the experience in the field of athletic injuries, especially as related to "concussion," indicates that loss of consciousness may be hard to discern and of variable import in injury severity.

In a survey of Swedish hospitals, Bellner et al. found wide variability in application of head injury diagnostic criteria, as indicated by International Statistical Classification of Diseases and Related Health Problems, 10th Edition, codes (Table 10).

In a report to the United States Congress, a committee reported on the epidemiology and prevention of mild head trauma. Their operational definition is presented in Table 11.

PAIN DISORDERS

The International Association for the Study of Pain defines *pain* as "an unpleasant sensory and emotional experience associated with actual or potential tissue damage, or described in terms of such damage."

Several aspects of this definition are worth noting. Pain is linked to the concept of consciousness, in terms of the words "unpleasant experience." This definition also puts the concept of pain squarely in terms

Table 12
Diagnostic Criteria for Pain Disorder

- Pain in one or more anatomic sites is the predominant focus of the clinical presentation and is of sufficient severity to warrant clinical attention.
- The pain causes clinically significant distress or impairment in social, occupational, or other important areas of functioning.
- Psychological factors are judged to have an important role in the onset, severity, exacerbation, or maintenance of the pain.
- The symptom or deficit is not intentionally produced or feigned (as in factitious disorder or malingering).
- The pain is not better accounted for by a mood, anxiety, or psychotic disorder and does not meet criteria for dyspareunia.

Code as follows:
Pain disorder associated with psychological factors: Psychological factors are judged to have the major role in the onset, severity, exacerbation, or maintenance of the pain. (If a general medical condition is present, it does not have a major role in the onset, severity, exacerbation, or maintenance of the pain.) This type of pain disorder is not diagnosed if criteria are also met for somatization disorder.
Specify if:
Acute: duration of less than 6 months.
Chronic: duration of 6 months or longer.
Pain disorder associated with both psychological factors and a general medical condition: Both psychological factors and a general medical condition are judged to have important roles in the onset, severity, exacerbation, or maintenance of the pain. The associated general medical condition or anatomic site of pain is coded on Axis III.
Specify if:
Acute: duration of less than 6 months.
Chronic: duration of 6 months or longer.

Adapted from American Psychiatric Association. Diagnostic and Statistical Manual of Mental Disorders, 4th rev. ed. Washington, DC: American Psychiatric Association, 1994.

Table 13

Diagnostic Criteria for Second-Impact Syndrome

Criteria	Definition
(a)	Medical review after a witnessed first impact
(b)	Documentation of ongoing symptoms following the first impact up to the time of the second impact
(c)	Witnessed second head impact with a subsequent rapid cerebral deterioration
(d)	Neuropathological or neuroimaging evidence of cerebral swelling without significant intracranial hematoma or other cause for edema

Definite second-impact syndrome (SIS): (a), (b), (c), and (d).
Probable SIS: (c) and (d) and either (a) or (b).
Possible SIS: (c) and (d) only.
Not SIS: (c) or (d) absent.

Adapted from McCrory PR, Berkovic SF. Second-impact syndrome. Neurology 1998;50:677–683, with permission from Lippincott, Williams, and Wilkins.

of the patient's perception. It does not specify any objective correlate in terms of physiological functioning or evidence of tissue damage. Understanding the concept may help some trainees and practitioners in evaluation of individuals presenting with pain. Implicit in the diagnosis is a central component of pain, whose biological basis involves multiple levels of the neuraxis and inputs from multiple neurotransmitter systems. However, the definition does not specify how this may change as related to the chronicity of the pain.

Several discrete pain syndromes have been described and are listed in Table 12.

SECOND-IMPACT SYNDROME

A syndrome of diffuse cerebral swelling with catastrophic results after a second head injury. It is seen most commonly in children and adolescents, particularly in the setting of sports injuries with a brief concussion, when a second impact occurs before the symptoms of the first injury have cleared, resulting in more severe cerebral injury.

SOURCES

Cancer-Related Fatigue

Cella D, Peterman A, Passik S, et al. Progress toward guidelines for the management of fatigue. Oncology 1998;12:S369–S377.
Cella D, Davis K, Breitbart W, et al. Cancer-related fatigue: prevalence of proposed diagnostic criteria in a United States sample of cancer survivors. J Clin Oncol 2001;19:3385–3391.

Chronic Fatigue Syndrome

Fukuda K, Straus SE, Hickey I, et al. The chronic fatigue syndrome: a comprehensive approach to its definition and study. Ann Intern Med 1994;121:953–959.
Holmes G, Kaplan J, Gantz N, et al. Chronic fatigue syndrome: a working case definition. Ann Intern Med 1988;108:387–389.
Reeves WC, Lloyd A, Vernon SD, et al. Identification of ambiguities in the 1994 chronic fatigue syndrome research case definition and recommendations for resolution. BMC Health Serv Res 2003;3:25.
Sharpe MC, Archard L, Banatvala JE, et al. A report—chronic fatigue syndrome: guidelines for research. J R Soc Med 1991;84:118–121.

Complex Regional Pain Syndrome

Bruehl S, Harden RN, Galer BS, et al. External validation of IASP diagnostic criteria for complex regional pain syndrome and proposed research diagnostic criteria. Pain 1999;81:147–154.
Hassantash SA, Afrakhteh M, Maier RV. Causalgia: a meta-analysis of the literature. Arch Surg 2003;138:1226–1231.
Stanton-Hicks M, Janig W, Hassenbusch S, Haddox JD, Boas R, Wilson P. Reflex sympathetic dystrophy: changing concepts and taxonomy. Pain 1995;63:127–133.

Fatigue in Multiple Sclerosis

MS Council for Clinical Practice Guidelines. Fatigue in Multiple Sclerosis. Washington, DC: Paralyzed Veterans Association, 1998.

Fibromyalgia

Wolfe F, Smythe HA, Yunus MB, et al. The American College of Rheumatology 1990 criteria for the classification of fibromyalgia: report of the multicenter criteria committee. Arthritis Rheum 1990;33:160–172.

Minor Head Injury

Bellner J, Jensen S-M, Romner B. Diagnostic criteria and use of ICD-10 codes to define and classify minor head injury. J Neurol Neurosurg Psychiatr 2003;74:351–352.
Centers for Disease Control and Prevention, National Center for Injury Prevention and Control. Report to Congress on mild traumatic brain injury in the United States: steps to prevent a serious public health problem. September 2003. Available via http://www.cdc.gov/Migrated_Content/Report/TBI_Report_to_Congress_on_MTBI_Sept_2003.pdf).

Pain Disorders

American Psychiatric Association. Diagnostic and Statistical Manual of Mental Disorders, 4th rev. ed. Washington, DC: American Psychiatric Association, 1994.
Fishbain DA, Goldberg M, Meagher BR, Steele R, Rosomoff H. Male and female chronic pain patients categorized by DSM-III psychiatric diagnostic criteria. Pain 1986;26:181–197.

Second-Impact Syndrome

McCrory PR, Berkovic SF. Second impact syndrome. Neurology 1998;50:677–683.

Sleep Disorders

NARCOLEPSY

Narcolepsy is a sleep disorder with prominent sleep attacks as a form of excessive daytime somnolence. The other associated features of narcolepsy occur with varying frequency. These include cataplexy, hypnagogic and hypnopompic hallucinations, and sleep paralysis.

The laboratory method of diagnosis is the multiple sleep latency test. Narcoleptics will show sleep-onset rapid eye movement with short latency. Biochemical markers such as human leukocyte antigen DQB1*0602 or DR2 type have very high sensitivity but low specificity. Cerebrospinal fluid analysis may show low levels of the protein hypocretin, but the diagnostic utility of this is unclear.

A number of diagnostic criteria have been developed. *The Diagnostic and Statistical Manual of Mental Disorders, 4th edition*, relies on clinical criteria alone. The American Academy of Sleep Medicine's most recent revision of the International Classification of Sleep Disorders adds sleep lab parameters to the diagnosis. Silber et al., citing the ambiguity and complexity of the International Classification of Sleep Disorders criteria and the lack of validation of these two guidelines, have proposed revised criteria. However, their nomenclature is cumbersome for routine clinical use, and likely will find value primarily among sleep researchers.

From a practical standpoint, it is important to diagnose narcolepsy adequately. Many patients have endured numerous evaluations, leading to delays in diagnosis. The sleep attacks may make work or driving an automobile dangerous, and lead to significant disability. Treatment options include allowing for frequent naps, amphetamines, or modafinil. The first two treatments may themselves be associated with interference of work activities or the need to take stimulants on a chronic basis.

RESTLESS LEGS SYNDROME

Restless legs syndrome (RLS) features nocturnal involuntary limb movements that can cause insomnia because of frequent sleep disruption, and often affects bed partners because of frequent myoclonic-type jerking. It generally begins in early adulthood and affects from 2 to 5% of the population. RLS may run in families, with susceptibility genes identified on chromosomes 12q and 14q. RLS has also been associated with Parkinson's disease, pregnancy, end-stage renal disease, iron deficiency anemia, peripheral neuropathy, and diabetes.

Treatment of RLS is based on individual patient needs, age, and comorbid conditions. Dopaminergic drugs are generally used for initial treatment. Anticonvulsants, opioids, and sedative/hypnotics may also be effective in treating RLS.

SLEEP APNEA SYNDROME

Sleep apnea syndrome is a common cause of excessive daytime somnolence. Aside from its association with obesity and smoking, obstructive sleep apnea has also been associated with increased risk for many other disorders, including cardiovascular and cerebrovascular disease. The detailed diagnostic

From: *Current Clinical Neurology: Diagnostic Criteria in Neurology*
Edited by: A. J. Lerner © Humana Press Inc., Totowa, NJ

Table 1
Diagnostic and Statistical Manual of Mental Disorders, 4th Revised Edition, Diagnostic Criteria for Narcolepsy

A. Irresistible attacks of refreshing sleep that occur daily over at least 3 months.
B. The presence of one or both of the following:
    a. Cataplexy (i.e., brief episodes of sudden bilateral loss of muscle tone, most often in association with intense emotion).
    b. Recurrent intrusions of elements of rapid eye movement sleep into the transition between sleep and wakefulness, as manifested by either hypnopompic or hypnagogic hallucinations or sleep paralysis at the beginning or end of sleep episodes.
C. The disturbance is not because of the direct physiological effects of a substance (e.g., a drug of abuse, a medication) or another general medical condition.

Adapted from American Psychiatric Association. Diagnostic and Statistical Manual of Mental Disorders, 4th rev. ed. Washington, DC: American Psychiatric Association, 1994.

Table 2
American Academy of Sleep Medicine Diagnostic Criteria: Narcolepsy

A. The patient has a complaint of excessive sleepiness or sudden muscle weakness.
B. Recurrent daytime naps or lapses into sleep occur almost daily for at least 3 months.
C. Sudden bilateral loss of postural muscle tone occurs in association with intense emotion (cataplexy).
D. Associated features include:
    1. Sleep paralysis.
    2. Hypnagogic hallucinations.
    3. Automatic behaviors.
    4. Disrupted major sleep episode.
E. Polysomnography demonstrates one or more of the following:
    1. Sleep latency <10 minutes;
    2. Rapid eye movement sleep latency <20 minutes;
    3. A multiple sleep latency test that demonstrates a mean sleep latency of <5 minutes; and
    4. Two or more sleep-onset rapid eye movement periods.
F. Human leukocyte antigen typing demonstrates DQB1*0602 or DR2 positivity.
G. No medical or mental disorder accounts for the symptoms.
H. Other sleep disorders (e.g., periodic limb movement disorder or central sleep apnea syndrome) may be present but are not the primary cause of the symptoms.
Minimal criteria: B plus C, or A plus D plus E plus G.
Severity criteria:
Mild: Mild sleepiness or rare cataplexy (less than once per week).
Moderate: Moderate sleepiness or infrequent cataplexy (less than daily).
Severe: Severe sleepiness or severe cataplexy (daily).
Duration criteria:
Acute: 6 months or less.
Subacute: More than 6 months but less than 12 months.
Chronic: 12 months or longer.

Adapted from The International Classification of Sleep Disorders, Revised: Diagnostic and Coding Manual. Rochester: American Sleep Disorders Association, 1997.

criteria for both obstructive and varieties of central sleep apnea are located in the section on sleep in the criteria adapted from the *American Sleep Disorders Associations International Classification of Sleep Disorders: Diagnosis and Coding Manual.*

SLEEP DISORDERS

Tables 11–62 have been adapted from the *American Sleep Disorders Association's International Classification of Sleep Disorders: Diagnosis and Coding Manual.*

Table 3
Narcolepsy Diagnostic Criteria by Silber et al.

Diagnostic criteria
Category A. Definite narcolepsy
History of excessive daytime sleepiness.
History of cataplexy, defined as definite bilateral weakness of brief duration brought on by emotion.
Mean initial sleep latency of 8 minutes on multiple sleep latency test (MSLT).[a]
Two or more sleep-onset rapid eye movement periods (SOREMP) on MSLT,[a] or one SOREMP on MSLT[a] and one SOREMP on the preceding nocturnal polysomnography (PSG).
Apnea–hypopnea index (AHI): 10/hour on nocturnal PSG preceding the MSLT.[a]
(The last three criteria can be replaced by cataplexy witnessed by a physician with documented recoverable areflexia, or cataplexy recorded by PSG and video recording.)
Category B. Probable narcolepsy (laboratory confirmation)
Subgroup B1
History of excessive daytime sleepiness.
A history of cataplexy, defined as definite bilateral weakness of brief duration brought on by emotion.
Mean initial sleep latency of 8 minutes on MSLT.[a]
One or fewer SOREMP on MSLT[a] or on the preceding nocturnal PSG.
AHI: 10/hour on the nocturnal PSG preceding the MSLT.[a]
Subgroup B2
History of excessive daytime sleepiness.
No history of cataplexy.
Mean initial sleep latency of 8 minutes on MSLT.[a]
Two or more SOREMP on MSLT or one SOREMP on the MSLT[a] and one SOREMP on the preceding nocturnal PSG.
AHI: 10/hour on the nocturnal PSG preceding the MSLT.[a]
Category C. Probable narcolepsy (clinical)
History of excessive daytime sleepiness.
History of cataplexy, defined as definite bilateral weakness of brief duration brought on by emotion.
No or inadequate sleep studies performed.

[a]MSLT performed under standard conditions, including a total sleep time of 6 hours on the preceding night PSG.
(Adapted from Silber MH, Krahn LE, Olson EJ. Diagnosing narcolepsy: validity and reliability of new diagnostic criteria. Sleep Med 2002;3:109–113, with permission of Elsevier.)

Table 4
Summary of Diagnostic Criteria for Narcolepsy According to Silber et al.

Category	Cataplexy	Laboratory confirmation of sleepiness	SOREM periods
A	Yes	Yes	Yes
B1	Yes	Yes	No
B2	No	Yes	Yes
C	Yes	No	No

SOREM, sleep-onset rapid eye movement periods.
(Adapted from Silber MH, Krahn LE, Olson EJ. Diagnosing narcolepsy: validity and reliability of new diagnostic criteria. Sleep Med 2002;3:109–113, with permission of Elsevier.)

Table 5
Essential Diagnostic Criteria for Restless Legs Syndrome

1. An urge to move the legs, usually accompanied or caused by uncomfortable and unpleasant sensations in the legs. (Sometimes, the urge to move is present without the uncomfortable sensations and sometimes the arms or other body parts are involved in addition to the legs.)
2. The urge to move or unpleasant sensations begin(s) or worsen(s) during periods of rest or inactivity, such as lying or sitting.

(Continued)

Table 5 *(Continued)*

3. The urge to move or unpleasant sensations are relieved partially or totally by movement, such as walking or stretching, at least as long as the activity continues.
4. The urge to move or unpleasant sensations are worse in the evening or night than during the day or only occur in the evening or night. (When symptoms are very severe, the worsening at night may not be noticeable but must have been previously present.)

Adapted from Allen RP, Picchietti D, Hening WA, Trenkwalder C, Walters AS, Montplaisi J. Restless legs syndrome: diagnostic criteria, special considerations, and epidemiology. A report from the restless legs syndrome diagnosis and epidemiology workshop at the National Institutes of Health. Sleep Med 2003;4:101–119, with permission of Elsevier.

Table 6
Supportive Clinical Features of Restless Leg Syndrome

Family history:
The prevalence of restless leg syndrome (RLS) among first-degree relatives of people with RLS is three to five times greater than in people without RLS.

Response to dopaminergic therapy:
Nearly all people with RLS show at least an initial positive therapeutic response to either L-DOPA or a dopamine-receptor agonist at doses considered very low in relation to the traditional doses of these medications used for the treatment of Parkinson's disease. This initial response is not, however, universally maintained.

Periodic limb movements (during wakefulness or sleep):
Periodic limb movements in sleep (PLMS) occur in at least 85% of people with RLS; however, PLMS also commonly occur in other disorders and in the elderly. In children, PLMS are much less common than in adults.

Adapted from Allen RP, Picchietti D, Hening WA, Trenkwalder C, Walters AS, Montplaisi J. Restless legs syndrome: diagnostic criteria, special considerations, and epidemiology. A report from the restless legs syndrome diagnosis and epidemiology workshop at the National Institutes of Health. Sleep Med 2003;4:101–119, with permission from Elsevier.

Table 7
Restless Legs Syndrome in Cognitively Impaired Elderly

Essential criteria for the diagnosis of probable restless leg syndrome in the cognitively impaired elderly (all five are necessary for diagnosis).

1. Signs of leg discomfort, such as rubbing or kneading the legs, and groaning while holding the lower extremities are present.
2. Excessive motor activity in the lower extremities, such as pacing, fidgeting, repetitive kicking, tossing and turning in bed, slapping the legs on the mattress, cycling movements of the lower limbs, repetitive foot tapping, rubbing the feet together, and the inability to remain seated, are present.
3. Signs of leg discomfort are exclusively present or worsen during periods of rest or inactivity.
4. Signs of leg discomfort are diminished with activity.
5. Criteria 1 and 2 occur only in the evening or at night or are worse at those times than during the day.

Adapted from Allen RP, Picchietti D, Hening WA, Trenkwalder C, Walters AS, Montplaisi J. Restless legs syndrome: diagnostic criteria, special considerations, and epidemiology. A report from the restless legs syndrome diagnosis and epidemiology workshop at the National Institutes of Health. Sleep Med 2003;4:101–119, with permission of Elsevier.

Table 8
Supportive or Suggestive Criteria for the Diagnosis of Probable Restless Leg Syndrome in the Cognitively Impaired Elderly

1. Dopaminergic responsiveness.
2. Patient's past history—as reported by a family member, caregiver, or friend—is suggestive of restless leg syndrome.
3. A first-degree, biological relative (sibling, child, or parent) has restless leg syndrome.

(Continued)

Table 8 *(Continued)*

4. Observed periodic limb movements while awake or during sleep.
5. Periodic limb movements in sleep recorded by polysomnography or actigraphy.
5. Significant sleep-onset problems.
6. Better quality sleep in the day than at night.
7. The use of restraints at night (for institutionalized patients).
8. Low serum ferritin level.
9. End-stage renal disease.
10. Diabetes.
11. Clinical, electromyographic, or nerve-conduction evidence of peripheral neuropathy or radiculopathy.

Adapted from Allen RP, Picchietti D, Hening WA, Trenkwalder C, Walters AS, Montplaisi J. Restless legs syndrome: diagnostic criteria, special considerations, and epidemiology. A report from the restless legs syndrome diagnosis and epidemiology workshop at the National Institutes of Health. Sleep Med 2003;4:101–119, with permission of Elsevier.

Table 9
Criteria for the Diagnosis of Definite Restless Leg Syndrome in Children

1. The child meets all four essential adult criteria for restless leg syndrome (RLS); and
2. The child relates a description in his or her own words that is consistent with leg discomfort. (The child may use terms such as "oowies," "tickle," "spiders," "boo-boos," "want to run," and "a lot of energy in my legs" to describe symptoms. Age-appropriate descriptors are encouraged.)

   or

1. The child meets all four essential adult criteria for RLS; and
2. Two of the three following supportive criteria are present.
   Supportive criteria for the diagnosis of definite RLS in children
   a. Sleep disturbance for age.
   b. A biological parent or sibling has definite RLS.
   c. The child has a polysomnographically documented periodic limb movement index of 5 or more per hour of sleep.

Adapted from Allen RP, Picchietti D, Hening WA, Trenkwalder C, Walters AS, Montplaisi J. Restless legs syndrome: diagnostic criteria, special considerations, and epidemiology. A report from the restless legs syndrome diagnosis and epidemiology workshop at the National Institutes of Health. Sleep Med 2003;4:101–119, with permission of Elsevier.)

Table 10
Criteria for the Diagnosis of Probable Restless Leg Syndrome in Children

1. Adult criterion no. 4 in Table 5 (the urge to move or sensations are worse in the evening or at night than during the day),

   and

2. The child has a biological parent or sibling with definite restless leg syndrome.

   Or[a]

1. The child is observed to have behavior manifestations of lower extremity discomfort when sitting or lying, accompanied by motor movement of the affected limbs, the discomfort has characteristics of adult criteria nos. 2, 3, and 4 (i.e., is worse during rest and inactivity, relieved by movement, and worse during the evening and at night);

   and

2. The child has a biological parent or sibling with definite restless leg syndrome.

[a]This last probable category is intended for young children or cognitively impaired children who do not have sufficient language to describe the sensory component of restless leg syndrome.
(Adapted from Allen RP, Picchietti D, Hening WA, Trenkwalder C, Walters AS, Montplaisi J. Restless legs syndrome: diagnostic criteria, special considerations, and epidemiology. A report from the restless legs syndrome diagnosis and epidemiology workshop at the National Institutes of Health. Sleep Med 2003;4:101–119, with permission of Elsevier.)

Associated With Behavioral/Psychophysiological Disorders

Table 11
Diagnostic Criteria for Adjustment Sleep Disorder

1. Complaint of insomnia or excessive sleepiness.
2. Complaint is a reaction temporarily associated with an identifiable stressing event.
3. The disorder is expected to remit if the stress is reduced or the level of adaptation is increased.

Table 12
Diagnostic Criteria for Psychophysiological Insomnia

1. Complaint of insomnia combined with a complaint of diminished performance during waking hours.
2. Learned associations that prevent sleep are identified:
   a. Forcing sleep, which suggests inability to sleep at the desired time, but with the ability to sleep in the course of other relatively monotonous activities, such as watching television or reading.
   b. Awakenings conditioned by the room or sleep-related activities, indicated by poor sleeping at home, but improved sleeping away from home or when no room routines are performed.

Table 13
Diagnostic Criteria for Inadequate Sleep Hygiene

Complaint of insomnia or excessive sleepiness
Presence of at least one of the following:

1. Daytime naps at least twice a week.
2. Variable bedtime or awakening hours.
3. Frequent episodes (two to three times a week) of extended time in bed.
4. Routine use of products containing alcohol, tobacco, or caffeine in the period preceding bedtime.
5. Performance of exercise near bedtime.
6. Plans to become implicated in exciting or emotionally bothersome activities near bedtime.
7. Frequent use of the bed for unrelated activities (e.g., to watch television, read, study, eat, etc.).
8. Sleeps in an uncomfortable bed (mattress in poor condition, inadequate bed linen, etc.).
9. Allows the room to be too bright, poorly ventilated, untidy, too warm, too cold or otherwise conditioned to preclude sleep induction.
10. Carries out activities requiring high levels of concentration shortly before bedtime.
11. Allows mental activities in bed, such as thinking, planning, remembering, etc.

Table 14
Diagnostic Criteria for Limit-Setting Sleep Disorder

1. Evasive or refuses to go to bed at appropriate time.
2. Once sleep period has started, sleeping is of normal quality and duration.

Table 15
Diagnostic Criteria for Sleep-Onset Association Disorder

1. Complaint of insomnia.
2. Complaint is temporarily associated with the absence of certain conditions (e.g., being picked up in arms, moved or breastfed, listening to radio or watching television, etc.).
3. With the particular association present, sleep is normal in terms of onset, duration, and quality.
4. No evidence of significant underlying medical or psychiatric disorder able to account for complaint.
5. No other criteria for other sleep disorders able to cause difficulties in falling asleep (e.g., limit-setting sleep disorder).

Table 16
Diagnostic Criteria for Nocturnal Eating/Drinking Syndrome

1. Frequent and recurrent awakenings in order to eat or drink.
2. Following food or drink intake, sleep onset is normal.

Associated With Psychiatric Disorders

Table 17
Diagnostic Criteria for Sleep Disorder With Psychoses

1. Complaint of insomnia or excessive sleepiness.
2. Clinical diagnosis of schizophrenia, schizophrenia-like disorder, or some other functional psychosis.

Table 18
Diagnostic Criteria for Sleep Disorder With Mood Disorders

1. Complaint of insomnia or excessive sleepiness.
2. Complaint is temporally associated with diagnosis of mood disorder.

Table 19
Diagnostic Criteria for Sleep Disorder With Anxiety Disorders

1. Complaint of insomnia or excessive sleepiness.
2. Presence of long-term generalized anxiety disorder or some other anxiety disorder.
3. The sleep disorder has followed the course of the psychiatric problem without significant prolonged periods of remission.

Table 20
Diagnostic Criteria for Sleep Disorder With Panic Disorders

1. Complaint of sudden awakening or insomnia.
2. Presence of panic disorder with or without agoraphobia.
3. The sleep disorder has followed the course of the psychiatric problem without significant prolonged periods of remission.

Table 21
Diagnostic Criteria for Sleep Disorder With Alcoholism

1. Complaint of insomnia or excessive sleepiness.
2. Diagnosis of alcoholism.

Associated With Environmental Factors

Table 22
Diagnostic Criteria for Environmental Sleep Disorder

1. Complaint of insomnia or excessive sleepiness.
2. Complaint is temporally associated with the introduction of an environmental stimulus or circumstance that alters sleep and is physically measurable.
3. The physical properties of the environmental factor explain the sleep complaint; the psychological significance of the environmental factor does not account for the complaint.
4. Withdrawal of the causal environmental factor leads to immediate or gradual resolution with a return to normal sleep.
5. The disorder has been present for more than 3 weeks.

Table 23
Diagnostic Criteria for Food Allergy Insomnia

1. Complaint of insomnia.
2. Complaint is temporally associated with the introduction of a concrete food or drink.
3. Withdrawal of the agent restores normal sleep and waking, either immediately or in the course of about 4 weeks. The diurnal behavior may improve before the sleep model.
4. Recurrence of altered sleep and diurnal behavior when the suspected allergen is reintroduced in the diet.

Table 24
Diagnostic Criteria for Toxin-Induced Sleep Disorder

1. Complaint of insomnia or excessive sleepiness.
2. Complaint is temporally associated with the presence of an environmental or ingested toxic agent (e.g., heavy metals or organic toxins, etc.).
3. No evidence of any other medical or psychiatric disorder other than that associated with the toxicity accounting for the complaint.
4. The diagnostic criteria for any other sleep disorder causing complaints of insomnia or excessive sleepiness are not met.

Associated With Drug Dependencies

Table 25
Diagnostic Criteria for Hypnotic-Dependent Sleep Disorder

1. Complaint of insomnia or excessive sleepiness.
2. Use of hypnotics practically daily for at least 3 weeks.
3. Withdrawal of the hypnotic is associated with exacerbation of the primary complaint, which is often judged as being worse than the original sleep problem.

Table 26
Diagnostic Criteria for Stimulant-Dependent Sleep Disorder

1. Complaint of insomnia or excessive sleepiness.
2. Complaint is temporally associated with the use or withdrawal of a stimulant medication.
3. Use of stimulant medication alters the habitual sleep period, or more than one attempt to withdraw the stimulant induces symptoms of excessive sleepiness.

Table 27
Diagnostic Criteria for Alcohol-Dependent Sleep Disorder

1. Complaint of insomnia or excessive sleepiness.
2. Complaint is temporally associated with more than one attempt to withdraw alcohol consumption before bedtime.

Associated With Sleep-Induced Respiratory Impairment

Table 28
Diagnostic Criteria for Obstructive Sleep Apnea Syndrome

1. Complaint of insomnia or excessive sleepiness. The patient may occasionally be unaware of clinical facts that are nevertheless apparent to others.
2. Frequent episodes of obstructed breathing during sleep.
3. The associated conditions include:
   a. Heavy snoring.
   b. Dry mouth on awakening.
   c. Chest retraction during sleep in young children.

Table 29
Diagnostic Criteria for Central Sleep Apnea Syndrome

1. Complaint of insomnia or excessive sleepiness. The patient may occasionally be unaware of clinical facts that are nevertheless apparent to others.
2. Frequent episodes of shallow breathing or absence of breathing during sleep.
3. Polysomnography shows central apneic pauses lasting more than 10 seconds (20 seconds in infancy), with one of the following:

(Continued)

Table 29 *(Continued)*

a. Frequent awakening from sleep associated with apnea.
b. Bradycardia or tachycardia.
c. Oxygen desaturation associated with the apneic episodes (criteria included in the International Classification of Sleep Disorders).
d. Multiple sleep latency test exhibiting a mean sleep latency of less than 10 minutes.

Table 30
Diagnostic Criteria for Central Alveolar Hypoventilation Syndrome

1. Complaint of insomnia or excessive sleepiness. The patient may occasionally be unaware of clinical facts that are nevertheless apparent to others, such as hypoventilation during sleep.
2. Frequent episodes of shallow breathing or absence of breathing during sleep.
3. Absence of primary lung disease, skeletal malformations, or neuromuscular disorders affecting respiration.
4. Polysomnography shows episodes of shallow breathing lasting more than 10 seconds, associated with oxygen desaturation and one or more of the following:
    a. Frequent awakening from sleep associated with the breathing alterations.
    b. Bradycardia or tachycardia.
    c. Multiple sleep latency test exhibiting a mean sleep latency of less than 10 minutes.

Table 31
Diagnostic Criteria for Sleep Disorder Associated With Chronic Obstructive Pulmonary Disease

1. Complaint of insomnia or excessive sleepiness.
2. Complaint is temporally associated with the presence of chronic obstructive pulmonary disease.

Table 32
Diagnostic Criteria for Sleep-Related Asthma

1. Complaint of insomnia or excessive sleepiness, and cough or dyspnea.
2. Complaint is temporally associated with the presence of asthma.

Table 33
Diagnostic Criteria for Altitude Insomnia

1. Complaint of insomnia.
2. Complaint is temporally associated with elevations typically higher than 4000 m.

Insomnias Associated With Movement Disorders

Table 34
Sleep Starts (Hypnic Jerks)

1. Complaints of difficulties falling asleep, or of intense bodily movements at start of sleep.
2. Sudden, brief jerks at start of sleep, affecting mainly arms or legs.

Table 35
Diagnostic Criteria for Restless Leg Syndrome (see Table 5 for Full Criteria)

1. Complaint of unpleasant sensation in legs at night, or difficulty falling asleep.
2. Unpleasant slipping sensation within gastrocnemius region often associated with generalized pain and leg pain.
3. Discomfort is calmed with limb movements.

Table 36
Diagnostic Criteria Periodic Limb Movement Disorder

1. Complaint of insomnia or excessive sleepiness. Occasionally the patient is asymptomatic, and the movements are observed by another person.
2. Repetitive and highly stereotyped limb muscle movements, characterized in the leg by extension of the big toe in combination with partial flexion of the ankle, knee, and occasionally the hip.

Table 37
Diagnostic Criteria for Nocturnal Leg Cramps (Nocturnal Myoclonus)

1. Complaint of painful sensation in the leg associated with muscle stiffness or pressing feeling.
2. Recurrent awakenings associated with painful leg sensation.

Table 38
Diagnostic Criteria for Rhythmic Movement Disorder

1. Rhythmic body movements occurring during sleepiness period or actual sleep.
2. At least one of the following alterations is present:
   a. The head moves strongly in an anterior–posterior direction (head banging).
   b. The head moves laterally when in dorsal decubitus (head rolling).
   c. The entire body moves in jerks while supported by hands and knees (body rocking).
   d. The entire body moves laterally when in dorsal decubitus (body rolling).

Table 39
Diagnostic Criteria for Rapid Eye Movement Sleep Behavior Disorder

1. Limb or body movements associated with dreaming.
2. At least one of the following:
   a. Hazardous or potentially hazardous sleep behaviors.
   b. Sleep appears to involve acting.
   c. The behaviors alter sleep continuity.

Table 40
Diagnostic Criteria for Nocturnal Paroxysmal Dystonia

1. Abnormal motor activity during sleep.
2. Dystonic or dyskinetic episodes occurring mainly during sleep.
3. Not associated with any underlying medical or psychiatric disorder capable of accounting for the symptom, e.g., frontal lobe epilepsy.
4. Does not meet the diagnostic criteria for other sleep disorders, such as rapid eye movement sleep behavior disorder or night terror.

Associated With Alterations of the Sleep–Wake Cycle Temporal Model

Table 41
Diagnostic Criteria for Time-Zone Change (Jet-Lag) Syndrome

a. Complaint of insomnia or excessive sleepiness.
b. Symptom started 1-2 days after air travel across at least two time-zones.

Table 42
Diagnostic Criteria for Shift-Work Sleep Disorder

a. Primary complaint of insomnia or excessive sleepiness.
b. Primary complaint is temporarily associated with a work period (normally at night) taking place during normal sleeping period.

Table 43
Diagnostic Criteria for Delayed Sleep-Phase Syndrome

a. Complaint of inability to fall asleep at desire time, or inability to spontaneously wake up at desired time, or excessive tiredness.
b. Delay in main sleep phase with respect to desired sleeping time.
c. Symptoms present for at least 1 month.

(Continued)

Table 43 *(Continued)*

d. When no strict sleep model is required (e.g. during holidays), the patient:
1. Has a habitual sleep period that is deep and of normal quality and duration.
2. Wakes up spontaneously.
3. Maintains stable coupling to the 24-hour sleep-waking model, though with a phase delay.
4. Evidence of temporal delay of habitual sleep period in sleep diaries, for a period of at least 2 weeks.

Table 44
Diagnostic Criteria for Advanced Sleep-Phase Syndrome

a. Inability to stay awake until the desired bedtime, or inability to continue sleeping until the desired waking up time.
b. The symptoms are present for at least 3 months.
c. Evidence of time-advance in habitual sleeping period, as evidenced by polysomnographic monitoring over a period of 24–36 hours.
d. The diagnostic criteria for any other sleep disorder causing inability to maintain sleep or excessive sleepiness are not met.

Table 45
Diagnostic Criteria for Non-24-Hour Sleep–Wake Disorder

a. Principal complaint of difficulty falling asleep or waking up.
b. Progressive delays in start and end of sleep, with inability to maintain stable entrainment of a 24-hour sleep–waking model.
c. Presence of the sleep–waking model for at least 6 weeks.

Table 46
Diagnostic Criteria for Irregular Sleep–Wake Pattern

a. Complaint of insomnia or excessive sleepiness.
b. Irregular model of at least three sleep episodes in the course of a 24-hour period.
c. Presence of the sleep model for at least three months.
d. Evidence of altered chronobiological rhythmicity attributable to any of the following:
Demonstration of loss of normal sleep–waking model via continuous polysomnographic monitoring for at least 24 hours.
Demonstration of normal temperature model loss via continuous polysomnographic monitoring for at least 24 hours.

Table 47
Diagnostic Criteria for Confusional Awakenings (Sleep Drunkenness)

a. Complaint by patient or some observer of recurrent mental confusion with micro-awakening or full awakening.
b. Spontaneous confusional episodes can be induced by forced awakening.
c. Not associated with other medical disorders such as complex partial epilepsy.
d. The diagnostic criteria for any other sleep disorder causing the complaint (e.g., night-time fears, sleepwalking) are not met.

Associated With Parasomnias

Table 48
Diagnostic Criteria for Confusional Awakenings (Sleep Drunkenness)

1. Complaint by patient or some observer of recurrent mental confusion with microawakening or full awakening.
2. Spontaneous confusional episodes can be induced by forced awakening.
3. Not associated with other medical disorders such as complex partial epilepsy.
4. The diagnostic criteria for any other sleep disorder causing the complaint (e.g., nighttime fears, sleepwalking) are not met.

Table 49
Diagnostic Criteria for Night Terrors (Pavor Nocturnus, Incubus Attacks)

1. A sudden episode of intense terror during sleep.
2. The episodes usually occur within the first third of the night.
3. Produces partial or total amnesia of the events during the episode.

Table 50
Diagnostic Criteria for Nightmares

1. At least one episode of sudden awakening from sleep with intense fear, anxiety, and imperative harm sensation.
2. Immediate recall of terror contents of sleep.
3. Alertness is complete immediately after awakening, with little confusion or disorientation.
4. The associated conditions include at least one of the following:
   a. Return to sleep after the episode is delayed and not rapid.
   b. The episode occurs during the last half of the habitual sleep period.

Associated With Disorders of the Central Nervous System

Table 51
Diagnostic Criteria for Sleep Disorder With Parkinsonism

1. Frequent awakenings or episodes of daily sleeping with or without motor activity during the sleep period.
2. Diagnosis of parkinsonism.
3. Dementia.
4. Frequent awakening, daily sleeping episodes, or nocturnal confusion associated with the diagnosis of dementia (e.g., Alzheimer's disease).
5. Degenerative brain disease
   a. Complaint by patient or some observer of insomnia or excessive sleepiness. There may be abnormal body movements or alterations in the number of movements during sleep.
   b. Associated with the diagnosis of degenerative central nervous disease (e.g., Huntington's disease).
   c. The symptom is not associated with psychiatric disorders.

Table 52
Diagnostic Criteria for Sleep-Related Epilepsy

1. Complaint of one of the following:
   a. Sudden awakening at night.
   b. Unaccounted urinary incontinence.
   c. Abnormal movements during sleep.
2. More than 75% of the episodes occur at night.
3. At least two of the following conditions are present:
   a. Generalized tonic–clonic movements of the limbs.
   b. Focal limb movement.
   c. Automatisms (lip sucking, sheet-grasping maneuvers, etc.)
   d. Urinary incontinence.
   e. Tongue biting.
   f. Forced expiratory epileptic crying.
   g. Poststroke lethargy and confusion.

Table 53
Diagnostic Criteria for Fatal Familial Insomnia[a]

1. Insomnia complaint initially present.
2. Autonomous hyperactivity with pyrexia, excessive salivation, hyperhidrosis or anhidrosis, and cardiac and respiratory dysfunction.
3. Familial model present.
4. Progression to stupor, coma, and death in about 24 months.
5. Not the result of some other medical or psychiatric disorder, e.g., Alzheimer's dementia, Creutzfeldt-Jakob syndrome, or schizophrenia.

   [a]*See* "Creutzfeldt-Jakob Disease" in Chapter 3.

Associated With Indeterminate Sleep Disorders

Table 54
Diagnostic Criteria for Sleep State Misperception

1. Complaint of insomnia.
2. Normal duration and quality of sleep.

Table 55
Diagnostic Criteria for Sleep Choking Syndrome

1. Sudden awakening during sleep.
2. Frequent (almost daily) episodes of choking or suffocation during sleep.
3. The associated conditions include at least one of the following:
   a. Tachycardia.
   b. Intense anxiety.
   c. Imminent death sensation.

Idiopathic Insomnia

Table 56
Diagnostic Criteria for Idiopathic Insomnia

1. Complaint of insomnia, associated with complaint of diminished performance during waking hours.
2. Insomnia is of prolonged duration, typically commencing in early infancy or even after birth.
3. No evidence of any other medical or psychiatric disorder capable of accounting for the early onset of insomnia.

Other Causes Of Insomnia

Table 57
Diagnostic Criteria for Sleep-Related Gastroesophageal Reflux

1. Complaint of recurrent awakening. The disorder may occasionally be asymptomatic.
2. Episodes of chest discomfort or burning and substernal pain sensation during sleep.
3. Other conditions occurring during sleep include one or more of the following:
   a. Sour or bitter taste in mouth.
   b. Cough or choking.
   c. Heartburn.
4. Polysomnographic monitoring shows:
   a. Awakenings during sleep.
   b. The monitoring of pH reveals acid gastroesophageal reflux during sleep related to polysomnographic monitoring.

Table 58
Diagnostic Criteria for Fibrositis[a]

1. Complaint of nonrestorative sleep and muscle pain.
2. Muscle pain is not associated with other musculoskeletal disorders.
3. Hard and tender zones are palpated in the muscles, particularly in the neck and shoulders.

[a]*See* "Fibromyalgia" and "Chronic Fatigue Syndrome" in Chapter 13.

Table 59
Diagnostic Criteria for Menstrual-Associated Sleep Disorder

1. Complaint of insomnia or excessive sleepiness.
2. Complaint of insomnia or excessive sleepiness is temporally associated with menstrual cycle, or insomnia complaint is temporally related to menopause.
3. The disorder is present for at least 3 months.

Table 60
Diagnostic Criteria for Pregnancy-Associated Sleep Disorder

1. Complaint of insomnia or excessive sleepiness.
2. The sleep disorder begins with, and is present during, pregnancy.

Table 61
Diagnostic Criteria for Terrifying Hypnagogic Hallucinations

1. Sudden awakening at the start of sleep, with immediate recall of terrifying hallucinations.
2. Alertness is present immediately after awakening, with little confusion or disorientation.

Table 62
Diagnostic Criteria for Sleep-Related Laryngospasm

1. Sudden awakening during sleep.
2. Stridor associated with laryngeal spasm.

SOURCES

Narcolepsy

American Academy of Sleep Medicine. International Classification of Sleep Disorders, Revised: Diagnostic and Coding Manual. Chicago: American Academy of Sleep Medicine, 2002.

American Psychiatric Association. Task force on DSM-IV. Diagnostic and statistical manual of mental disorders, 4th ed. Washington, DC: American Psychiatric Association, 1994.

Silber MH, Krahn LE, Olson EJ. Diagnosing narcolepsy: validity and reliability of new diagnostic criteria. Sleep Med 2002;3:109–113.

Restless Legs Syndrome

Allen RP, Picchietti D, Hening WA, Trenkwalder C, Walters AS, Montplaisi J. Restless legs syndrome: diagnostic criteria, special considerations, and epidemiology. A report from the restless legs syndrome diagnosis and epidemiology workshop at the National Institutes of Health. Sleep Med 2003;4:101–119.

Garcia-Borreguero D, Odin P, Schwarz C. Restless legs syndrome: an overview of the current understanding and management. Acta Neurol Scand 2004;109:303–317.

Lesage S, Hening WA. The restless legs syndrome and periodic limb movement disorder: a review of management. Semin Neurol 2004;24:249–259.

Montplaisir J. Abnormal motor behavior during sleep. Sleep Med 2004;5:S31–S34.

Taheri S. The genetics of sleep disorders. Minerva Med 2004;95:203–212.

Zucconi M, Ferini-Strambi L. Epidemiology and clinical findings of restless legs syndrome. Sleep Med 2004;5:293–299.

Sleep Disorders

Estivill A, Bov A, Garca-Borreguero J, et al. Consensus on drug treatment, definition and diagnosis for insomnia. Clin Drug Invest 2003;23:351–385.

Index